Chassin's Operative Strategy in Esophageal Surgery

Carol E.H. Scott-Conner, MD, PhD, MA

Professor of Surgery, Department of Surgery
University of Iowa Hospitals and Clinics
Iowa City, Iowa

Editor

Chassin's Operative Strategy in Esophageal Surgery

Illustrations by Caspar Henselmann

With 210 Illustrations

Springer

Carol E.H. Scott-Conner, MD, PhD, MA
Professor of Surgery
Department of Surgery
University of Iowa Hospitals and Clinics
Iowa City, IA 52242
USA

ISBN 978-1-4419-2074-4 e-ISBN 978-0-387-32181-3

Printed on acid-free paper.

Softcover reprint of the hardcover 1st edition 2006

Reprinted from Scott-Conner, *Chassin's Operative Strategy in General Surgery: An Expositive Atlas*, third edition, copyright 2002, 1994, 1984 (vol. 2), 1980 (vol. 1) Springer Science+Business Media.

9 8 7 6 5 4 3 2 1

springeronline.com

To Harry

Carol E.H. Scott-Conner

To Charlotte

Jameson L. Chassin

Preface

The first volume of *Chassin's Operative Surgery in General Surgery* was published in 1980. That volume included three unusually rich and detailed chapters on esophageal surgery. As a senior resident in surgery, I immediately bought a copy that I used as a reference for several years. Many years passed before the second volume of that first edition was published. In due time, second and third editions followed. The ample coverage of esophageal surgery was maintained and, in fact, expanded. The esophageal section of the third edition had grown to thirteen chapters and included minimal access surgical approaches.

Times, however, change, and in the 25 years since publication of that first volume, esophageal surgery has become a specialty in itself—one shared by general surgeons, surgical oncologists and thoracic surgeons. This volume, a reprint of the Esophageal Section of the third edition, is offered as a service to those surgeons and surgeons in training who are more narrowly focused than the general surgeons of Dr. Jameson Chassin's day. I hope that you find it valuable and useful.

Carol E.H. Scott-Conner, MD, PhD, MA

Contents

1 Concepts in Esophageal Surgery

Thomas H. Gouge

Advances in diagnostic studies, perioperative management, and the techniques of esophageal surgery have greatly reduced mortality, morbidity, and length of hospital stay. Multidisciplinary approaches have even begun to improve the long-term results of treatment for esophageal malignancy. Long-term survival following resection of a carcinoma of the esophagus is usually limited to patients without regional spread whose tumors are confined to the wall of the esophagus. Successful esophageal surgery still requires knowledge of the anatomy and physiology of the esophagus and attention to the details of the operative technique.

CARCINOMA OF THE CARDIA REGION

Resection of lesions of the distal esophagus and gastric cardia with esophagogastric anastomosis is no longer an operation with high mortality, significant complications, and intractable reflux esophagitis. Resection with an overall mortality of 2% should be routine, and anastomotic leakage should be a rare event today. Operation without an intensive care unit stay, with early ambulation, return to oral intake within 48 hours, and hospitalizations of 1 week are achievable even for patients over age 70. Continuing epidural analgesia with patient control after surgery has been an important advance. Although return of normal appetite and meal volume is slow, most patients have no dietary restrictions after the early narrowing of the anastomosis due to edema has resolved.

Important concepts are resection with adequate margins of normal esophagus and stomach, resection of the fibroareolar tissue around the tumor to ensure local circumferential margins, and adequate lymphadenectomy for adequate staging. The stomach must be well mobilized with preserved vascularity and esophagogastric continuity restored with an end-to-side anastomosis. The gastroepiploic arcade must be carefully preserved and the esophageal hiatus widened to prevent a tourniquet effect with obstruction to venous outflow. Properly performed, esophagogastrectomy is a safe operation with good symptomatic and nutritional results.

If a tumor extends into the stomach a significant distance along the lesser curvature or into the fundus, a significant proximal gastrectomy is necessary for adequate tumor margin. If resection of more than 50% of the stomach is required for tumor margins or if the anastomosis is less than 10 cm from the pylorus, a total gastrectomy with roux-Y esophagojejunostomy gives a much more satisfactory result. Intraabdominal esophagogastric anastomoses near the pylorus permit too small a gastric remnant to construct a satisfactory end-to-side anastomosis. Such end-to-end anastomoses have a higher leak rate and severe problems with uncontrolled bile reflux esophagitis.

Laparotomy with right thoracotomy can be used for lesions at any level of the thoracic esophagus, and transhiatal esophagectomy is an option for lesions in the distal 10 cm of the esophagus. I continue to prefer a left thoracoabdominal approach with the patient in the lateral position for tumors whose proximal extent on computed tomography (CT) are clearly below the carina. One-stage mobilization and anastomosis shortens the operating time, provides superb exposure to both esophagus and stomach, and decreases blood loss. Although the upper extent of the tumor should be known with accuracy with CT imaging, the need for additional proximal length can easily be addressed. The surgeon can simply mobilize the esophagus from under the aortic arch and make the anastomosis as high in the pleural space as necessary.

CARCINOMA OF THE MIDDLE AND UPPER ESOPHAGUS

The operation of choice for lesions in the mid-thoracic esophagus is subtotal resection by right thoracotomy following full mobilization of the stomach through a midline laparotomy. I routinely place a feeding jejunostomy as part of the abdominal phase. The anastomosis should be constructed with an end-to-side technique at the apex of the right chest or in the neck. A stapled anastomosis at the apex of the chest usually provides at least as much esophageal margin as a cervical anastomosis. The same considerations of blood supply and lack of tension apply. Good vascularity ensured by preservation of the gastroepiploic arcade, enlargement of the hiatus to prevent compression, and wide mobilization of the stomach and duodenum to eliminate tension are essential to a satisfactory anastomosis. With appropriate preparation the laparotomy and subsequent right thoracotomy approach can be done safely with resultant good digestive function and little or no reflux problems. The tumor must be staged as completely as possible prior to operation to ensure resectability because the surgeon cannot assess local fixation until after completion of the abdominal mobilization if the thoracic phase is done second. Bronchoscopy and endoscopic ultrasonography are the most accurate studies to determine the extent of invasion for these tumors. Doing the thoracic mobilization first has the advantage of evaluating the local condition early in the operation but adds substantially to the operating time.

I prefer dissection under direct vision through a posterolateral thoracotomy for these lesions even though the same thing can be accomplished by the transhiatal approach. The use of video-assisted surgery may prove to be a good alternative. I use a transhiatal approach only for mid-esophageal lesions that were clearly confined to the wall of the esophagus to avoid injury to major vessels and the trachea. Wide resection around the esophagus is not as feasible in the mid and upper esophagus as it is in the lower third and cardia because of the adjacent respiratory and vascular structures.

My preference has been for a high intrathoracic anastomosis when the location of the tumor permits rather than using a cervical anastomosis on principle. Anastomosis in the neck has a higher leak rate than intrathoracic anastomosis. As the incidence of anastomotic failure in the intrathoracic anastomoses has been reduced to a rarity, the previous arguments about safety have lost their force. Cervical leaks do not necessarily remain localized. If it does not drain anteriorly, a cervical leak can track down and cause thoracic mediastinitis. Cervical leaks, however, often cause strictures that require dilation and can be difficult to manage. The amount of esophagus resected with an anastomosis in the neck is minimally (if any) longer than for an anastomosis at the apex of the thorax. Cervical anastomosis has improved neither local recurrence nor long-term survival.

UNRESECTABLE CARCINOMA

Patients whose lesions appear locally unresectable on initial evaluation by CT scan or ultrasonography should be treated with radiation and chemotherapy and then reevaluated for surgical treatment after completing the course of neoadjuvant therapy. For patients with significant invasion beyond the esophageal wall, a multimodality approach with radiation and chemotherapy has the potential to reduce significantly or even eliminate the tumor mass. Resection may be feasible for palliation or even with curative intent after such neoadjuvant treatment.

Tumors that invade the aorta or the tracheobronchial tree must be approached with extreme caution. It is doubtful that heroic measures can prove more beneficial than a palliative approach, and the chance of creating an unsalvageable situation is great.

Distant metastases are not a contraindication to palliative resection of a locally resectable tumor. The patient's condition and the potential benefit must be carefully weighed when deciding whether to resect for palliation. A suitable patient is one whose tumor has caused obstruction or bleeding and who can easily withstand the operation. For such a patient, the ability to swallow can significantly enhance the quality of life. A palliative resection can be accomplished during a short hospitalization in appropriately selected patients.

Although it is feasible to interpose a colon segment between the proximal esophagus and the stomach for palliation of obstruction caused by an unresectable carcinoma, the operation has a high mortality rate and provides poor palliation for the short expected survival of such patients. The development of new techniques including endoscopic treatment with dilators, lasers, and stents provides a much more acceptable means of palliation.

CARCINOMA OF THE ESOPHAGUS: TRANSHIATAL OR TRANSTHORACIC APPROACH

Each approach to resection of esophageal cancers has had strong proponents. Each also has advantages and disadvantages, and no series has demonstrated a clear superiority of one over the others. Although the left-sided approach I favor for distal lesions has been widely accepted, some have reported excessive mortality and leak rates. We have not had this experience, and others have also noted exceedingly low mortality and complication rates. Akiyama [1], Ellis et al. [2], and Mathiesen et al. [3] have reported the same experience we have had with complications and mortality, both in the 2% range or lower. With a large experience, Orringer et al.'s [4] results with transhiatal resections are similar.

Each operative approach requires knowledge of the anatomy, appropriate staging and preparation of the patient, a well orchestrated team approach in the operating room and afterward with meticulous and delicate surgical technique, careful anesthetic technique and monitoring, and devoted postoperative care to achieve comparable results.

REPLACING OR BYPASSING THE ESOPHAGUS: STOMACH, COLON, OR JEJUNUM

The stomach is the closest we have to the ideal esophageal replacement. When fully mobilized and based on the gastroepiploic arcades, the apex of the stomach reaches the nasopharynx. When the stomach is stretched out to reach the neck, it becomes a tubular organ of modest diameter, with the fundus at its apex and the site of the gastroesophageal junction one-third of the way down the lesser curvature side. Its arterial supply and venous drainage are reliable and difficult to compromise even if the lesser curvature arcades are divided to gain length. The stomach is thick-walled and resistant to trauma when passed up to the neck by any route. Restoration of continuity to the esophagus or pharynx is straightforward and requires only a single anastomosis.

Although end-to-side anastomosis and creation of a partial antireflux "fundoplication" by wrapping or "inkwelling" the anastomosis help decrease the amount of reflux, all patients with esophagogastrostomies have abnormal gastroesophageal reflux. Significantly symptomatic reflux, however, is seen primarily with low anastomoses and rarely with cervical anastomoses. Deprived of vagal innervation, the stomach acts as a passive conduit, but its function is usually satisfactory. High anastomoses (in the neck or apex of the pleural space) help minimize the amount of reflux. I believe this improvement is on a purely mechanical basis. The complete vagotomy that occurs as part of an esophageal resection makes acid secretion minimal. Bile is the main culprit. A long, thin gastric tube helps minimize pooling in the intrathoracic stomach and facilitate emptying, thereby decreasing the amount of bile reflux. When the stomach is available I have used it and reserved intestinal interposition for special circumstances. I have not had the opportunity to use the gastric tube technique described by Gavrilu [5] and Heimlich [6] and prefer other techniques in adults.

The use of the jejunum or colon to replace a resected segment of esophagus preserves a functioning stomach intact. Although less used today than previously, colon or jejunal interposition is an essential technique if the stomach is diseased or was previously resected. Most of the benign strictures formerly treated by short segment colon interposition are now managed without resection. The colon is easily mobilized and can be supported on one of several major vascular pedicles and the marginal arcades. The transverse and descending colon based on the ascending branches of the left colic artery in isoperistaltic position is the appropriate size and length for substernal or intrathoracic interposition. The arterial supply is reliable and the venous pedicle short and less prone to kinking or twisting. Although sufficient length of colon can usually be achieved to reach the neck, use of the colon presents some special problems. The colon serves as a passive conduit and does not have effective peristalsis. Gastrocolic reflux occurs routinely, and the refluxate is slowly cleared; but the reflux is seldom symptomatic. The transit time for a bolus of food to pass into the stomach is invariably slow but variably symptomatic. Benign or malignant disease of the colon may preclude its use; and the mesenteric vascular arcade is variable, especially on the right. The interposed colon is also subject to venous infarction by trauma to the colon mesentery or compression at the hiatus.

The jejunum retains effective peristalsis when used to replace a segment of the esophagus. Short segment jejunal interposition has been used effectively as a salvage operation to prevent reflux when multiple direct operations on the gastroesophageal junction for reflux esophagitis have failed. The shape of the jejunal mesentery limits the length of the interposition that can be achieved with a conventional technique. Without special techniques, the jejunum does not reach above the inferior pulmonary vein. Some of the limitations of jejunal interpositions have been solved by microvascular techniques, which allow either free transfer of jejunum to replace segments of the pharynx or proximal esophagus or interruption of the mesentery with a second proximal vascular anastomosis.

Even without microvascular techniques, the major objection to using jejunum or colon as an esophageal substitute has been the time involved in the additional dissection and the three required anastomoses. Mobilizing the bowel with careful preservation of both arterial and venous circulation can be difficult and time-consuming. Although experienced surgeons have reported excellent results with both colon and jejunum, higher mortality and morbidity rates are the rule. The higher complication rate for interposition operations likely reflects both the additional surgery required and the more complicated nature of the patients who require such an approach. When approaching a patient who needs an intestinal interposition, the surgeon must know as much as possible about the condition of the bowel and its vascular supply. Endoscopy, contrast studies, and vascular studies by angiography or magnetic resonance imaging (MRI) should be performed and the bowel prepared both mechanically and with antibiotics in every case. The surgeon must have alternatives well thought out if the originally selected segment of bowel is not usable or the adequacy of the blood supply is questionable.

Effective complete vagotomy is likely after any esophageal resection. Although it may not be necessary in more than one-third of cases, I routinely do a pyloromyotomy to facilitate gastric emptying. It is a simple maneuver if the patient does not have scarring from a chronic duodenal ulcer. I have not found it harmful, and it avoids the need for balloon dilation or reoperation. Although a matter of judgment, a pyloromyotomy or other drainage procedure should be done any time the pyloroduodenal segment is within the hiatus when the stomach is pulled up because reoperation in this area is extremely difficult.

HIATUS HERNIA AND REFLUX DISEASE

With the exception of traumatic diaphragmatic rupture, virtually all acquired diaphragmatic hernias enter the chest through the esophageal hiatus. Parahiatal hernia occurs but is a rare finding of no particular significance. On the other hand, it is essential for a surgeon to understand the difference between a sliding and a paraesophageal hiatus hernia and to differentiate them from posttraumatic hernias caused by blunt or penetrating trauma.

A sliding hiatus hernia may be thought of as a disease of the esophagus whose significance depends on the severity of associated gastroesophageal reflux and its consequences. A sliding hiatus hernia is sliding both in the anatomic sense (one wall of the hernia is made up of the visceral peritoneum covering the herniated stomach) and in the direction it herniates (the gastroesophageal junction migrates cephalad along the axis of the esophagus): hence the synonym axial hiatus hernia. The hiatus hernia must be reduced and the hiatus repaired as part of the operation to control reflux.

A paraesophageal hernia, also known as a rolling hiatus hernia, is best conceived as a disease of the diaphragm. In this case the gastroesophageal junction is in its normal position, and the stomach with the attached greater omentum and transverse colon herniates into the posterior mediastinum through an anterior widening of the hiatus. This hernia has a true sac of parietal peritoneum. The problems associated with paraesophageal hernias are the same as those with any abdominal wall hernia with the additional special problems of having the acid-secreting stomach involved. Patients with paraesophageal hernia are more often older and frequently have kyphoscoliosis. They usually do not have significant reflux but often have abnormal esophageal peristalsis. Many are entirely asymptomatic, and the diagnosis is suggested by the presence of a mediastinal air-fluid level on chest radiography. Unlike sliding hernias, all patients who have a significant paraesophageal hernia should undergo repair to avoid the mechanical complications of the hernia unless they are unfit candidates for general anesthesia. All symptomatic patients require surgical repair because this disease is caused by a mechanical problem for which there is no medical therapy. The essentials of the operation are reduction of the stomach and repair of the hiatus. Patients who do not have reflux do not benefit from an antireflux operation.

Complicating the matter is the combined hernia with features of both paraesophageal hernia and sliding hernia with reflux. These hernias are usually large and symptomatic. They should be repaired anatomically and to control reflux. They require an anatomic repair *and* an antireflux procedure.

A posttraumatic hernia may involve any injured portion of the diaphragm. Deceleration injuries from blunt trauma usually involve the apex of the left hemidiaphragm. These hernias are usually large and are detected soon after injury from a fall or motor vehicle accident. Posttraumatic hernias involving penetrating trauma, on the other hand, can be small and miss initial detection. Any atypical diaphragmatic hernia that appears to arise away from the hiatus should raise the suspicion of previous injury. Because these hernias do not have sacs, the abdominal contents are adherent to intrathoracic structures if time has passed between the time of injury and the time of repair. Consequently, all such hernias should be approached through the abdomen if repaired at the time of the injury and through the chest if operated late. Immediately after the trauma, the concern should be for the abdominal viscera; reduction should be a simple matter of traction. Late recognition of injury leads to incarceration of the viscera in the chest. The primary risk under these circumstances is injury to both the viscera and the lung. The abdominal contents are adherent to the edges of the diaphragmatic hernia, the lung, and the pleura and can much more safely be freed via the thoracic approach.

Complicated Paraesophageal Hiatus Hernia: Obstruction, Gastric Volvulus, and Strangulation

The patient with a large paraesophageal hernia may have a large portion of the stomach in the chest. As more and more stomach herniates, the fixed ends at the pylorus and the esophagogastric junction come close together, and volvulus becomes likely with intermittent obstruction. More complete volvulus leads to the rare but lethal complication of strangulation with necrosis and perforation. Much more commonly patients develop gastric ulcer with bleeding or obstruction with pain. An incarcerated hernia usually causes severe substernal or epigastric pain, often with an inability to vomit because of obstruction at the esophagogastric junction. All patients with these symptoms should have surgery as soon as the diagnosis has been confirmed with a chest radiograph and contrast esophagram unless the obstruction can be relieved. It may be hazardous to insert a nasogastric tube for the same reason the patients cannot vomit. If the patient is vomiting a tube can be passed safely, but in either case it should be inserted carefully with the distances measured out prior to insertion. Endoscopy or fluoroscopy should be used if there is any resistance to avoid perforation.

Surgical repair of a paraesophageal hernia should include resection of the sac, closure of the hiatus, and fixation of the anterior wall of the stomach in the abdomen if the esophagogastric junction is in normal position. The esophagogastric junction should be reduced and fixed in the abdomen if it has migrated cephalad.

Sliding Hiatus Hernia

The presence of a sliding hiatus hernia is not an indication for operation. An asymptomatic patient with a sliding hernia who has normal sphincter pressures and no significant reflux cannot be made better by medical or surgical therapy. The patient without a hiatus hernia who has significant reflux and esophagitis may be greatly improved by medical therapy or operation. It is generally agreed that medical management is the treatment of choice for patients who have symptomatic reflux with minimal esophagitis. Surgery is most clearly indicated for patients with reflux that causes significant esophagitis and its complications of ulceration and stricture. Patients whose symptoms are completely relieved or greatly improved by modern medical management are also excellent candidates for surgery if their symptoms recur after the withdrawal of therapy (as is likely but not certain). Patients whose reflux symptoms cannot be controlled even by escalating doses of proton pump inhibitors should be carefully evaluated prior to operation to exclude other causes for their symptoms. Atypical symptoms not clearly related to reflux episodes are rarely improved by antireflux operations. The use of antireflux surgery for patients with Barrett's esophagus (columnar-lined esophagus with intestinal metaplasia) is an unresolved issue at this time. Although Barrett's esophagus is clearly a premalignant lesion, it is less clear that it can be eliminated by antireflux surgery. Comparisons of medical and surgical treatment in controlled studies have proven the superiority of surgical control of reflux during every era of medical treatment: antacids, H_2-blockers, and proton pump inhibitors [7]. Surgical control of reflux also has the advantage of controlling all the refluxate—duodenal as well as gastric—whereas medical therapy at best reduces only the amount of acid refluxed.

The minimal preoperative evaluation of a patient with gastroesophageal reflux disease (GERD) and classic symptoms should include esophagoscopy with biopsy to confirm the presence of esophagitis and a barium contrast foregut study. A timed esophageal pH study confirms the relation of symptoms to episodes of acid reflux. Manometry is useful for defining any abnormalities of sphincter location and pressure. It is also essential to position the pH probe at the proper place. Manometry can define the strength and regularity of the contractions of the body of the esophagus and can exclude defined motility disorders such as achalasia. It is not clear, however, how the surgeon can use manometric information to modify antireflux surgery. I have been able to plan antireflux surgery much more effectively by looking at the results of a standard barium meal, which clearly demonstrates the size and reducibility of the sliding hiatus hernia, the amount of shortening, and the effectiveness of peristalsis in the body of the esophagus.

Minimally invasive approaches can clearly replicate open antireflux surgery, and the short-term results with laparoscopy are excellent, although significant additional time must pass before long-term results are confirmed. At present, patients with early-stage disease seem best suited for minimally invasive surgery. With the availability of effective acid reduction, fewer patients have peptic stricture, severe ulceration, or dramatic shortening of the esophagus. I continue to recommend open operations to patients with peptic stricture, nonreducing hernias, or an esophagus shortened enough that the gastroesophageal junction never returns to the abdomen. Further advances in laparoscopy will likely make minimally invasive surgery available to increasing numbers of patients with reflux disease.

Antireflux Operations

The multiple operations developed to prevent gastroesophageal reflux were developed empirically and only later validated. They have in common the principles of successful antireflux surgery, which seek to reproduce normal reflux control.

1. Reduce the gastroesophageal junction into the abdomen to restore the intraabdominal segment of esophagus
2. Narrow the esophageal hiatus posteriorly to increase the intraabdominal length of esophagus and prevent the development of an iatrogenic paraesophageal hernia
3. Restore the lower esophageal sphincter mechanism by creating a high pressure zone in the distal esophagus with a fundoplication

They differ in the degree of fundoplication, the method of fixation, and the approach required. Although known by the name of one or more of a technique's primary developers, it is preferable for the surgeon to define the operation by what is done than by the use of an eponym, as the current operation may little resemble the original description.

A complete (360°) fundoplication done by either the abdominal or thoracic approach is termed a Nissen-type operation [8]. Lesser degrees of anterior fundoplication follow the models of Hill [9], Watson et al. [10], or Dor et al. [11], which can only be done by the abdominal approach, or that of Belsey [12], which can only be done by the thoracic approach. Partial posterior fundoplication is termed a Toupet [13] procedure. It can be done effectively only through the abdomen. All these operations have been done by minimally invasive and open techniques.

Personal preference aside, the more complete the fundoplication, the more complete is control of reflux. The advantages of greater reflux control are offset by the more numerous postfundoplication symptoms created by the complete fundoplication. Fundoplications are associated with a reduced gastric reservoir and more rapid emptying of the stomach in addition to the abolition of both physiologic and pathologic reflux. The patient experiences postfundoplication symptoms as a result of these changes. Most patients have symptoms of early satiety, diarrhea, and increased flatus, which are usually mild and resolve over weeks to months. Some patients have a sensation of upper abdominal pressure or fullness, called the gas bloat syndrome. These symptoms are related to the changes created by the fundoplication and the habit of frequent swallowing or aerophagia common to refluxers. As the reflux resolves, so too do the postfundoplication symptoms.

The inevitable results of surgery to control reflux must be distinguished from the consequences of surgery done incorrectly. Dysphagia and the inability to belch or vomit are often listed as postfundoplication symptoms. I believe they are most often the result of too long or too tight a fundoplication and are rarely seen with appropriate narrowing of the hiatal opening, full mobilization of the fundus with division of both the short gastric vessels and posterior gastropancreatic folds, and a floppy fundoplication. Whichever operation is chosen, the fundoplication should be kept to the physiologic length and too tight a closure of the hiatus is avoided to minimize the undesirable effects of the antireflux surgery. The most reproducible operation with the best combination of durability and reflux control is the complete, loose (floppy) fundoplication done with posterior crural closure and complete mobilization of the fundus.

Benign Reflux Stricture

The most important step when dealing with a stricture in a patient with reflux is to be certain that the stricture is benign. Most carcinomas of the cardia present with symptoms of obstruction. The possibility of Barrett's esophagus with malignancy must be considered especially in white men over age 50 who have a long history of heartburn. If carcinoma can be excluded, the patient should undergo aggressive medical treatment with proton pump inhibitors and at least 40F sequential dilation prior to surgery. Almost all strictures regress with this treatment, and surgery is then greatly simplified. All patients who are good candidates for operation should undergo this initial treatment followed by antireflux surgery. Strictures that do not respond to acid reduction therapy and that cannot be dilated preoperatively with available techniques have a substantial chance of being malignant. When operating for such lesions, the surgeon must be prepared to resect the stricture, as for carcinoma. If the strictured esophagus splits open during aggressive dilation, resection is the only option. Some strictures that appear resistant to dilation dilate readily at operation with the esophagus mobilized. In my experience, all strictures not dilatable in the operating room or that split during operative dilation proved to be malignant.

The approach used when operating for stricture depends on the level of the stricture and the degree of esophageal shortening. In most cases with sliding hiatus hernia the shortening is more apparent than real, and I would approach those cases by laparotomy. Mobilization through the hiatus allows the surgeon to have the stricture under vision and in hand when dilators of increasing size are passed through the mouth to dilate the stricture. After dilation, an ample length of intraabdominal esophagus can ordinarily be restored. In the unusual case where mobilization does not allow reduction of the esophagogastric junction into the abdomen without tension, an esophageal lengthening procedure such as the standard Collis gastroplasty [14] or the uncut Collis gastroplasty described by Demos [15] can be used.

With long-standing reflux and columnar-lined esophagus, the stricture may be in the mid-esophagus and the shortening real. Such cases are best approached by thoracotomy with plans for an esophageal lengthening procedure. The surgeon must always be prepared to resect the esophagus under these circumstances. The bowel should be prepared to allow for colon or jejunal interposition as well as gastric advancement in all cases when an esophageal lengthening operation is done. Dilation is safest when it can be done with the esophagus completely mobilized using soft, tapered, mercuryfilled, rubber (Maloney) bougies. With the stricture in hand, the surgeon can see and feel the stricture and dilator and can then guide the dilator precisely into the stricture and assess the pressure required to achieve dilation. Only when the esophagus is pliable and easily reducible after mobilization should transthoracic fundoplication alone be done. All other patients should have a Collis gastroplasty combined with fundoplication.

Intrathoracic fundoplication is a potentially dangerous condition. Incomplete intrathoracic fundoplications do not prevent reflux. A complete intrathoracic fundoplication is an incarcerated paraesophageal hernia and has all the associated complications of that condition including ulceration and perforation. The intraabdominal segment of tubular esophagus should be restored in all cases, and the fundoplication should always be comfortably in the abdomen. Patients with these complications have advanced reflux disease and should always be treated with a complete, short, loose (Nissen) fundoplication to control their reflux.

Failed Antireflux Operation

Secondary operations for reflux are a challenge at best and are associated with increased mortality and failure rates. After abdominal operation, the decisions to reoperate and by what technique can be difficult. Following thoracic antireflux surgery an abdominal approach may provide relatively easy access for successful fundoplication provided the esophagus is not significantly shortened or adherent to the mediastinum. Likewise, following abdominal antireflux operations a transthoracic approach has the advantage of going through a previously unoperated body cavity. In general this plan has merit, but the surgeon must be prepared to use the alternative approach of a thoracoabdominal operation or another type of surgery when dealing with this clinical problem. For the abdominal surgeon the secondary approach should be a diversion procedure [16]. Distal gastrectomy and Roux-en-Y gastrojejunostomy prevents reflux of either acid or bile into the esophagus if the defunctionalized limb is 40–50 cm long. This operation usually provides relief of symptoms at minimal surgical risk. Especially in poor risk patients, it has much to recommend it over extensive operations, such as thoracoabdominal reoperation with resection and interposition. If a resection has been done previously, a complete vagotomy can be correctly assumed. Even if vagal trunks remain, an adequate distal gastrectomy prevents marginal ulcer formation. The possibility of delayed gastric emptying following the Roux-en-Y reconstruction is a concern that has been overstated. An individualized decision based on the situation and the surgeon's expertise should be used because of the complex nature of the disease and the understandable lack of consensus among experts.

PHARYNGOESOPHAGEAL DIVERTICULUM

Normal swallowing is an elegant, complex series of events coordinated by the swallowing center in the medulla. In the peristaltic sequence, both the upper and lower esophageal sphincters must relax to ensure proper timing to allow the bolus to pass. The upper esophageal sphincter—the cricopharyngeus muscle and the adjacent upper cervical esophagus—and the lower esophageal high pressure zone are physiologic sphincters. They are in a state of contraction in the resting state and then relax on stimulation. A pharyngoesophageal (Zenker's) diverticulum develops in the posterior midline just above the cricopharyngeus muscle. The pathophysiology appears to be a lack of coordination in the relaxation of the upper sphincter with a resultant false diverticulum through the weak area of the distal pharyngeal constrictor. Whatever the cause, Zenker's diverticulum is a progressive disorder with no known medical treatment that should be corrected by surgery when diagnosed. The operation is simple and straightforward with the use of surgical staplers. The diverticulum almost always projects toward the left, so it is best approached through a left cervical incision. Although the operation can be performed under local anesthesia, it is far better done under general anesthesia to control the airway and allow intubation of the esophagus. It is well tolerated in elderly, poor risk patients who characteristically have this disease.

The size of the diverticulum is not predictive of the severity of the patient's symptomatology. Small diverticula can be associated with severe dysphagia. Both that and the average length of the upper sphincter of >3 cm make combining myotomy and diverticulectomy the only logical operation for both the more common Zenker's diverticula, which are easily diagnosed radiographically, and those rare patients with dysphagia caused by upper esophageal sphincter disorders and so-called cricopharyngeal achalasia, which are related to neurologic dysfunction and which must be manometrically proven.

PERFORATIONS AND ANASTOMOTIC LEAKS

"Conservative" Management

Untreated, esophageal perforations are uniformly fatal. Expectant or nonoperative management of esophageal perforations is hardly "conservative." Although nonoperative treatment has a place in highly selected situations such as small perforations of the pharynx from endoscopy and clinically insignificant anastomotic leaks, its use must be confined to those settings in which the leak is proven to be small, contained or adequately drained, and minimally symptomatic with no sign of systemic sepsis. The posterior mediastinum has no compartments and poor defenses against the spread of infection. Perforation of the cervical esophagus can track through the mediastinum and into the retroperitoneum. A radiographically "small" thoracic perforation can cause a fulminant mediastinitis and lead to hydropneumothorax and empyema. Any pleural air or fluid is a contraindication to continued expectant management.

The essentials for treating perforations are as follows:

1. Early identification of the perforation
2. Accurate localization of the site of perforation
3. Control of the airway and pulmonary decompression
4. Adequate drainage of the leak
5. Broad-spectrum antibiotic coverage
6. Supportive care
7. Operation for débridement and closure of the perforation whenever it is appropriate and possible

Adequate drainage can be accomplished surgically or by radiographically guided intervention. Adequate drainage implies that the drain goes to the site of the perforation and completely controls the leakage. Débridement of devitalized mediastinal tissues and decortication of the pleural space are necessary to restore pulmonary function and treat the infection.

The mixture of digestive enzymes and foreign material characteristic of traumatic and postemetic perforations creates a fertile ground for microbial growth. Antibiotic therapy should cover aerobic and anaerobic bacteria and yeasts. Although proximal perforations contain mouth organisms generally sensitive to penicillin, the bacterial flora quickly changes to resemble that in the colon, so an antibiotic regimen suitable for a colon perforation should be used. The esophagus also contains large numbers of yeast, especially *Candida* species, which are more of a problem the longer the perforation is untreated.

Supportive care must include enteral or parenteral nutritional support. A feeding jejunostomy should be done in most cases.

Surgical Repair

Suture or stapled repair alone is unwise unless the perforation occurs during operation, occurs in normal tissue, and can be immediately repaired. Even under those circumstances, buttress of the repair with viable tissue is a logical approach. For all other circumstances, the surgeon should always buttress the repair with viable tissue and provide adequate drainage [17]. Parietal pleura, intercostal muscle, pericardium, diaphragm, and stomach have all been used successfully, and the choice depends on location and available tissue. Successful repair can still be achieved more than 48 hours after perforation with a buttress of viable tissue so long as the esophagus was normal prior to perforation and there is no distal obstruction [18]. Proximal and distal tube decompression are useful adjuncts but are not substitutes for an adequate repair.

When the esophagus is abnormal, resection is the best treatment. The resection can be done by a cervical approach combined with an abdominal and transhiatal or a transthoracic approach. The most effective proximal esophageal diversion is total thoracic esophagectomy with end-cervical esophagostomy. Primary anastomosis is usually unwise in this setting. The esophagogastric junction should be closed and the stomach decompressed with a gastrostomy. Reconstruction with stomach or colon can follow at an appropriate interval. In the special case of perforation following balloon dilation for achalasia, a complete myotomy of the distal sphincter must be done along with the buttressed repair.

ESOPHAGEAL PERFORATION AT VARIOUS ANATOMIC LEVELS

Cervical Esophagus

The cervical esophagus may be perforated during endoscopy, during endotracheal intubation, by swallowing a foreign body, or by external trauma. Although endoscopic perforations of the pharynx can almost be managed with antibiotics and usually do not need drainage, cervical perforations below the cricopharyngeal sphincter are a much more serious matter. The esophageal perforation in this location may be several centimeters long, and prompt surgical exploration should be the rule. Exploration of this area is a simple procedure, and adequate drainage prevents spread of the contamination into the thoracic mediastinum. All patients who are febrile or have tenderness or swelling in the neck should undergo exploration and drainage of the retropharyngeal space. All cervical esophageal perforations should be repaired. Repair of pharyngeal perforations is usually neither feasible nor necessary.

Thoracic Esophagus

Perforation by Instrumentation: Dilator or Endoscope

Pain, crepitation, fever, leukocytosis, mediastinal emphysema, and pneumothorax or hydropneumothorax are evidence of esophageal perforation following instrumentation as under other circumstances, but these findings develop gradually over 12–24 hours. When selecting the proper treatment for a patient with an iatrogenic perforation diagnosed within a few hours of the event, remember that the patient may look quite well during the first few hours only to collapse hours later with fulminating mediastinitis. Water-soluble contrast can define the presence and location of a perforation in almost all cases, but the study cannot accurately define the size of the perforation or the extent of spread of contamination in the mediastinum. If the signs and symptoms suggest a perforation but the contrast study is negative, CT or barium should be used to confirm the absence of perforation. Flexible endoscopy has only a limited role. Although normal esophageal mucosa excludes perforation, if a perforation is present insufflation can lead to tension pneumothorax. Therefore flexible endoscopy should be used only after decompressive thoracostomy or negative contrast studies.

All patients with instrumental perforation should be treated by exploration and drainage. Closed-tube thoracostomy is ineffective as definitive therapy. Buttressed repair or resection should be done depending on the pathology of the esophagus. Obstruction of the esophagus must be relieved if treatment is to be successful.

Barotrauma: Boerhaave Syndrome and External Pressure

Postemetic perforations of the thoracic esophagus are dangerous because they occur in a patient with a full stomach. Vomiting against a closed glottis floods the mediastinum with food, microbes, and digestive secretions. Rapidly developing, fulminant mediastinitis is the result, and patients often present late for medical care. Diagnosis is often further delayed because esophageal perforation is not considered. A missed diagnosis is common after the patient presents for emergency care. Mediastinal emphysema on the chest radiograph is diagnostic and should lead to a water-soluble contrast study to confirm the diagnosis and location even though the site of perforation is almost always in the distal esophagus with extension into the left pleura with Boerhaave syndrome. With a blast injury from external pressure, the perforation may be anywhere in the esophagus. In the absence of trauma, hydropneumothorax is diagnostic of esophageal perforation.

After resuscitation, chest decompression, and control of the airway, thoracotomy for decortication, repair of the esophagus with a parietal pleural flap, and adequate drainage is almost always successful even if the delay to operation is more than 24 hours. Although primary closure without leak is not achieved in every case, the fistula can be well controlled by the flap and drainage; and spontaneous closure occurs within weeks [19]. After completion of the thoracic phase, a separate laparotomy to place a gastrostomy and jejunostomy should be done in all patients.

ANASTOMOTIC LEAKS

Patients who develop a leak following a cervical anastomosis respond well to drainage so long as the interposition is viable, especially if drainage was established at surgery. Although an anastomotic stricture may develop secondary to the leak, systemic or mediastinal sepsis is unusual and recovery is expected. These strictures usually respond to sequential dilations.

Anastomotic failure following intrathoracic anastomosis is a far more serious occurrence. Although most patients survive, their hospitalizations are usually long and complicated. Without prompt, adequate treatment, death from sepsis and organ failure is probable. I believe that virtually all anastomotic leaks result from technical errors at operation. They are present but not clinically apparent early when the defect could be corrected by reoperation. The best time to check for leakage is in the operating room. In addition to inspection of the anastomosis, insufflation through the nasogastric tube distends the stomach and reveals gross defects in a stapled or sutured anastomosis. In the past, we conducted studies at 5–7 days, if at all, before allowing oral intake. For the past several years I have been doing contrast studies on all patients on the first postoperative day. The study is done first with a small amount of water-soluble contrast and then with barium if the first part of the swallow shows no leak. If the study is normal, patients are allowed liquids immediately. If the study is equivocal, a CT scan is obtained to look for extraluminal contrast. If none is seen, I leave the chest tube in place to maintain the seal of the lung around the anastomosis and withhold oral intake until a repeat study is normal. If a leak is demonstrated, the patient can be returned to the operating room for repair with a viable tissue buttress and wide drainage before extensive tissue reaction and infection limit the chance of success. Even if the leak is not completely sealed, the resulting lateral fistula is well controlled and closes spontaneously. If a jejunostomy was not done at the original operation, it should be done at this time.

If a leak is recognized late, reoperation should be done as soon as the patient can be prepared for anesthesia. Débridement, decortication, and closure can be attempted if the defect is small; but the realistic goal is creation of a controlled fistula and control of sepsis. Antibacterial and antifungal therapy is essential under these circumstances. Enteral feeding by jejunostomy is a necessary part of management.

Nonoperative treatment is a tenable plan only if strict criteria are met [18]. The leak must be an insignificant radiographic finding. It must be a small, localized sinus that drains completely back into the lumen and does not involve the pleural space. The presence of pneumothorax or significant effusion mandates exploration, as does any sign of systemic toxicity. CT scanning is essential to confirm that the sinus is behaving like a diverticulum, which would promptly resolve by itself. Broad-spectrum antibiotics and parenteral or enteral nutrition by jejunostomy should be used until healing is confirmed by a contrast study. Oral intake should await proof that no leak is present.

In the catastrophic situation of complete anastomotic dehiscence or necrosis of the interposition, the source of sepsis must be completely eliminated to avoid death from multiple organ failure. All nonviable tissue must be débrided. Decortication and wide pleural drainage help the antibacterial and antifungal therapy clear the sepsis. The anastomosis should be resected and the esophagus exteriorized as an end-esophagostomy. The stomach should be returned to the abdomen, closed, and drained with a gastrostomy. Reconstruction usually requires colon interposition and can be done at an appropriate time.

Occult perforation is a problem during esophageal surgery, especially with minimally invasive approaches. Hence testing for leaks should be done in the operating room and on the first postoperative day in all patients who undergo resection, myotomy, and fundoplication.

ACHALASIA

Achalasia, an acquired disease of unknown etiology, is characterized by denervation pathology. The ganglion cells of the myenteric plexus are lost, and the patient develops a hypertonic, nonrelaxing distal esophageal sphincter with an aperistaltic body of the esophagus that progressively dilates and then elongates. In the long term, patients with achalasia have an increased risk of epidermoid carcinoma. Their nutrition is usually well preserved, and patients typically present with a long history of eating slowly and dysphagia to liquids more than solids that is not progressive. All treatment modalities rely on ablation of the lower esophageal sphincter mechanism to allow more normal but passive emptying of the esophagus. In all cases, the striated muscle proximal to the esophagus retains its normal size and contraction. The methodologies available today include temporary paralysis of the muscle of the sphincter with botulinum toxin, disruption of the muscle by balloon dilation, and surgical myotomy. Botulinum injection has had a predictably transient effect. The only difference between surgical and balloon myotomy is that the modified Heller myotomy is more controlled and more effective than the balloon procedure. The availability of minimally invasive surgical approaches has largely rendered balloon myotomy irrelevant. Because of the possibility of perforation, all patients with balloon disruption of the sphincter should have surgical backup, and all should have follow-up contrast studies as soon as possible to exclude perforation.

All patients should be studied with radiography, manometry, and endoscopy to confirm the diagnosis and to exclude other causes of pseudoachalasia in even the most typical cases. When the diagnostic combination of an aperistaltic body of the esophagus with a nonrelaxing distal sphincter is present, the surgeon must chose among the available surgical approaches. The sphincter can be approached to perform a myotomy from the left chest or from the abdomen. The surgeon may use either a minimally invasive or open technique with or without an antireflux fundoplication. Although a complete myotomy can be done by any of the approaches, only a myotomy done by an expert through a left thoracotomy can be done accurately enough to complete the myotomy and not have an unacceptable amount of reflux [20]. Approached through the left chest, the pattern of vessels that mark the cephalad margin of the stomach can be identified as the lower limit of the sphincter and of the myotomy without disrupting the anatomy of the cardia. This anatomic landmark cannot be visualized adequately by thoracoscopy or through the abdomen. The most important principle is to complete the division of the sphincter. To do so by any of the other approaches, the myotomy must be carried down well onto the stomach, and the operation must include a partial circumference fundoplication to minimize reflux. At present, a laparoscopic myotomy with anterior, partial fundoplication is the operation most acceptable to patients and physicians and most easily done by many surgeons. The integrity of the mucosa must be ensured in the operating room and should be confirmed by a contrast study within 24 hours to identify incomplete myotomy and exclude perforation.

The morbidity associated with laparotomy is little different than that seen with laparoscopy for myotomy and fundoplication. The surgeon must exercise good judgment when choosing the approach best suited to the individual patient. Extensive previous abdominal surgery may make a laparotomy or thoracic approach a better choice for such a patient. Reoperative surgery for achalasia can be challenging. For patients with failed operations for achalasia and for end-stage disease with sigmoidization of the esophagus, resection with gastric interposition and esophagogastrostomy in the neck or at the apex of the right thorax is an effective, durable option.

OTHER MOTILITY DISORDERS

Diverse motility disorders of the esophagus—diffuse esophageal spasm, corkscrew esophagus, nutcracker esophagus, and others—have been described. They are poorly understood disorders of the body of the esophagus that do not affect the distal sphincter. The various diseases can be diagnosed and distinguished from achalasia and reflux by motility and pH studies. In the past, there has been enthusiasm for surgical procedures such as long myotomy of the body of the esophagus, but the results are mediocre at best. Although there may be a place for long myotomy in carefully selected patients who have failed medical therapy, almost all these patients should be treated pharmacologically.

REFERENCES

1. Akiyama H. Surgery for Cancer of the Esophagus. Baltimore, Williams & Wilkins, 1980.
2. Ellis FH Jr, Gibb SP, Watkins E Jr. Esophagogastrectomy: a safe, widely applicable, and expeditious form of palliation for patients with carcinoma of the esophagus and cardia. Ann Surg 1983;198:531.
3. Mathiesen DJ, Grillo HC, Wilkins EW, et al. Transthoracic esophagectomy: a safe approach to carcinoma of the esophagus. Ann Thorac Surg 1988;45:137.
4. Orringer MB, Marshall B, Stirling MC. Transhiatal esophagectomy for benign and malignant disease. J Thorac Cardiovasc Surg 1993;105:265.
5. Gavrilu D. Report on the procedure of reconstruction of the esophagus by gastric tube. Int Abstr Surg 1965;121:655.
6. Heimlich HJ. Esophagoplasty with reversed gastric tube: review of 53 cases. Am J Surg 1972;123:80.
7. Spechler SJ, Veterans Administration Reflux Disease Study Group. Comparison of medical and surgical therapy for complicated gastroesophageal reflux disease in veterans. N Engl J Med 1992;326:786.
8. Donahue PE, Samuelson S, Nyhus LM, Bombeck CT. The floppy Nissen fundoplication: effective long term control of pathologic reflux. Arch Surg 1985; 120:663.
9. Hill LD. An effective operation for hiatal hernia: an eight year appraisal. Ann Surg 1967;166:681.
10. Watson A, Jenkinson LR, Ball CS, Barlow AP, Norris TL. A more physiological alternative to total fundoplication for the surgical correction of resistant gastroesophageal reflux. Br J Surg 1991;78:1088.
11. Dor J, Humbert P, Paoli JM, et al. Traitement du reflus per la technique de Helle-Nissen modifiee. Presse Med 1967;75:2563.
12. Belsey R. Hiatal herniorrhaphy. In: Malt R (ed) Surgical Techniques Illustrated, vol 1, no. 2. Boston, Little Brown, 1976, p 5.
13. Toupet A. Technique d'oesophagogastroplastie avec phrenogastropexie appliquee dans la cure radicale des hernia hiatales et comme complement de l'operation de Heller dans les cardiospasms. Mem Acad Chir (Paris) 1963;89:374.

14. Pearson FG, Langer B, Henderson RD. Gastroplasty and Belsey hiatus hernia repair. J Thorac Cardiovasc Surg 1971;61:50.
15. Demos NJ. Stapled, uncut gastroplasty for hiatal hernia: 12 year follow-up. Ann Thorac Surg 1984;38:393.
16. Fekete F, Pateron D. What is the place of antrectomy with Roux-en-Y in the treatment of reflux disease? Experience with 83 total duodenal diversions. World J Surg 1992;16:349.
17. Richardson JD, Martin LF, Borzotta AP, Polk HC. Unifying concepts in the treatment of esophageal leaks. Am J Surg 1985;149:157.
18. Cameron JL, Kieffer RF, Hendrix TR, Mehigan DG, Baker RR. Selective nonoperative treatment of contained intrathoracic esophageal disruptions. Ann Thorac Surg 1979;27:404.
19. Gouge TH, DePan HJ, Spencer FC. Experience with the Grillo pleural wrap procedure in 18 patients with perforation of the thoracic esophagus. Ann Surg 1989;209:612.
20. Ellis FH Jr, Watkins E Jr, Gibb SP, Heatley GJ: Ten to 20 year clinical results after short esophagomyotomy without an antireflux procedure (modified Heller operation) for esophageal achalasia. Eur J Cardiothorac Surg 1992;6:86.

2 Esophagectomy

Right Thoracotomy and Laparotomy

INDICATIONS

Carcinoma of the esophagus

PREOPERATIVE PREPARATION

Institute nutritional rehabilitation by parenteral alimentation or nasogastric tube feeding in patients who have lost more than 10 lb.

Perform preoperative esophagoscopy and biopsy.

Use computed tomography (CT) and other staging studies, including preoperative bronchoscopy, to detect invasion of the tracheobronchial tree.

Improve oral and dental hygiene, if necessary.

Insist on smoking cessation.

Conduct pulmonary function studies.

Preoperative chemotherapy and radiation therapy is appropriate in selected cases.

Pass a nasogastric tube before operation.

Administer perioperative antibiotics.

PITFALLS AND DANGER POINTS

Hemorrhage from aorta

Perforation of trachea or bronchus

Anastomotic leak

Anastomotic stenosis

Inadvertent interruption of gastroepiploic arcade on greater curvature of the stomach

OPERATIVE STRATEGY

The right chest allows access to the upper esophagus with resection of associated lymphatic tissue. The stomach must be fully mobilized during the abdominal phase of the operation. With care to preserve the arterial supply and venous drainage, the stomach can be extended as far as the cervical esophagus. Anastomosis in the neck allows the greatest margin of safety if anastomotic leakage occurs.

Critical errors such as attempting to resect a tumor that has invaded adjacent structures (aorta, bronchus, trachea) can be avoided by accurate preoperative staging. Anastomotic leakage and postoperative stenosis may be minimized by adopting several techniques. Maintain the blood supply to the stomach by meticulous attention to the gastroepiploic arcade. *The esophageal hiatus must be enlarged sufficiently to prevent any element of venous compression, as obstruction of the venous circulation is as detrimental as arterial ischemia.* The end-to-side esophagogastric anastomosis described here has markedly reduced the incidence of anastomotic leaks in our experience (see Chapter 3).

Because the submucosal spread of esophageal carcinoma has been observed by microscopy to extend a considerable distance cephalad from the visible carcinoma, remove a 10 cm margin of apparently normal esophagus with the specimen. Check the upper limit of the specimen by frozen section examination. Ease of access to the proximal esophagus is one of the major advantages of this operative approach.

OPERATIVE TECHNIQUE

Incision and Position

Use a small sandbag to elevate the patient's right side 30°, with the right arm abducted and suspended from the "ether screen" cephalad to the surgical field. Turn the patient's head to the left in case the right cervical region has to be exposed for the esophagogastric anastomosis. Prepare the right neck, right hemithorax, and abdomen. Rotate the operating table slightly so the abdomen is parallel with the floor. After induction of one-lung endotracheal anesthesia, perform a

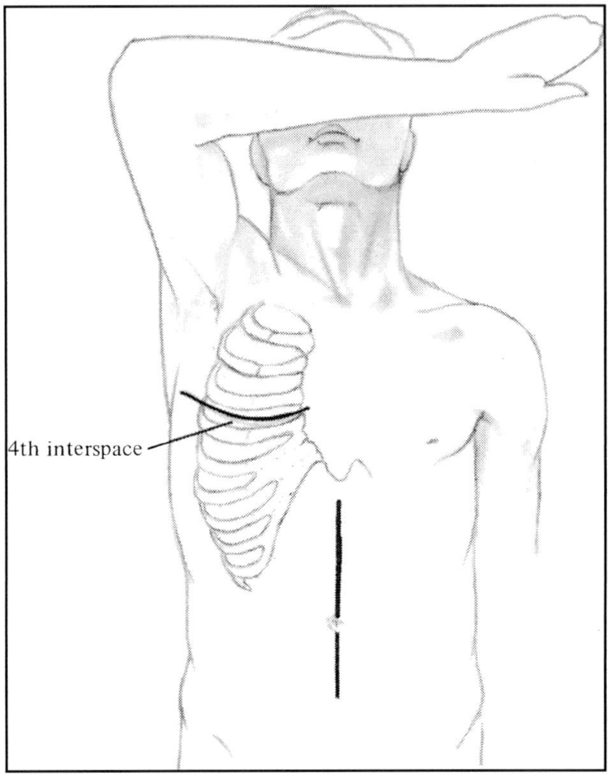

Fig. 2–1

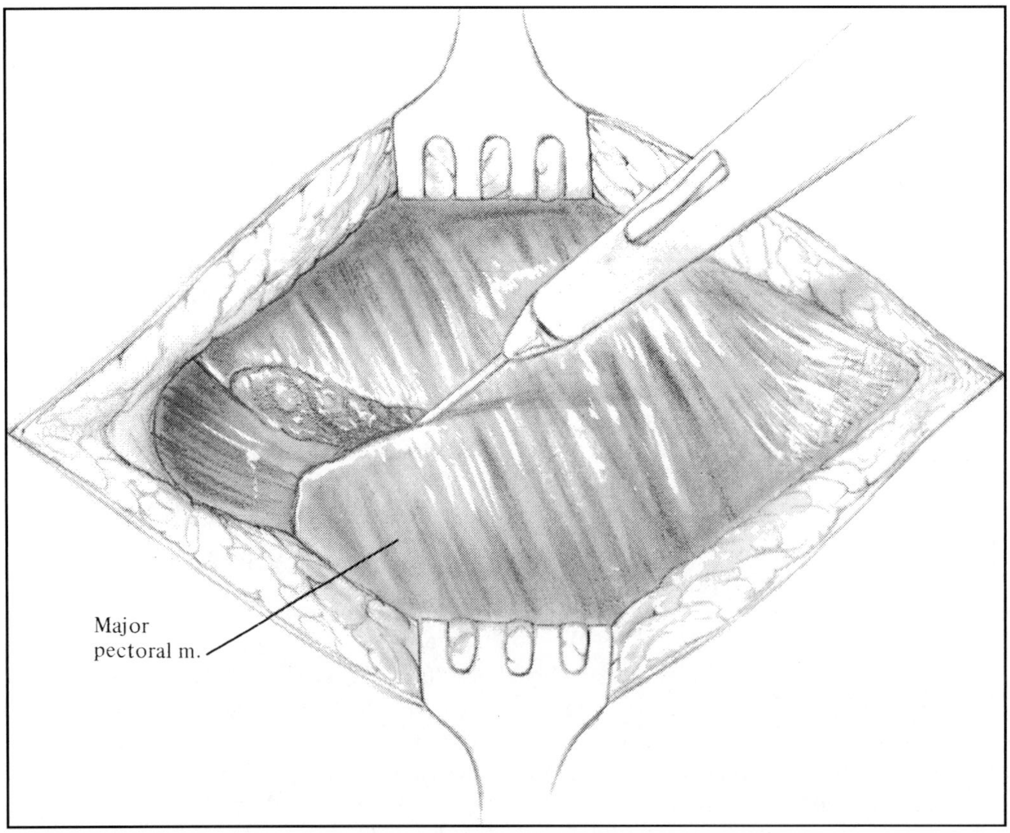

Fig. 2–2

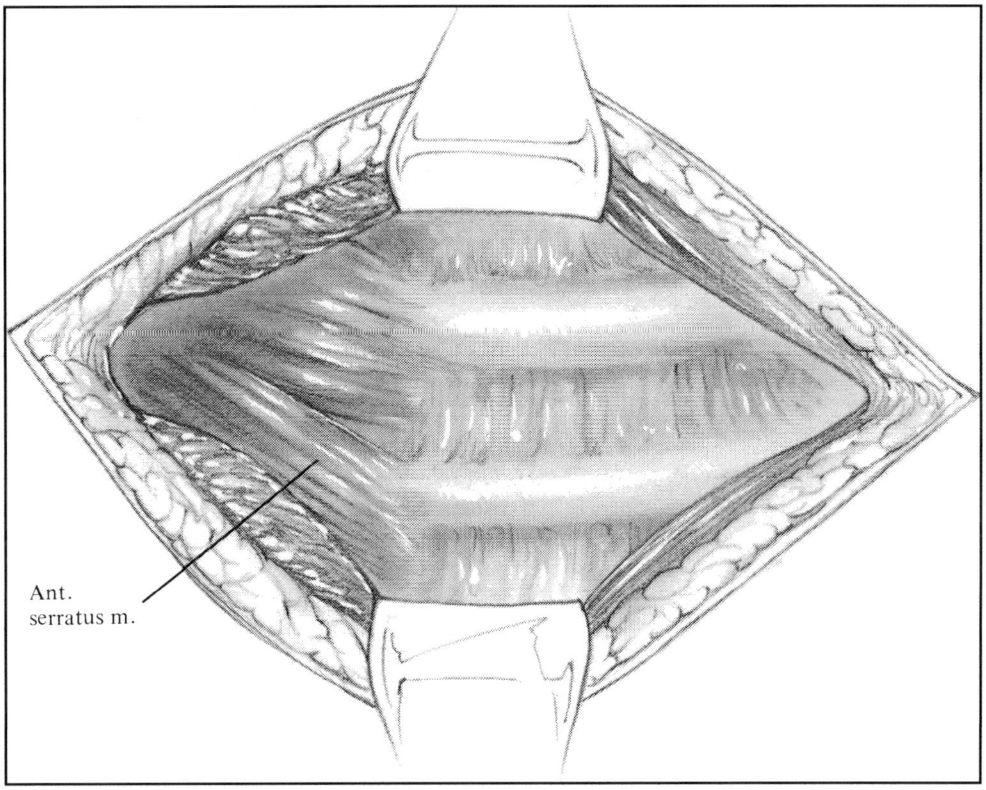

Fig. 2-3

midline upper abdominal incision for preliminary exploration of the liver and lower esophagus to help determine if resection should be attempted.

Then, in men, make an incision along the course of the fourth intercostal space from the sternum to the posterior axillary line **(Fig. 2–1)**. In women, make the skin incision in the inframammary fold. Incise the pectoral and anterior serratus muscles with electrocautery along the fourth interspace **(Figs. 2–2, 2–3)**. Similarly incise the intercostal muscles along the upper border of the fifth rib. Identify the internal mammary artery near the sternal margin, doubly ligate it, and divide it. Enter the pleura of the fourth intercostal space and then divide the cartilaginous portion of the fourth rib near its articulation with the sternum **(Fig. 2–4)**. Clamp the

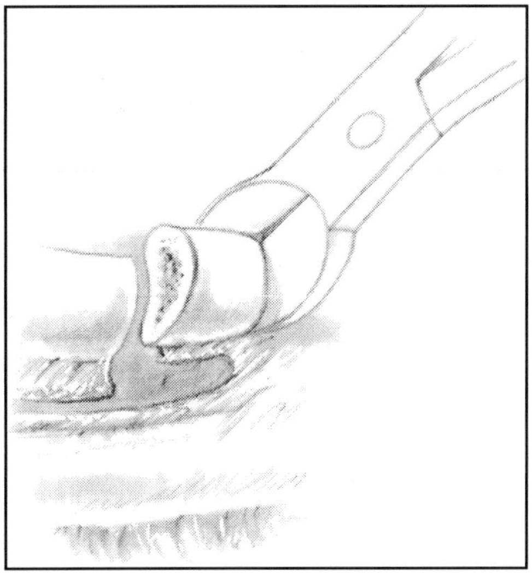

Fig. 2-4

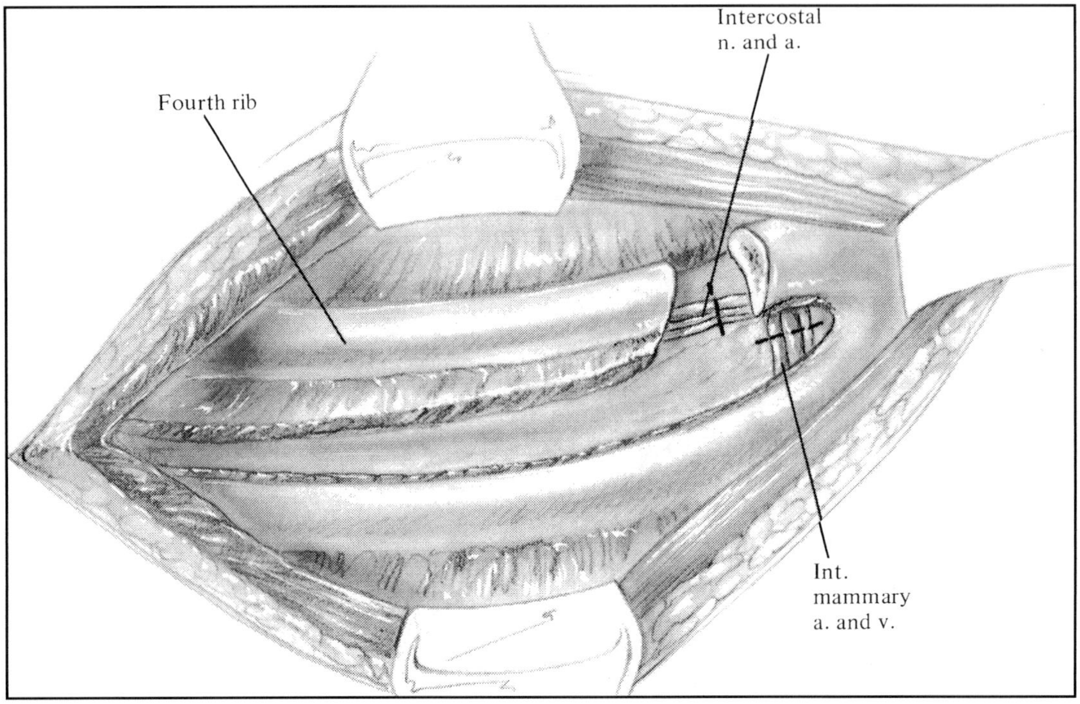
Intercostal
n. and a.
Fourth rib
Int.
mammary
a. and v.

Fig. 2-5

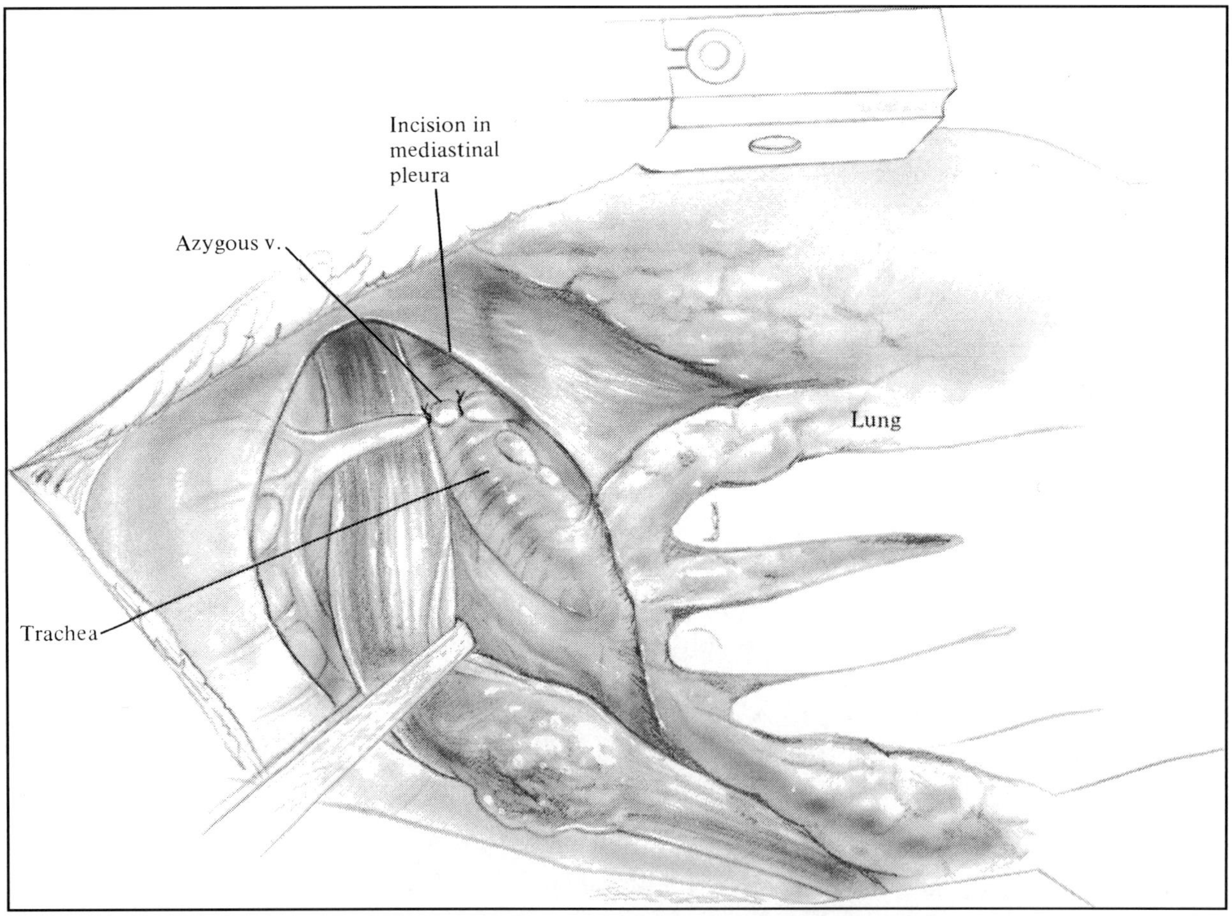
Incision in
mediastinal
pleura
Azygous v.
Lung
Trachea

Fig. 2-6

neurovascular bundle, divide it, and ligate with 2-0 silk **(Fig. 2–5)**.

Insert a Finochietto retractor over gauze pads and separate the ribs. If an additional costal cartilage requires division for adequate exposure, do not hesitate to perform this maneuver. Retract the lung anteriorly, cover it with gauze pads, and hold it with Harrington refractors.

Some surgeons prefer a posterolateral thoracotomy incision from the region of the paraspinal muscles to the sternum through the fourth or fifth interspace, but we have found the above exposure to be satisfactory. Using the anterior incision permits placing the patient in a position that is convenient for operating in the abdomen, the thorax, and even the neck, as necessary.

Mobilization of Esophagus

Make an incision in the mediastinal pleura, exposing the esophagus. Identify the azygous vein. Skeletonize, divide, and ligate it with 2-0 silk **(Fig. 2–6)**. Encircle the esophagus with the index finger at a point away from the tumor. The dissection reveals several small arterial branches to the esophagus. Divide each branch between hemostatic clips. Wherever the pericardium or pleura is adherent to the tumor, excise patches of these structures and leave them attached to the specimen. Include adjacent mediastinal lymph nodes in the specimen. Dissect the esophagus from the apex of the chest to the diaphragmatic hiatus; this maneuver requires division of the proximal vagal trunks. To minimize spillage of tumor cells, ligate the lumen of the esophagus proximal and distal to the tumor, utilizing narrow umbilical tapes or a 55 mm linear surgical stapler.

Remove the Harrington retractors and gauze pads, permitting the right lung to expand. Cover the thoracic incision with a sterile towel.

Mobilization of Stomach

Expose the abdominal incision. Use a Thompson retractor to elevate the sternum. Elevate the left lobe of the liver in a cephalad direction with the Weinberg blade of the Thompson retractor and incise the peritoneum overlying the abdominal esophagus. Circumferentially mobilize the lower esophagus. Transect the vagal trunks and surrounding phrenoesophageal ligaments **(Figs. 2–7, 2–8, 2–9)**. The cephalad portion of the gastrohepatic ligament, generally containing an accessory left hepatic artery, should be doubly clamped, divided, and ligated with 2-0 silk or Hemoclips **(Fig. 2–10)**. Insert the left hand behind the

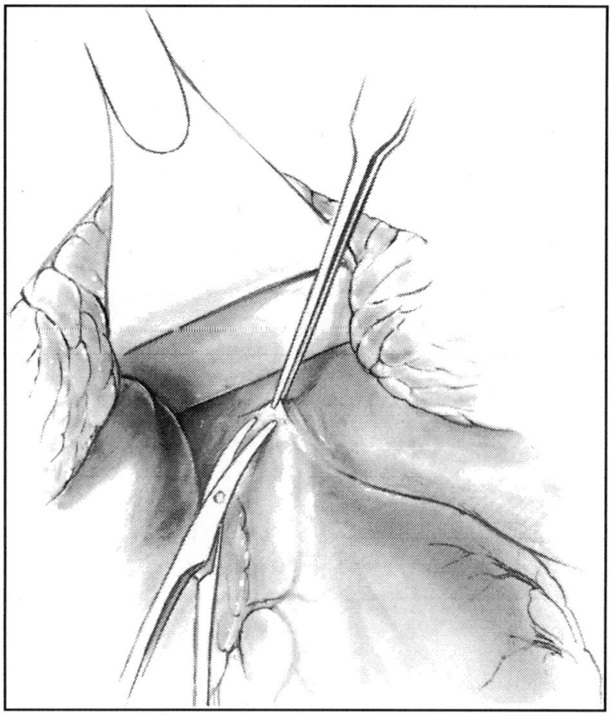

Fig. 2-7

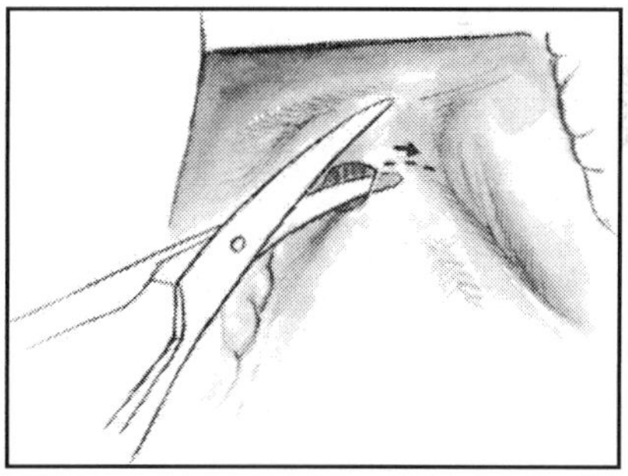

Fig. 2-8

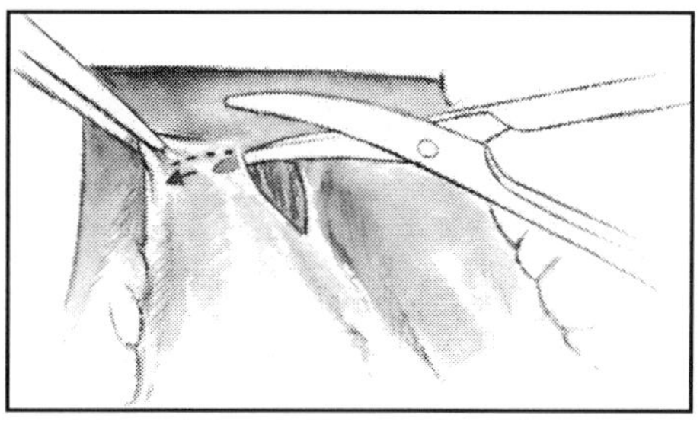

Fig. 2-9

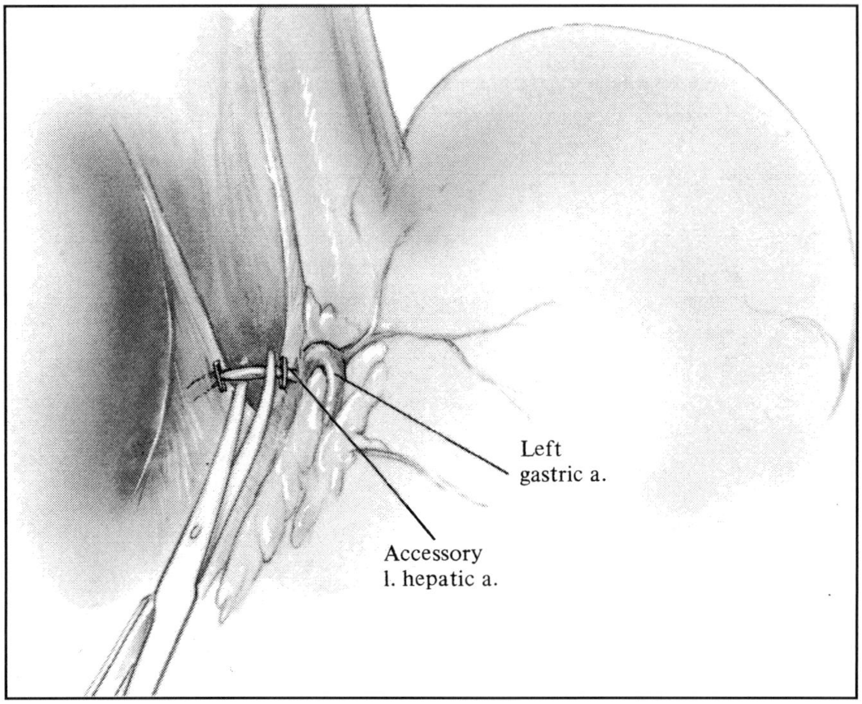

Fig. 2-10

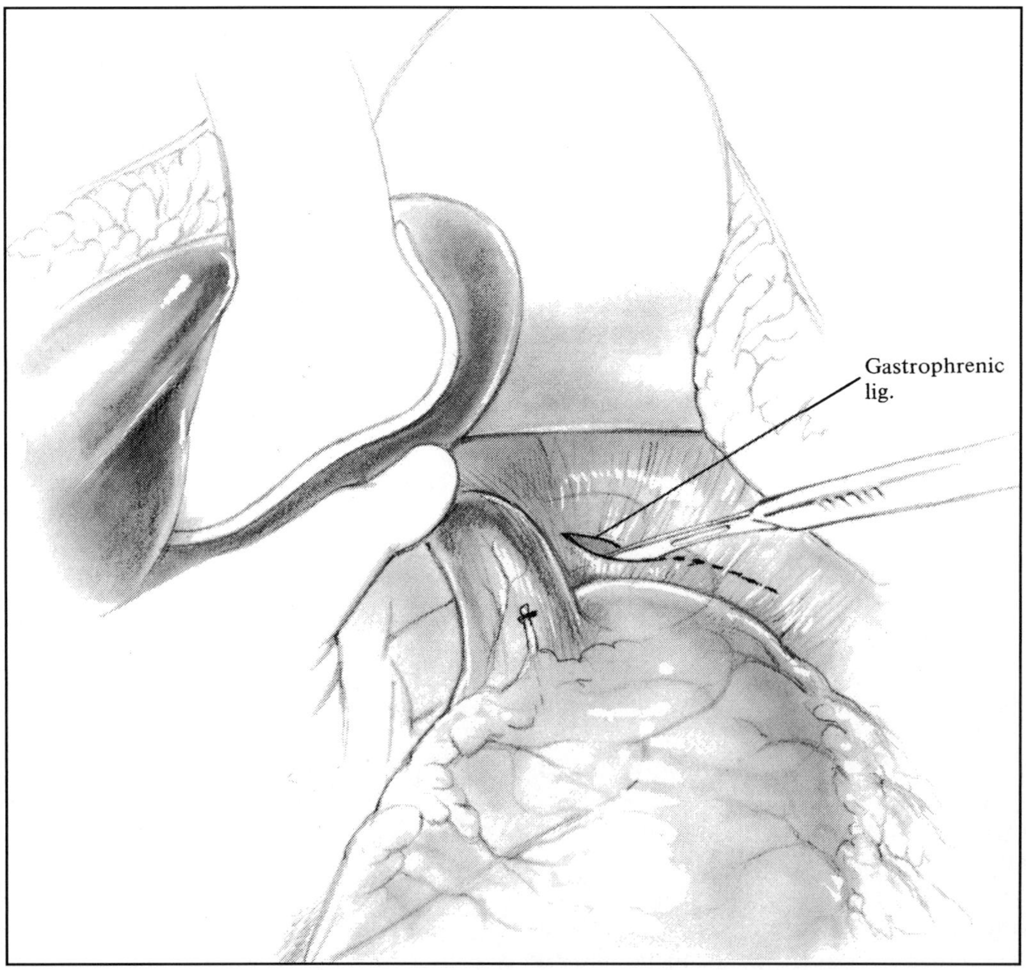

Fig. 2-11

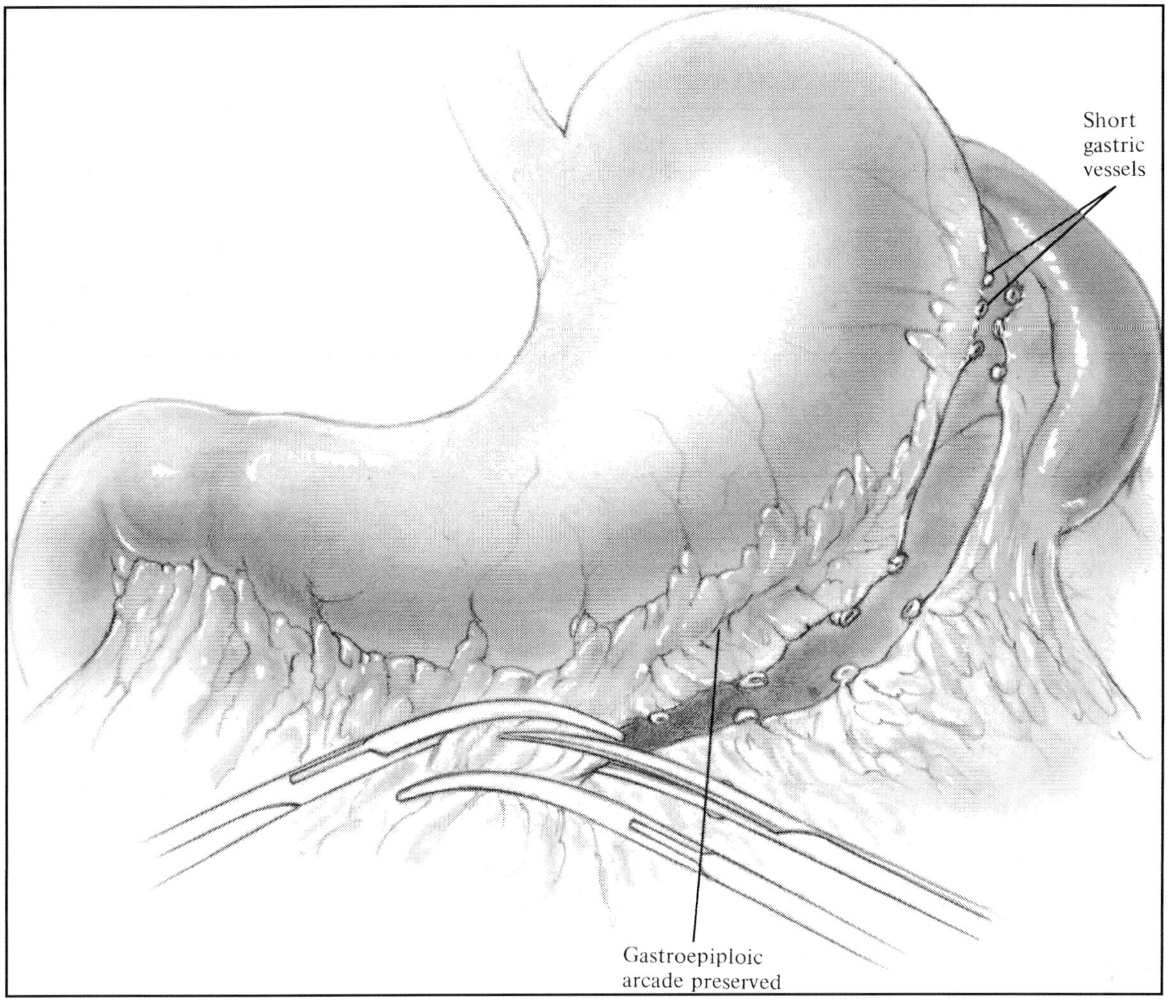

Fig. 2-12a

esophagus and cardia of the stomach, elevate the gastrophrenic ligaments on the index finger, and transect them **(Fig. 2–11)**. This dissection leads to the cephalad short gastric vessel; divide it between clamps and ligate it, along with the remaining short gastric vessels. The spleen need not be removed.

Divide and ligate the *left* gastroepiploic artery, but perform the remainder of the dissection *outside the gastroepiploic arcade, which must be kept intact and free of trauma*. This is accomplished by dividing the greater omentum serially between Kelly clamps, leaving 3–5 cm of omentum attached to the arcade as a margin of safety. Discontinue this dissection 6–8 cm proximal to the pylorus **(Fig. 2–12)**.

With the greater curvature of the stomach elevated, use palpation to identify the origin of the left

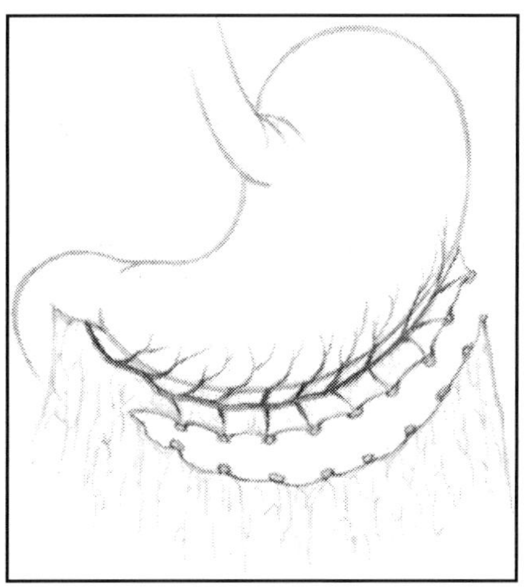

Fig. 2-12b

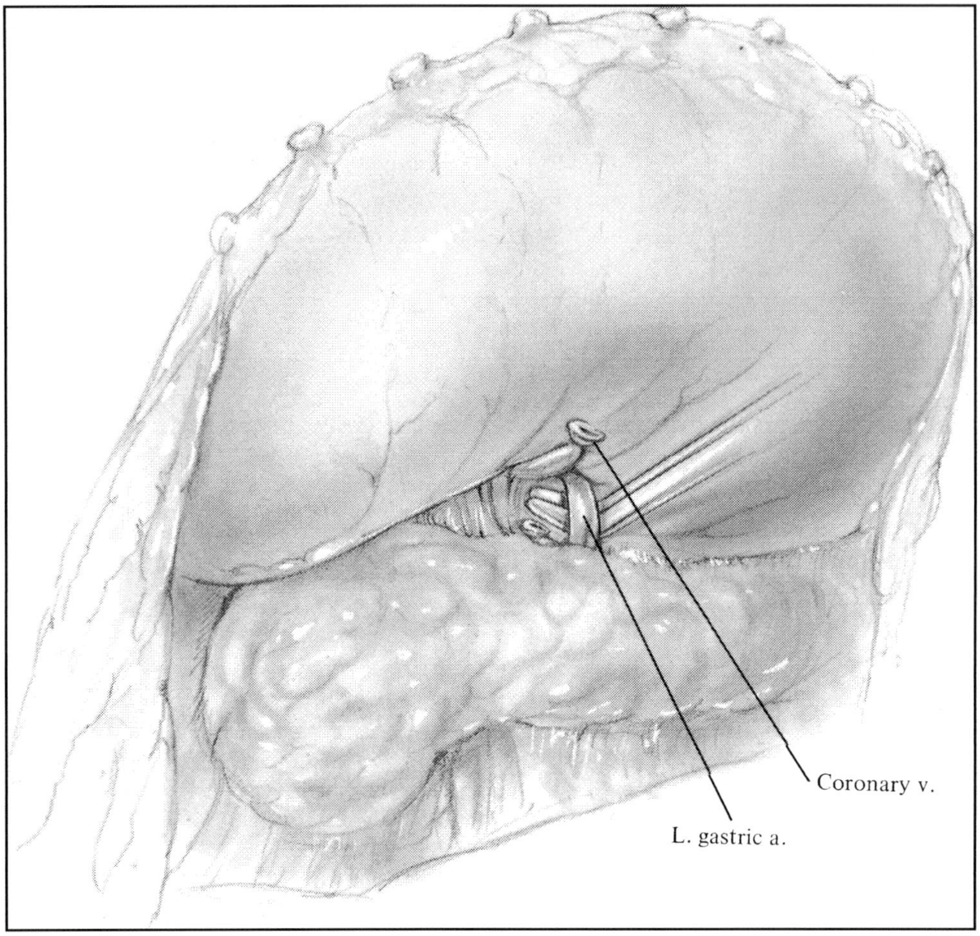

Fig. 2–13

gastric artery at the celiac axis. The coronary vein is situated just caudal to the artery. Clear it and encircle it with a Mixter clamp. Then divide it between 2-0 silk ligatures. Skeletonize the left gastric artery **(Fig. 2–13)** so two 2-0 ligatures can be placed on the proximal portion of the artery and one on the specimen side. Transect the vessel and follow with an extensive Kocher maneuver.

Kocher Maneuver

Make an incision in the peritoneum lateral to the proximal duodenum **(Fig. 2–14)**. Insert the left index finger behind the peritoneum and compress this tissue between fingertip and thumb, pushing retroperitoneal blood vessels and fat away. Incise the peritoneum on the index finger with scissors until the third portion of the duodenum is reached. Note that dividing the peritoneum alone is not sufficient to release the duodenum from its posterior attachments. There remains a ligamentous structure connecting the posterior duodenum to the region of Gerota's fascia. This ligamentous structure is easily delineated by inserting the left index finger behind

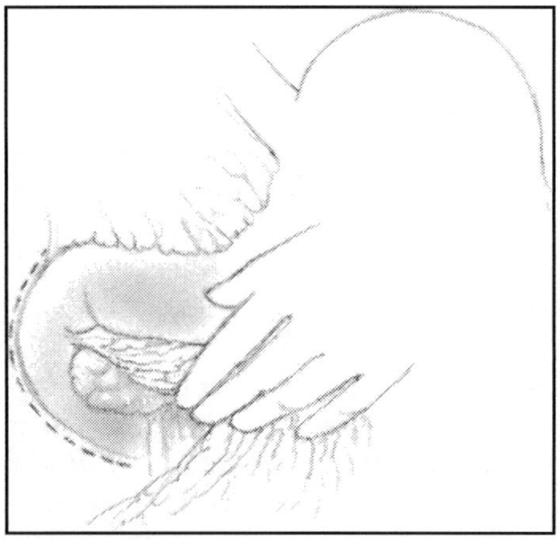

Fig. 2–14

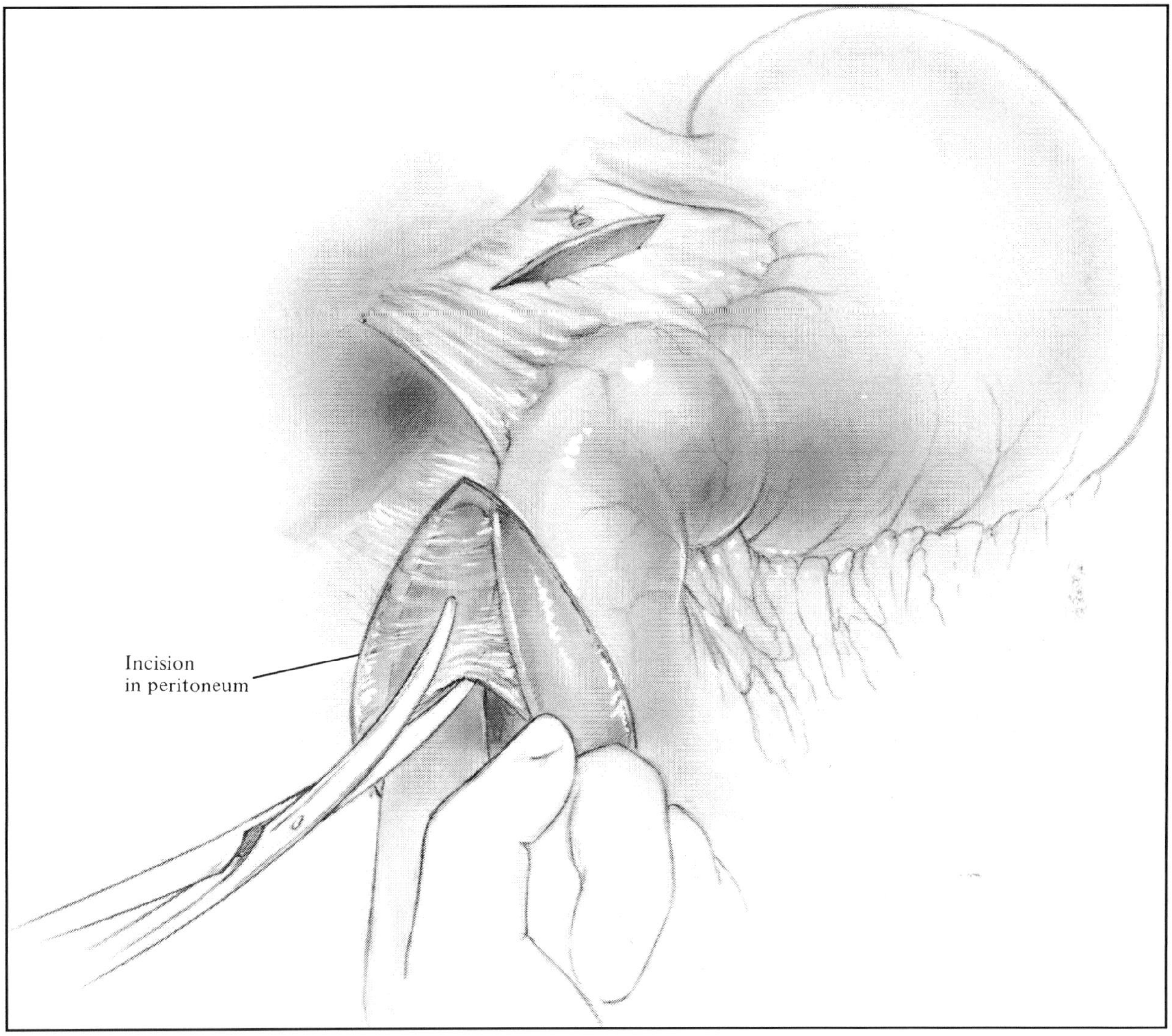

Fig. 2-15

the pancreas. Move the finger laterally, exposing a lateral duodenal "ligament" behind the descending duodenum. Again, pinch the tissue between fingertip and thumb, which leaves vascular and fatty tissue behind, allowing this ligamentous structure to be divided. Incise it with Metzenbaum scissors **(Fig. 2–15)**. Repeat this maneuver, going around the second and third portions of duodenum (behind the hepatic flexure); this leads to the point at which the superior mesenteric vein crosses over the duodenum. *Be careful*, as excessive traction with the index finger may tear this vessel.

For esophagogastric resection the Kocher maneuver need not be continued much beyond the junction of the second and third portions of the duodenum. At this point the left hand is easily passed behind the head of the pancreas, which should be elevated from the renal capsule, vena cava, and aorta **(Fig. 2–16)**. This permits the pyloroduodenal segment to be placed high in the abdomen, 8–10 cm from the esophageal hiatus, which in turn permits the gastric fundus to reach the thoracic apex, or neck, without tension.

Pyloromyotomy

Although in 80% of patients satisfactory results may be obtained without it, pyloromyotomy is generally performed at this point to prevent secondary operations for excessive gastric stasis due to vagotomy.

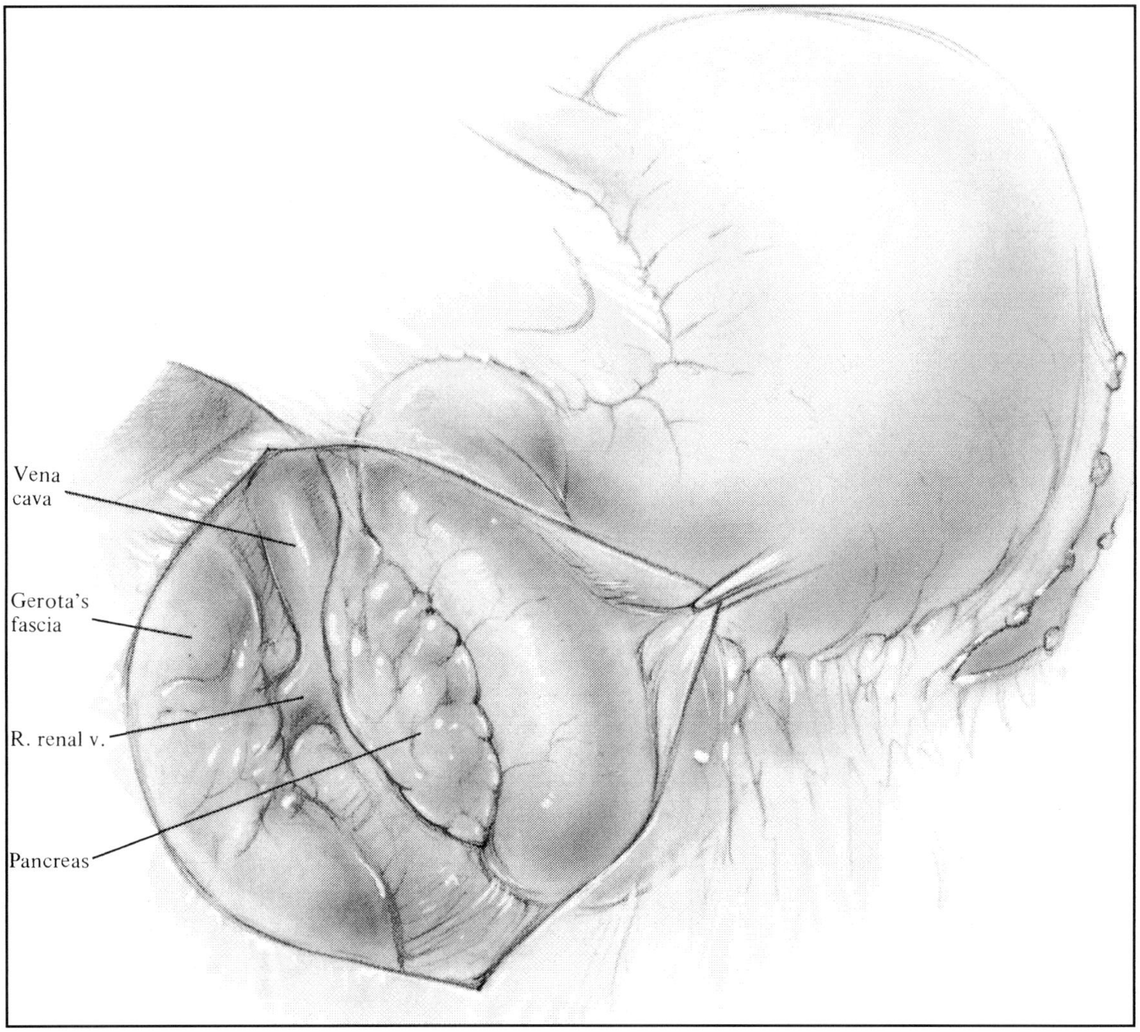

Fig. 2-16

Pyloromyotomy is accomplished by making a 1.5- to 2.0-cm incision across the anterior surface of the pyloric sphincter muscle **(Figs. 2–17, 2–18, 2–19)**. This maneuver is more difficult in an adult (who has only the normal thickness of muscle) than in an infant who suffers hypertrophic pyloric stenosis. Frequently, sharp dissection with a no. 15 scalpel blade must be done through most of the circular muscle. Separate the muscle fibers with a hemostat until the mucosa bulges out. This procedure may be expedited by invaginating the anterior gastric wall into the pyloric sphincter with the index finger to divide the few remaining circular muscle fibers. Exercise care not to perforate the mucosa, which is prone to such injury at the duodenal end of the incision.

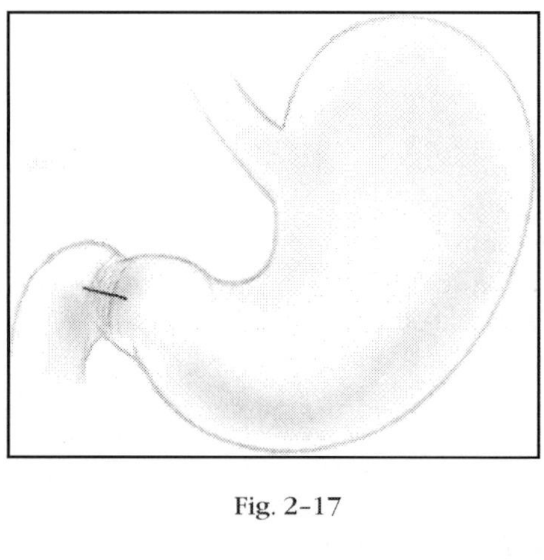

Fig. 2-17

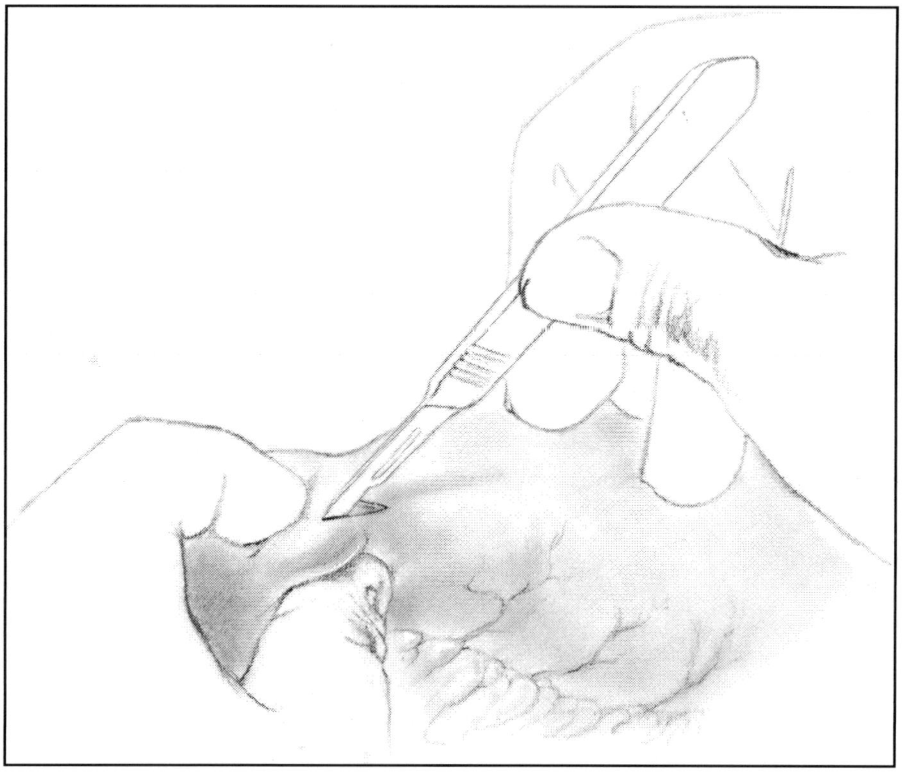

Fig. 2-18

Advancement of Stomach into Right Chest

Divide the right crux of the diaphragm transversely using electrocautery **(Fig. 2–20)** and further dilate the esophageal hiatus manually. Advance the stomach into the right hemithorax, which should again be exposed by expanding the Finochietto retractor. There must be *no constriction of the veins* in the vascular pedicle of the stomach at the hiatus. Suture the wall of stomach to the margins of the hiatus by means of interrupted 3-0 silk or Tevdek sutures spaced 2 cm apart to avoid postoperative herniation of bowel into the chest.

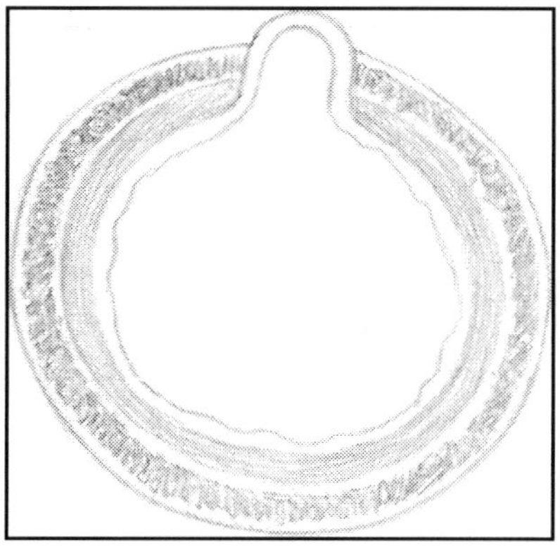

Fig. 2-19

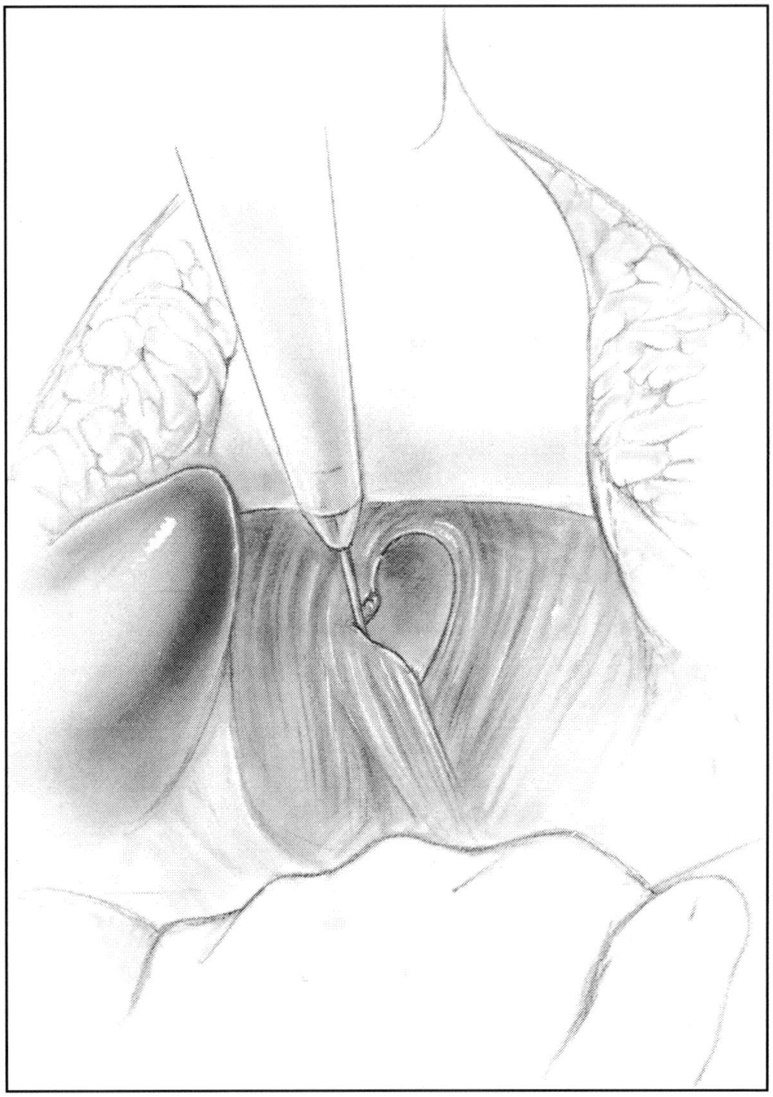

Fig. 2–20

With the right lung collapsed, expose the esophagogastric junction in the right chest. When the esophageal carcinoma is located in the middle or upper esophagus, it is not necessary to remove the lesser curvature of the stomach and the celiac lymph nodes.

After clearing the areolar tissue and the fat pad from the region of the esophagocardiac junction, apply a 55/4.8 mm linear stapler to the gastric side of this junction and fire the staples. Apply an Allen clamp to the esophagus, which should be transected flush with the stapler. Place a rubber glove over the divided esophagus and fix it in place with a narrow tape ligature. Lightly electrocoagulate the everted gastric mucosa and remove the stapling device **(Fig. 2–21)**. It is not necessary to invert this stapled closure with a layer of sutures. The fundus of the stomach should now reach the apex of the thorax without tension. Take care to avoid twisting the stomach and its vascular pedicle.

Esophagogastric Anastomosis

Select a point on the proximal esophagus 10 cm above the tumor for the anastomosis. Before removing the specimen, insert the posterior layer of sutures to attach the posterior esophagus to the anterior seromuscular layer of the stomach at a point 6–7 cm from the cephalad end of the fundus **(Fig. 2–22)**. The posterior layer should consist of about five interrupted atraumatic 4-0 silk Cushing sutures. Each bite should be 5 mm in width and deep enough to catch submucosa. The Stratte needle-holder may facilitate suture placement.

Transect the posterior wall of the esophagus with a scalpel at a point 6 mm beyond the first line of sutures. One can be certain that the esophageal

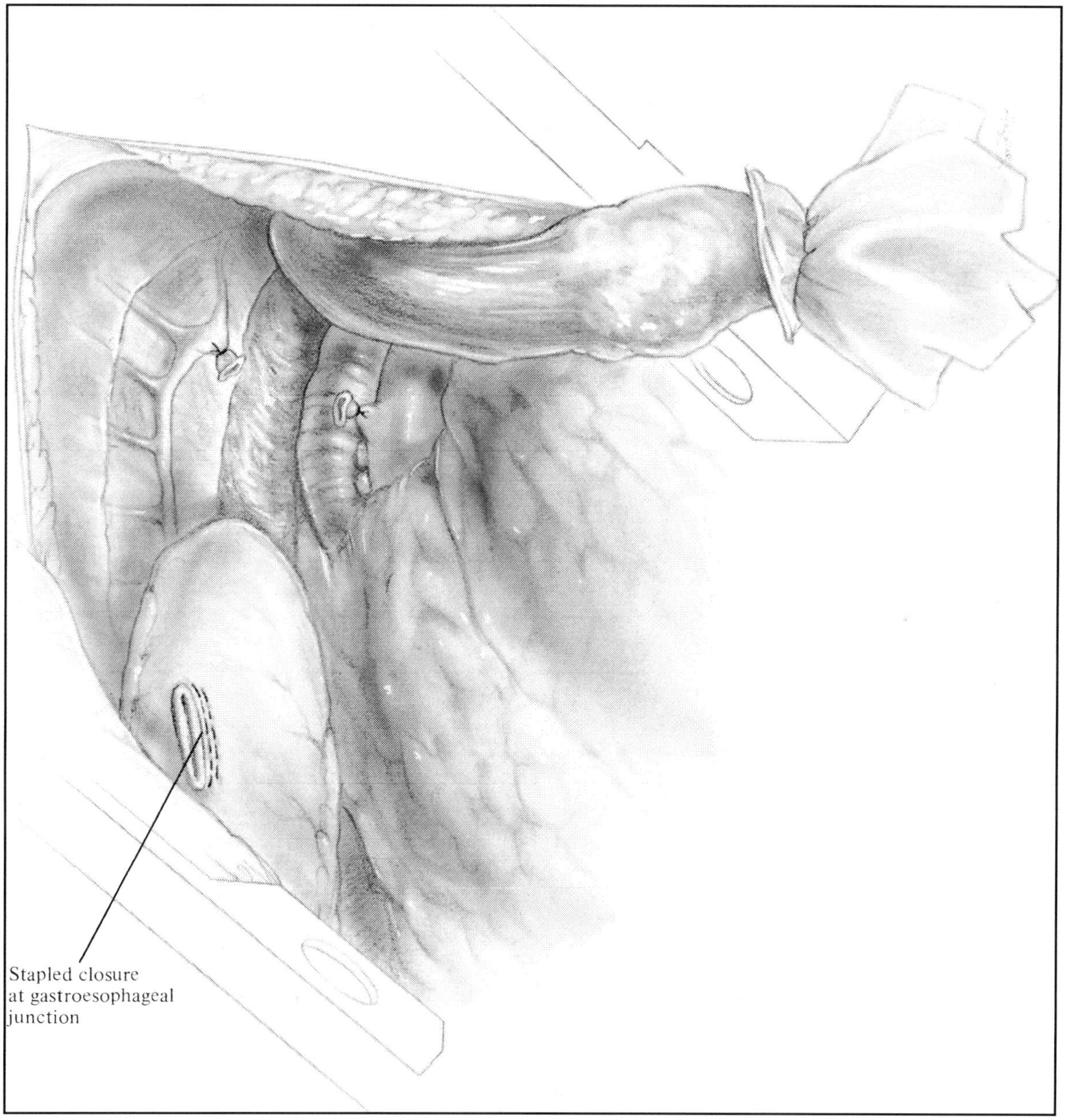

Fig. 2–21

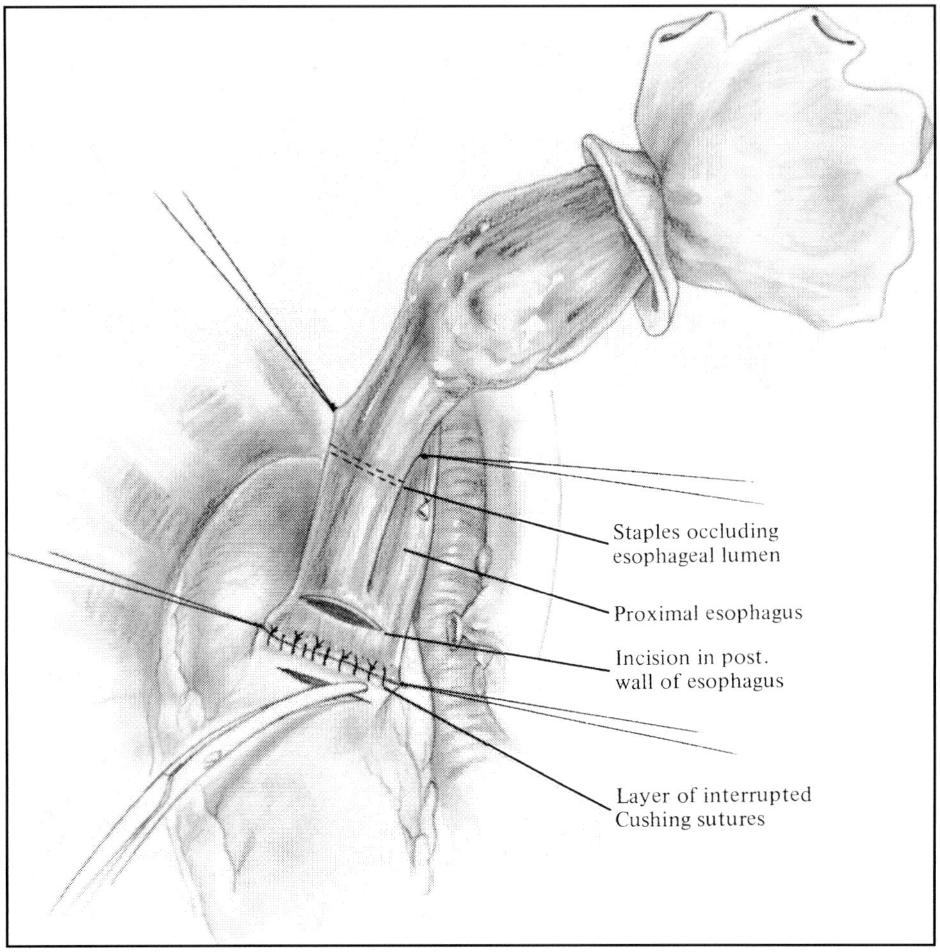

Fig. 2–22

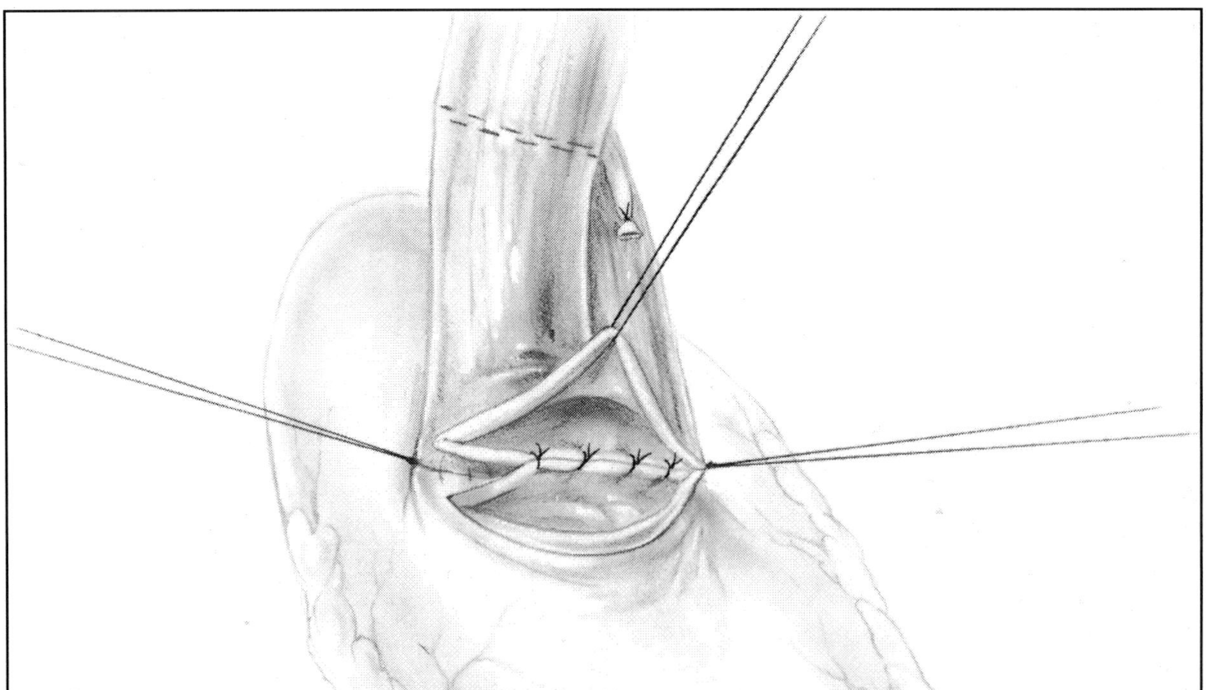

Fig. 2–23

mucosa has been transected when the nasogastric tube appears in the esophageal lumen. Now make a transverse incision in the stomach and control the bleeding points. This incision should be slightly longer than the diameter of the esophagus (Fig. 2–22).

Approximate the posterior mucosal layer by means of interrupted or continuous 5-0 atraumatic PG sutures, with the knots tied inside the lumen **(Fig. 2–23)**. Then pass the nasogastric tube from the proximal esophagus through the anastomosis into the stomach.

Detach the specimen by dividing the anterior wall of the esophagus with scissors in such fashion as to leave the anterior wall of the esophagus 1 cm longer than the posterior wall **(Fig. 2–24)**. This maneuver enlarges the stoma if the incision in the stomach is large enough to match that of the elliptical esophageal lumen.

Execute the anterior mucosal layer by means of interrupted sutures of 5-0 PG, with the knots tied inside the lumen thus inverting the mucosa **(Fig. 2–25)**. Accomplish the second anterior layer by means of interrupted Cushing sutures of 4-0 silk **(Fig. 2–26)**. Tie these sutures gently to approximate but not strangulate the tissue.

At this point some surgeons perform a Nissen fundoplication, which can be done if there is enough loose gastric wall to permit a wraparound without constricting the esophagus. Otherwise, a partial fundoplication may be accomplished by inserting several sutures between the outer walls of the esophagus and adjacent stomach. We have observed that even if fundoplication is not performed few patients develop reflux esophagitis following this operation so long as end-to-side esophagogastric anastomosis has been accomplished 6 cm or more below the cephalad margin of the gastric remnant.

Surgeons who lack wide experience with this anastomosis might find it wise to inflate the gastric pouch to test the anastomosis for leakage. A solution of methylene blue is injected into the nasogastric tube by the anesthesiologist for this purpose.

As a final, essential step in this operation, tension on the anastomosis is prevented by tacking the fundus of the stomach to the prevertebral fascia and mediastinal pleura at the apex of the thorax. Use interrupted sutures of 3-0 silk or Tevdek for this purpose (Fig. 2–26). These sutures must not penetrate the lumen of the stomach, lest a gastropleural fistula result.

As soon as the specimen has been removed, examine the proximal end of the esophagus by frozen section to see if there has been submucosal extension of the cancer. If the pathologist detects tumor cells in the esophageal margin, more esophagus should be resected.

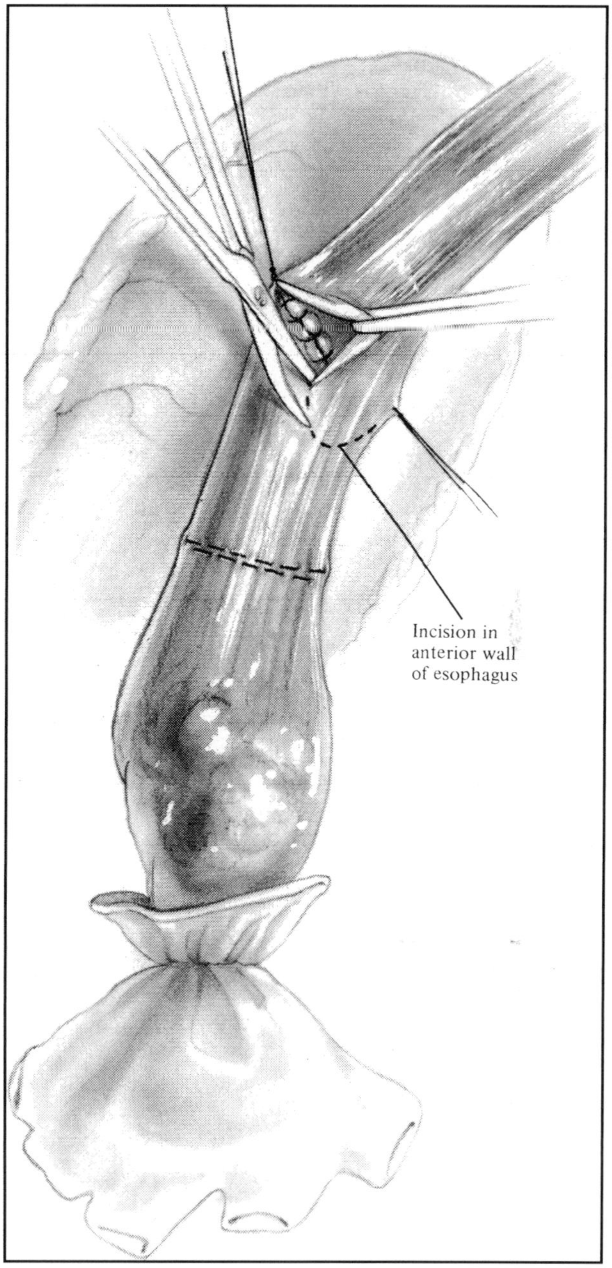

Fig. 2–24

Stapled Esophagogastric Anastomosis

Stapling techniques for this anastomosis are described in Chapter 3.

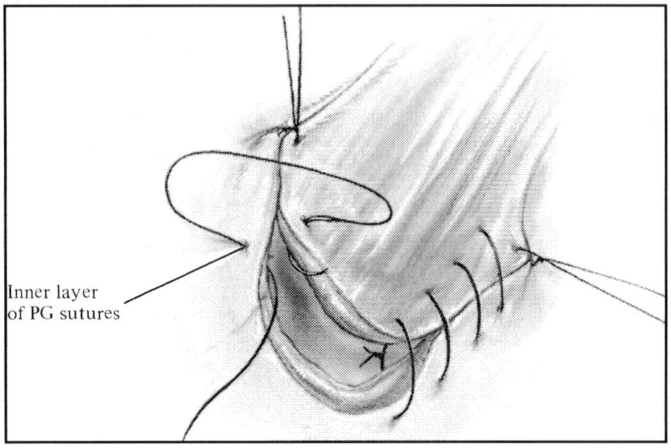

Fig. 2-25

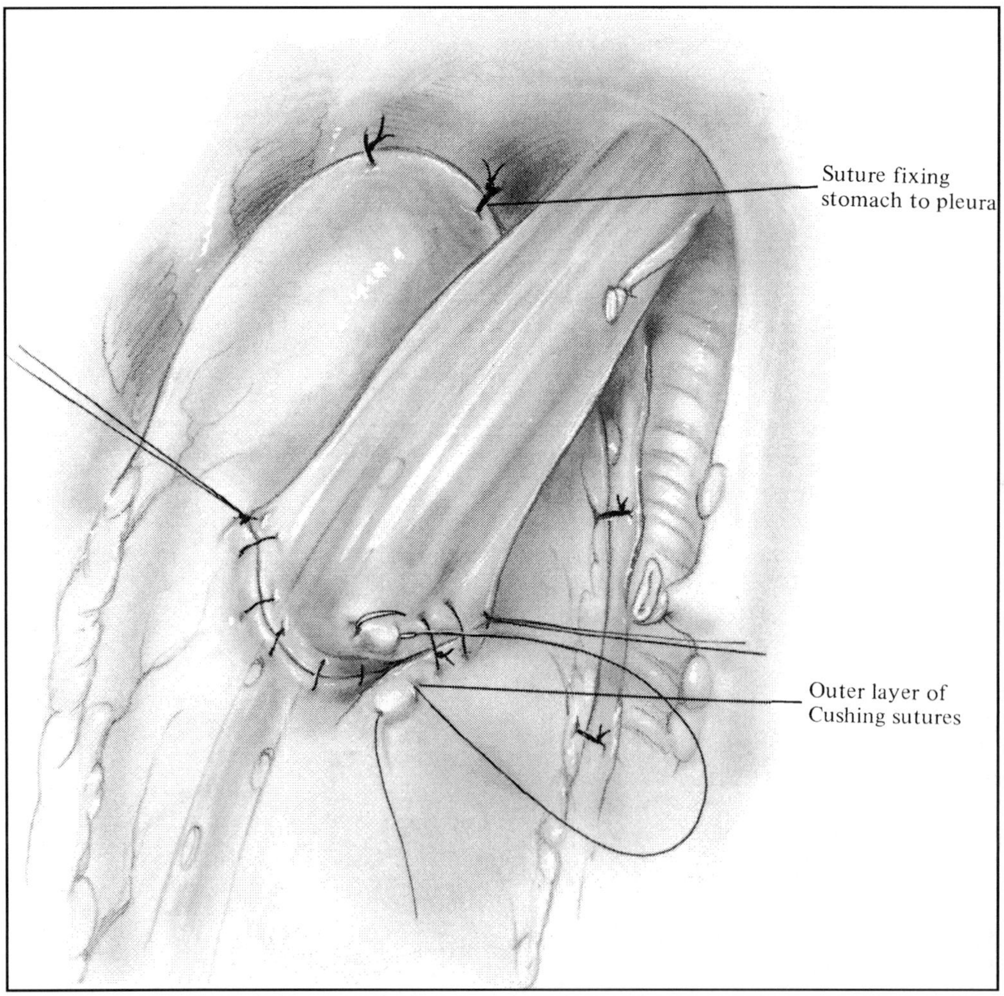

Fig. 2-26

Cervical Esophagogastric Anastomosis

When treating carcinoma of the mid-esophagus it is often necessary to resect the entire thoracic esophagus to obtain a sufficient margin of normal tissue above the tumor. This requires esophagogastric reconstruction in the neck.

With the patient's head turned slightly to the left, make an oblique incision along the anterior border of the right sternomastoid muscle **(Fig. 2–27)**. Carry the incision through the platysma. Identify **(Fig. 2–28)** and transect the omohyoid muscle. Retract the sternomastoid muscle and carotid sheath laterally and retract the prethyroid muscles medially, exposing the thyroid gland **(Fig. 2–29)**. The middle thyroid vein, when present, should be doubly ligated and divided. Put traction on the areolar tissue between the gland and the carotid sheath by upward and medial displacement of the thyroid. Excessive traction applied to the thyroid or larynx may injure the contralateral recurrent laryngeal nerve. Identify and skeletonize the inferior thyroid artery, which crosses the lower third of the surgical field in a transverse direction, by a Metzenbaum dissection toward the prevertebral fascia. Dissect it toward the thyroid gland until the recurrent laryngeal nerve can be seen. Then dissect the nerve upward to achieve thorough exposure, so it can be preserved (Fig. 2-29).

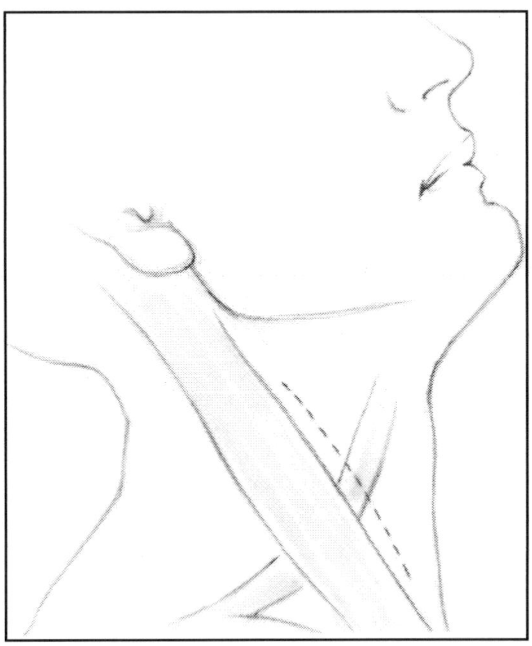

Fig. 2-27

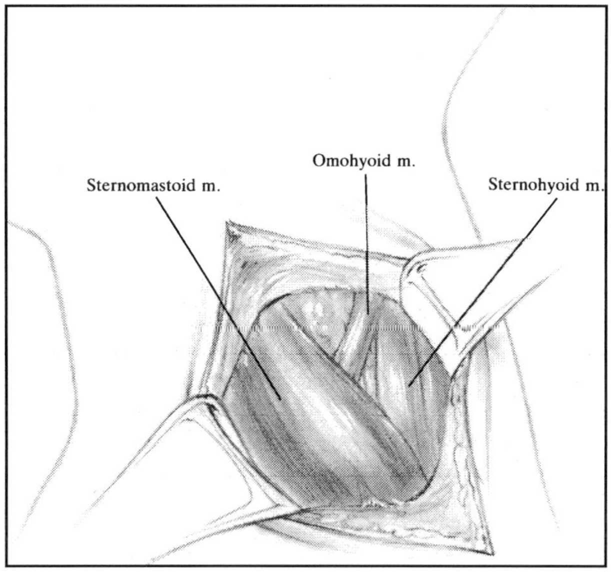

Fig. 2-28

At this point the tracheoesophageal groove is seen, and the cervical esophagus can be encircled by the surgeon's index finger, which should be passed between the esophagus and the prevertebral fascia and then between the esophagus and trachea. The finger should stay close to the esophageal wall; otherwise the *left* recurrent laryngeal nerve may be avulsed during this dissection. Although the inferior thyroid artery generally must be ligated and divided before the esophagus is mobilized, in some cases its course is low enough in the neck so it can be preserved.

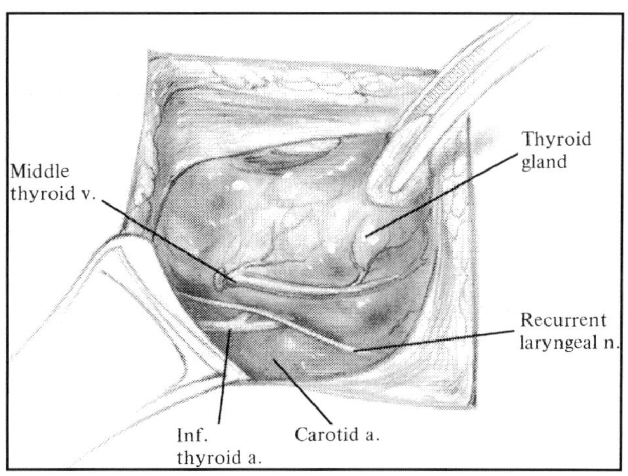

Fig. 2-29

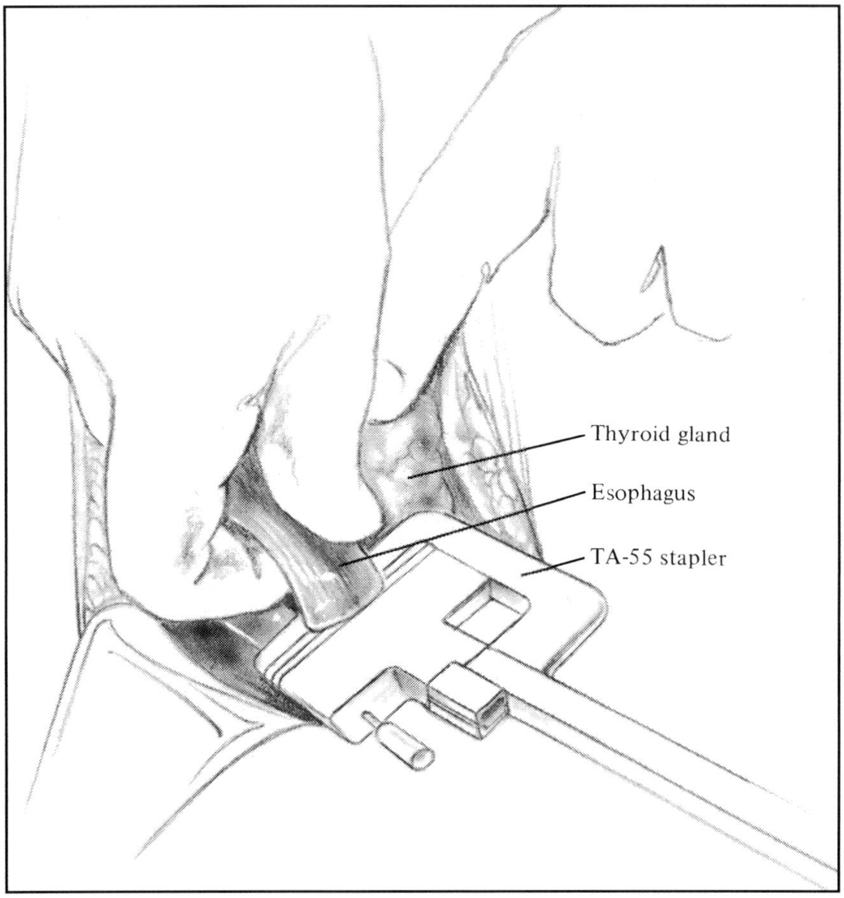

Fig. 2-30

Because the thoracic esophagus has been dissected up to the thoracic inlet, it is a simple matter to transect the esophagus low in the neck. When the proper point of transection of the esophagus has been selected, apply a 55 mm linear stapler to the specimen side **(Fig. 2–30)** and transect the esophagus flush with the stapler. Remove the specimen through the thoracic incision.

Now pass the fundus of the stomach (which has already been passed into the thorax) through the thoracic inlet into the cervical region. The fundus should reach the hypopharynx without tension. Anchor it to the prevertebral fascia with several 3-0 silk sutures. Then construct an end-to-side anastomosis by the same technique described above **(Figs.** 2-25, 2-26, **2–31, 2–32)**.

Lavage the operative site with an antibiotic solution and initiate wound closure by inserting a layer of interrupted 4-0 PG sutures, approximating the anterior border of the sternomastoid to the prethyroid strap muscles. Several similar sutures may be used loosely to approximate the platysma. Close the skin, generally by means of a continuous 4-0 PG subcuticular suture, leaving sufficient space to bring a latex drain out from the prevertebral region through the lower pole of the incision.

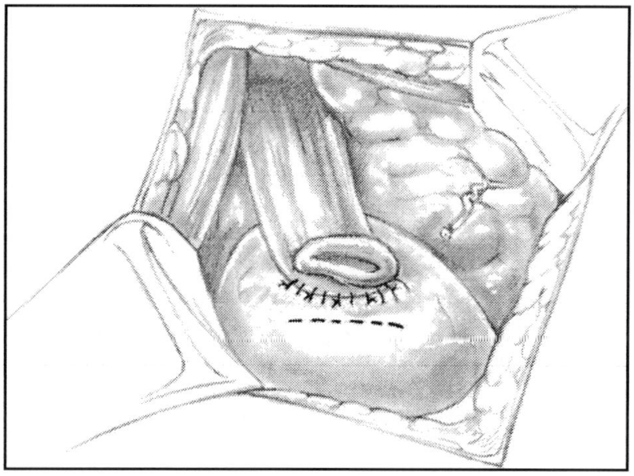

Fig. 2–31

Closure

Insert a 36F chest tube through a stab wound in the ninth intercostal space, and use 4-0 absorbable sutures to secure the catheter to the posterior pleura in the upper thorax. After thoroughly irrigating the thoracic and abdominal cavities with an antibiotic solution, approximate the ribs with four or five interrupted pericostal sutures of no. 1 PDS and approximate the serratus and pectoral muscles in layers by means of continuous 2-0 atraumatic PG **(Figs. 2–33, 2–34)**. Close the skin with continuous 3-0 nylon or subcuticular 4-0 PG. Consider inserting a needle-catheter feeding jejunostomy. Close the abdominal wall in the usual fashion by means of interrupted no. 1 PDS sutures.

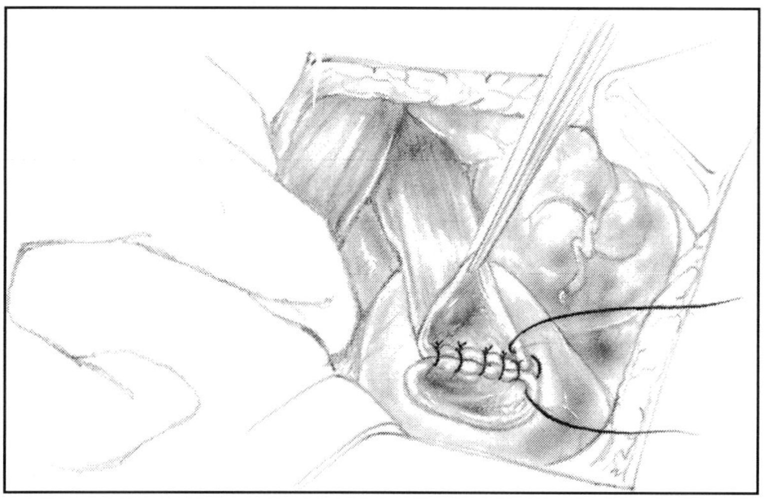

Fig. 2–32

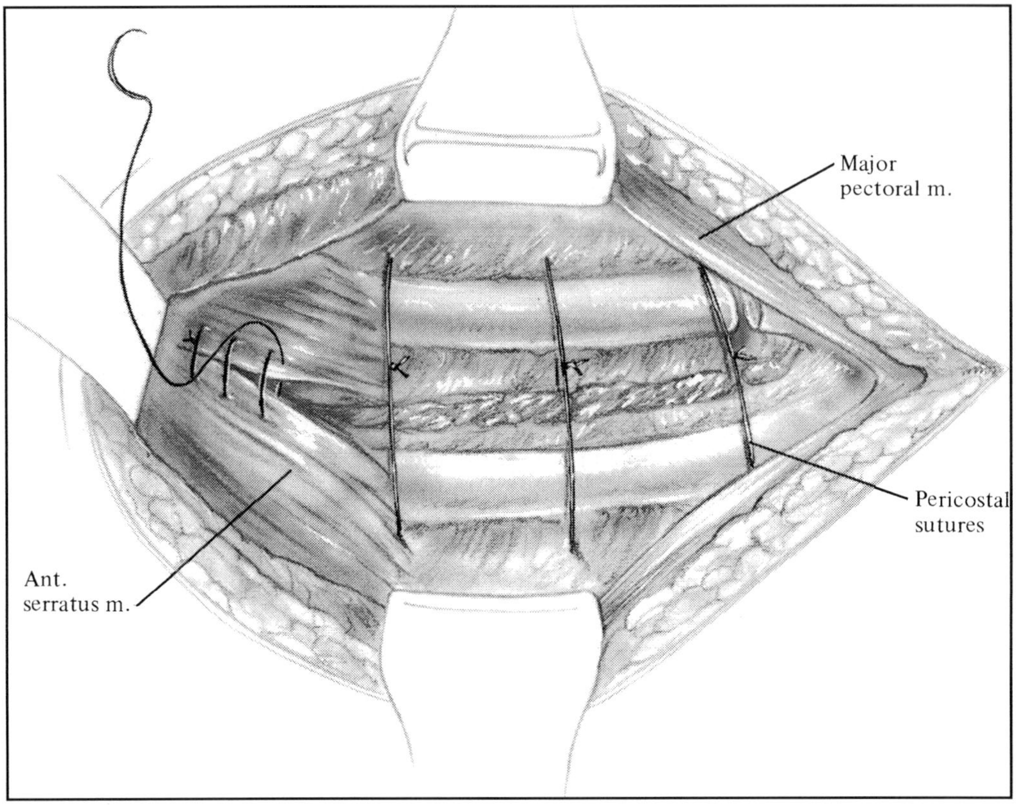

Fig. 2-33

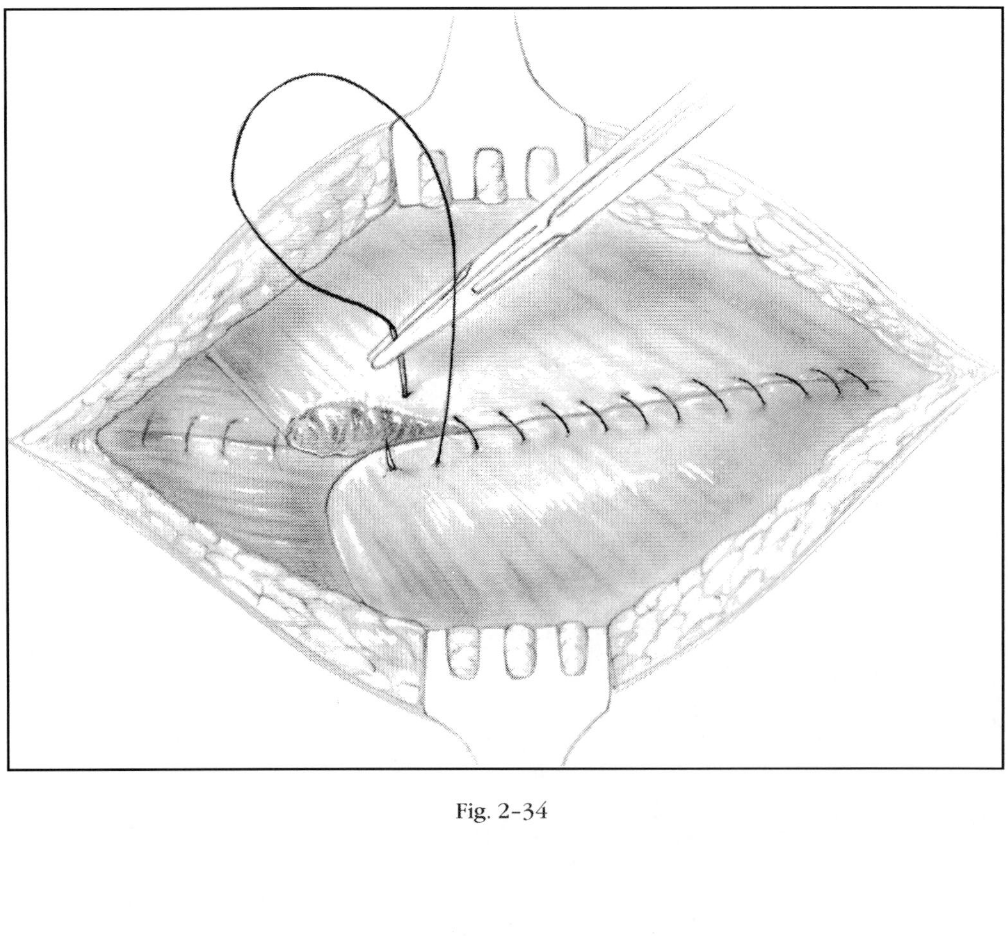

Fig. 2-34

POSTOPERATIVE CARE

Keep the nasogastric tube on low suction for 4–5 days. Permit nothing by mouth until a contrast study has demonstrated integrity of the anastomosis.

Obtain an esophagram with water-soluble contrast followed by thin barium on the seventh postoperative day. If no leak is demonstrated, the patient is given a liquid diet, which is advanced to a full diet within 3–5 days.

Attach the chest tube to underwater suction drainage for 4–5 days. Follow the routine steps for managing a postoperative thoracotomy patient, including frequent determinations of arterial blood gases and pH. Tracheal suction is used with caution to avoid possible trauma to the anastomosis. Ventilatory support is employed when necessary. Continue prophylactic antibiotics until removal of the chest tube. Use the needle-catheter jejunostomy for enteral alimentation beginning promptly after surgery.

COMPLICATIONS

Anastomotic leaks. Anastomotic leaks constitute by far the most important complication of this operation, but they are *preventable if proper surgical technique is used.* Although minor contained leaks may be treated nonoperatively, most leaks require operative drainage, diversion, repair, or a combination of these maneuvers (see Chapter 14).

Abscesses. A subphrenic or subhepatic abscess may follow an operation for an ulcerated malignancy because a necrotic gastric tumor often harbors virulent organisms. The incidence of this complication can be reduced by administering prophylactic antibiotics before and during the operation. Treatment is by computed tomography (CT)-directed or surgical drainage.

Pulmonary problems. Pulmonary complications were common in the past, but their incidence has been minimized by proper postoperative pulmonary care. Adequate pain control may require epidural analgesia.

Cardiac arrhythmias. Cardiac failure and arrhythmia are not uncommon in patients who are in their seventh or eighth decade of life. Generally, with careful monitoring and early detection these complications can be easily managed. Hemodynamic monitoring may be helpful.

Stenosis. In the absence of recurrent mediastinal cancer, stenosis of the anastomosis has not occurred in any of the cases Chassin managed and reported. When this complication does occur, repeated passage of Maloney bougies may reverse the condition.

REFERENCES

Bates BA, Detterbeck FC, Bernard SA, et al. Concurrent radiation therapy and chemotherapy followed by esophagectomy for localized esophageal carcinoma. J Clin Oncol 1996;14:156.

Chassin, JL. Esophagogastrectomy: data favoring end-to-side anastomosis. Ann Surg 1978;188:22.

Chu KM, Law SY, Fok M, Wong J. A prospective randomized comparison of transhiatal and transthoracic resection for lower-third esophageal carcinoma. Am J Surg 1997;174:320.

Lee RB, Miller JI. Esophagectomy for cancer. Surg Clin North Am 1997;77:1169.

Lerut T, Coosemans W, De Leyn P et al. Treatment of esophageal carcinoma. Chest 1999;116(suppl):463S.

Skandalakis JE, Ellis H. Embryologic and anatomic basis of esophageal surgery. Surg Clin North Am 2000;80:85.

Skinner DB, Little AG, Ferson MK, Soriano A. Selection of operation for esophageal cancer based on staging. Ann Surg 1986;204:391.

Stark SP, Romberg MS, Pierce GE, et al. Transhiatal versus transthoracic esophagectomy for adenocarcinoma of the distal esophagus and cardia. Am J Surg 1996;172: 478.

Sugarbaker DJ, Jaklitsch MT, Liptay MJ. Thoracoscopic staging and surgical therapy for esophageal cancer. Chest 1995;107(suppl):218S.

3 Esophagogastrectomy

Left Thoracoabdominal Approach

INDICATIONS

Carcinoma of the distal esophagus or proximal stomach

Distal esophageal stricture

PREOPERATIVE PREPARATION

See Chapter 2.

PITFALLS AND DANGER POINTS

Anastomotic failure.

Ischemia of gastric pouch. Pay meticulous attention to preserving the entire arcade of the right gastroepiploic artery and vein along the greater curvature of the stomach.

Hemorrhage. Occasionally, the left gastric artery is embedded in tumor via invasion from metastatic lymph nodes. Unless this vessel can be identified, transecting the artery through the tumor may produce hemorrhage that is difficult to control.

Pancreas. Trauma to the tail of the pancreas may cause a pancreatic fistula or acute hemorrhagic pancreatitis.

Sepsis. Some malignancies in the proximal portion of the stomach are ulcerated and bulky with areas of necrosis that contain virulent bacteria. These bacteria may produce postoperative subhepatic or subphrenic abscesses via operative contamination even without anastomotic leakage. Both enteral and parenteral antibiotics that cover colon flora should be used.

Inadequate cancer operation. Because gastric and esophageal malignancies can spread submucosally for some distance without being visible, frozen section studies of both proximal and distal margins of the excision are helpful.

Paralysis of the diaphragm. The diaphragm should be divided around the periphery to preserve phrenic innervation and prevent paralysis.

OPERATIVE STRATEGY

Objectives of Esophagogastrectomy

With operations done for cure, the objective is wide removal of the primary tumor, along with a 6- to 10-cm margin of normal esophagus in a proximal direction and a 6 cm margin of normal stomach below. Even if the stomach is not involved, when the tumor is situated low in the esophagus the proximal lesser curvature of the stomach should be included to remove the left gastric artery at its origin and the celiac lymph nodes. Splenectomy and removal of the lymph nodes at the splenic hilus may be required for large lesions of the proximal stomach and fundus. Any suspicious nodes along the superior border of the pancreas should also be removed.

Thoracoabdominal Incision with Preservation of Phrenic Nerve Function

When gastric cancer encroaches on the gastroesophageal junction, operations done by abdominal incision exclusively are contraindicated for several reasons. In the first place, this anastomosis frequently requires the surgeon's hand and the needle-holder to be in an awkward position and may result in leakage. Furthermore, the abdominal incision makes it difficult to perform wide excision of possible areas of invasion of the distal esophagus. We have seen some upper gastric lesions that extended into the esophagus as far as 10 cm.

The left thoracoabdominal incision, we have found, is both safe and efficacious. It is easy to divide all the muscles of the thoracic cage rapidly by electrocautery. Even patients in their eighties have tolerated this incision well when given adequate postoperative support. Epidural anesthesia minimizes pain and allows early mobilization.

Positioning the patient in the full lateral position with an incision through the fifth or sixth intercostal space gives wide exposure to the mediastinum, left pleural space, and left upper quadrant of the abdomen.

The diaphragm should *not* be incised radially from the costal margin to the esophageal hiatus because it would transect the phrenic nerve and paralyze the left diaphragm. Many patients who require gastric surgery for cancer are aged and have limited pulmonary reserve; moreover, because atelectasis is a common postoperative complication, it is better to make a circumferential incision in the periphery of the diaphragm to preserve phrenic and intercostal nerve function and normal diaphragmatic motion.

Postoperative pain at the site of the divided costal margin is allegedly common following a thoracoabdominal incision. In our experience proper resuturing of the costal margin with monofilament steel wire results in solid healing of this area. Neither pain nor costochondritis has been a problem.

Anastomotic Leakage

Delicacy and precision of anastomotic technique and adequate exposure are important for preventing anastomotic leaks. If a gastric or lower esophageal lesion has spread up the lower esophagus for a distance of more than 6–8 cm, the esophagogastric anastomosis should not be constructed high up under the aortic arch, as it is a hazardous technique. Instead, 1 cm posterior segments of two additional ribs are resected if necessary to give more proximal exposure, and the esophagus is liberated behind the arch of the aorta and passed out to an intrapleural, supra-aortic position. This exposure permits the anastomosis to be done in a manner less traumatic to the tissues than an anastomosis constructed high up under the aortic arch. Otherwise, the surgeon's hand and wrist are situated in an awkward position, which makes smooth manipulation of instruments difficult. Jerky suturing motions produce small tears in the esophagus, especially in the posterior layer, where access is difficult.

End-to-End versus End-to-Side Anastomosis

We showed that the end-to-end esophagogastric anastomosis carries with it a much higher rate of leakage and a higher mortality rate than the end-to-side variety (Chassin 1978). Explanations for the increased complication rate following end-to-end esophagogastrostomy are not difficult to find.

1. It is necessary to close a portion of the end of the stomach because of the disparity between the lumen of the stomach and that of the esophagus. This increases the technical difficulty of doing the end-to-end anastomosis **(Fig. 3–1a,b)**.

2. The blood supply of the gastric pouch at its proximal margin is inferior to that at the site of the end-to-side anastomosis.

3. Inserting the posterior layer of esophagogastric sutures may be difficult. Traction must be applied to the esophagus to improve exposure, and the surgeon's hand and the needle-holder may have to assume positions that are awkward for efficient, atraumatic suturing, which produces imperfections in the suture line.

4. As seen in **Figure 3–2a**, protection from posterior leakage is achieved in the end-to-side cases by the buttress effect of a 6- to 7-cm segment of gastric wall behind the esophagus. In end-to-end

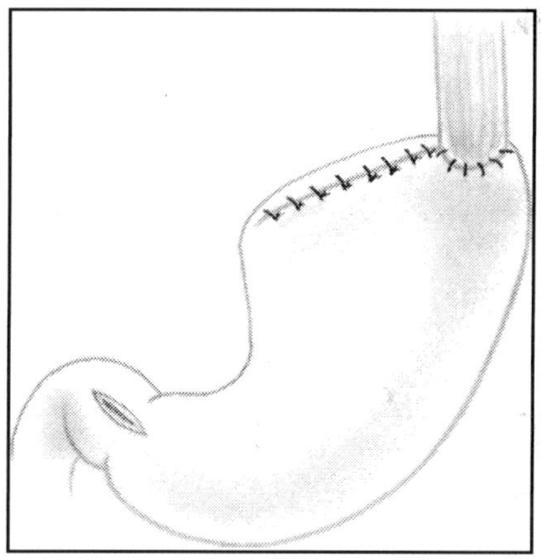

Fig. 3-1a

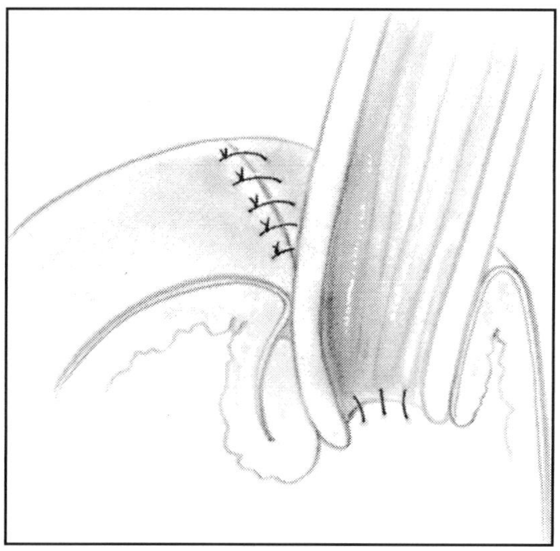

Fig. 3-1b

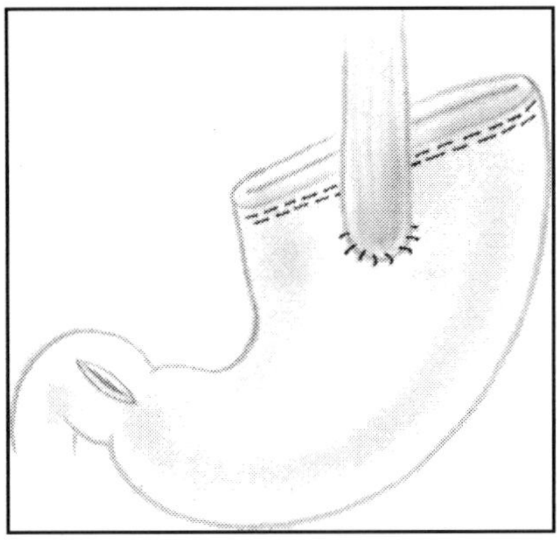

Fig. 3-2a

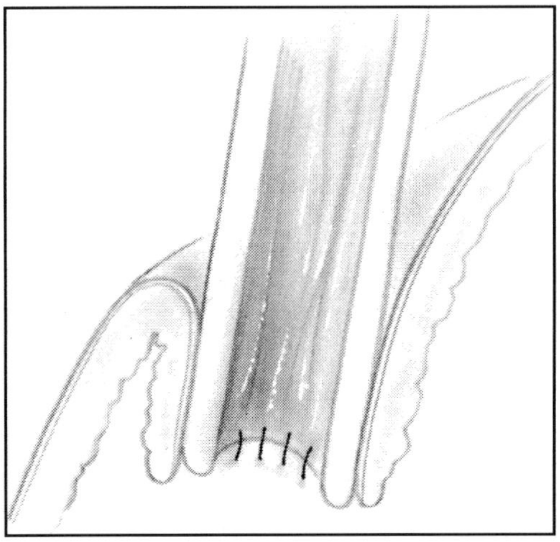

Fig. 3-2b

operations, however, there is no second line of defense against technical error.

5. Although the anterior layer of the end-to-end or the end-to-side esophagogastrostomy is much easier to construct without technical defects than the posterior layer, even here the end-to-side version offers advantages. **Figure 3–2b** illustrates how the anterior wall of the esophagus invaginates into the stomach for additional protection. If this were attempted with an end-to-end anastomosis, the large inverted cuff would produce stenosis at the stoma (Fig. 3-1b).

Additional protection against leakage from the anterior aspect of the end-to-side anastomosis can be achieved by performing a Nissen fundoplication around the anastomosis. This also helps prevent postoperative gastroesophageal reflux, but it requires the presence of a large gastric pouch and cannot be performed, unless modified, when the proximal stomach has been resected.

Avoiding Postoperative Reflux Esophagitis

Another serious drawback of an end-to-end esophagogastric anastomosis is the occurrence of reflux esophagitis in patients who achieve long-term survival. It can be avoided by implanting the end of the esophagus end-to-side into the stomach at least 6 cm beyond the proximal margin of the gastric pouch. This type of construction functions as a valve, probably because air in the gastric pouch behind the distal esophagus and above the esophagogastric anastomosis compresses the overlying esophagus. This is fortunate, as there is rarely enough remaining stomach to fashion an adequate "fundoplication" when the gastric fundus has been resected.

When the anastomosis is performed by the stapling method, the anastomosis should still be a comfortable distance from the proximal end of the gastric interposition for the same reason as elaborated for the sutured anastomosis.

Efficacy of Stapling Techniques for the Esophagogastric Anastomosis

We have developed a stapling technique for end-to-side esophagogastrostomy that can be done swiftly with an extremely low leak rate (Chassin 1978). After a long, sometimes complicated dissection, an accurate anastomosis that takes only 2–3 minutes of operating time constitutes a welcome epilogue, especially when treating poor-risk patients. Whereas 28 mm and 31 mm circular stapling cartridges produce a good anastomosis, use of the 25 mm cartridge results in a high incidence of anastomotic postoperative strictures requiring dilatation.

Postoperative Sepsis

To prevent postoperative sepsis, meticulously avoid spillage of the gastric content, which can contaminate the subhepatic or subcutaneous space. Any instruments that come into contact with the lumen of the stomach or esophagus should be treated as dirty and the area walled off wherever possible. During the operation intravenous antibiotics that cover a spectrum from lower mouth to skin to enteric organisms should be given at appropriate intervals to ensure that body fluid and tissue levels are maintained.

OPERATIVE TECHNIQUE

Incision and Position

Endobronchial (double-lumen) one-lung anesthesia permits atraumatic collapse of the left lung during the esophageal dissection. It is far preferable to advancing an endotracheal tube down the right mainstream bronchus.

With the aid of sandbags and wide adhesive tape across the patient's hips and left shoulder, elevate the patient's left side to a 60°–90° angle. Place the right arm straight on an arm board. Pad the patient's left arm and suspend it in a forward position **(Fig. 3–3)**.

Begin the incision at the umbilicus and continue it up the midline about halfway to the xiphoid, or use an oblique incision parallel to the right costal margin midway between the xiphoid and umbilicus. Explore the abdomen. The presence of metastasis of moderate degree to the celiac lymph nodes or to the liver does not constitute a contraindication to resection.

Redirect the incision to cross the costal margin into the sixth intercostal space and continue to it the region of the erector spinae muscle near the tip of the scapula. After the skin incision has been completed, use the coagulating current to divide the latissimus dorsi muscle in as caudal a location as possible **(Fig. 3–4)**. The index fingers of both the surgeon and

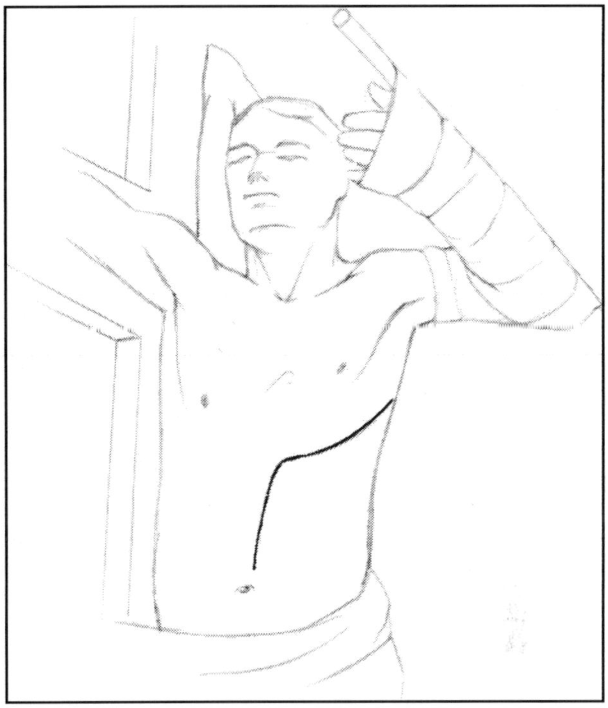

Fig. 3–3

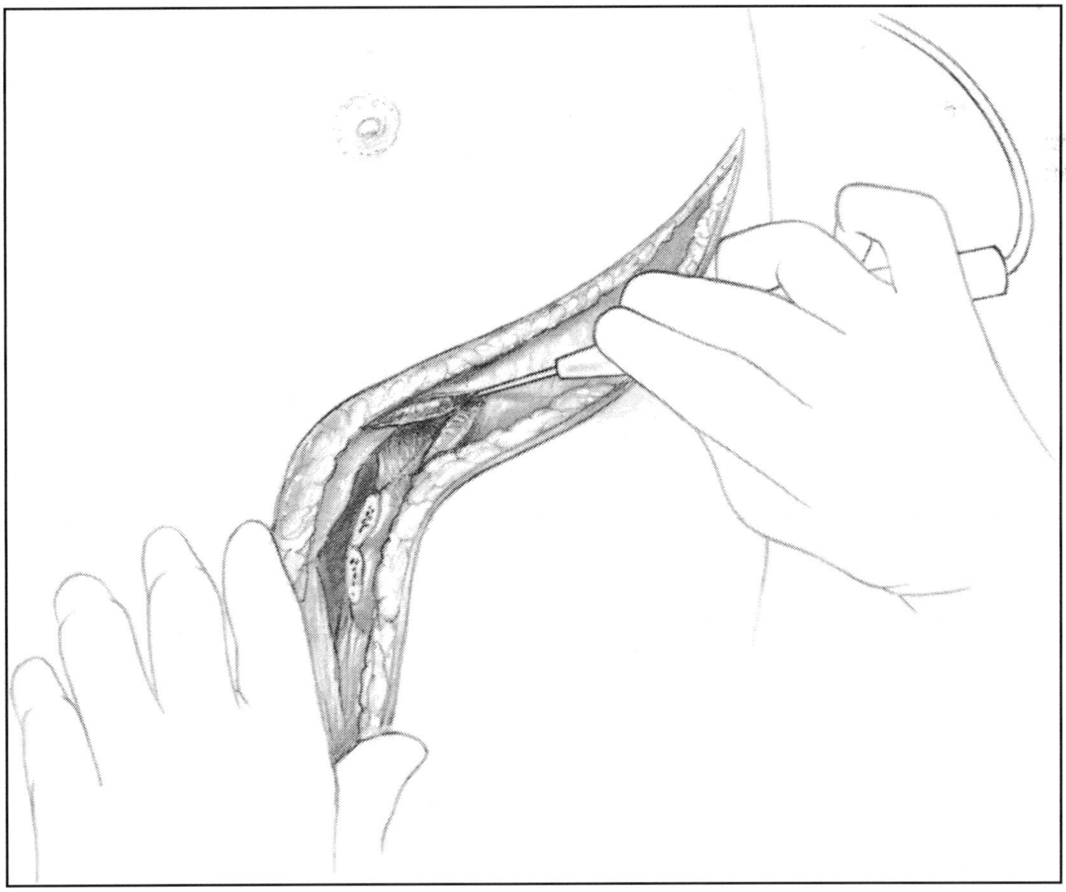

Fig. 3–4

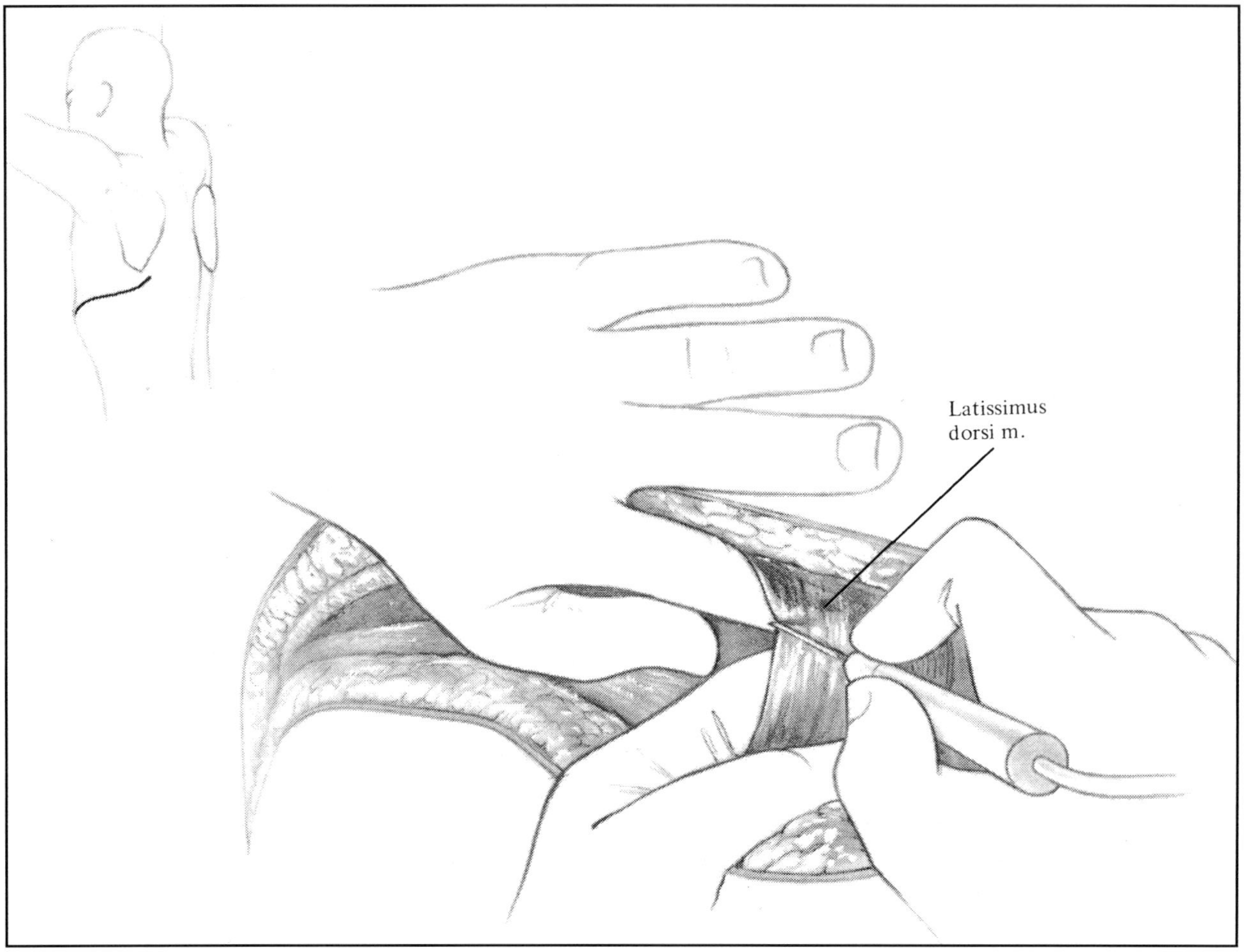

Fig. 3-5

first assistant should be inserted side by side underneath the latissimus muscle while the electrocautery divides the muscle **(Fig. 3–5)**. Divide the anterior serratus muscle in a similar fashion. The rhomboid muscles medial to the scapula need not be divided unless a supraaortic dissection proves necessary.

Next retract the scapula in a cephalad direction and count down the interspaces from the first rib to confirm the location of the sixth interspace. Divide the intercostal musculature by electrocautery along the superior surface of the seventh rib and enter the pleura **(Fig. 3–6)**. Divide the costal margin where it is a wide plate with a scalpel, heavy scissors, or rib cutter. Divide the internal mammary artery, deep and slightly lateral to the costal margin, ligate or electrocoagulate it **(Fig. 3–7)**.

Incise the diaphragm in a circumferential fashion **(Figs.** 3-7, **3–8)** along a line 3-4 cm from its insertion into the rib cage. Use electrocautery for this incision, which should extend laterally about 15 cm from the divided costal margin. Spread the intercostal incision by inserting a mechanical retractor. Use of a multiarm retraction system without a mechanical advantage allows retraction of the lung, diaphragm, and liver for both the thoracic and abdominal phases of the operation, and it avoids fracturing the ribs.

Liberation of Esophagus

Divide the inferior pulmonary ligament with electrocautery or long Metzenbaum scissors, progressing in a cephalad direction until the inferior pulmonary vein has been reached. Collapse the lung, cover it with moist gauze pads, and retract it in a cephalad and anterior direction with Harrington retractors.

Incise the mediastinal pleura from the aorta to the hiatus, beginning at a point above the tumor **(Fig. 3–9)**. Encircle the esophagus first with the index

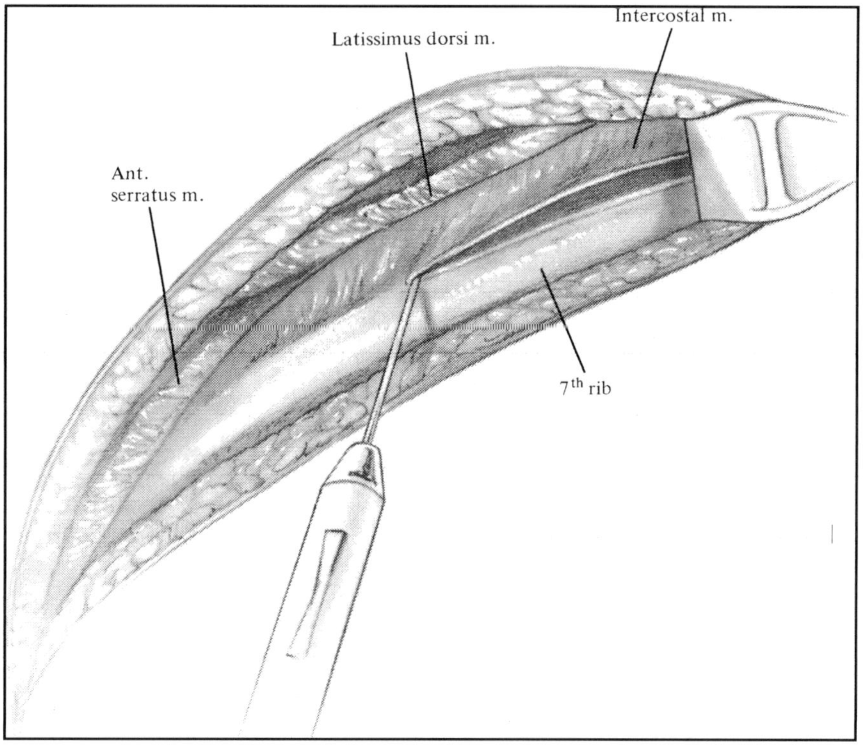
Intercostal m.
Latissimus dorsi m.
Ant.
serratus m.
7th rib

Fig. 3-6

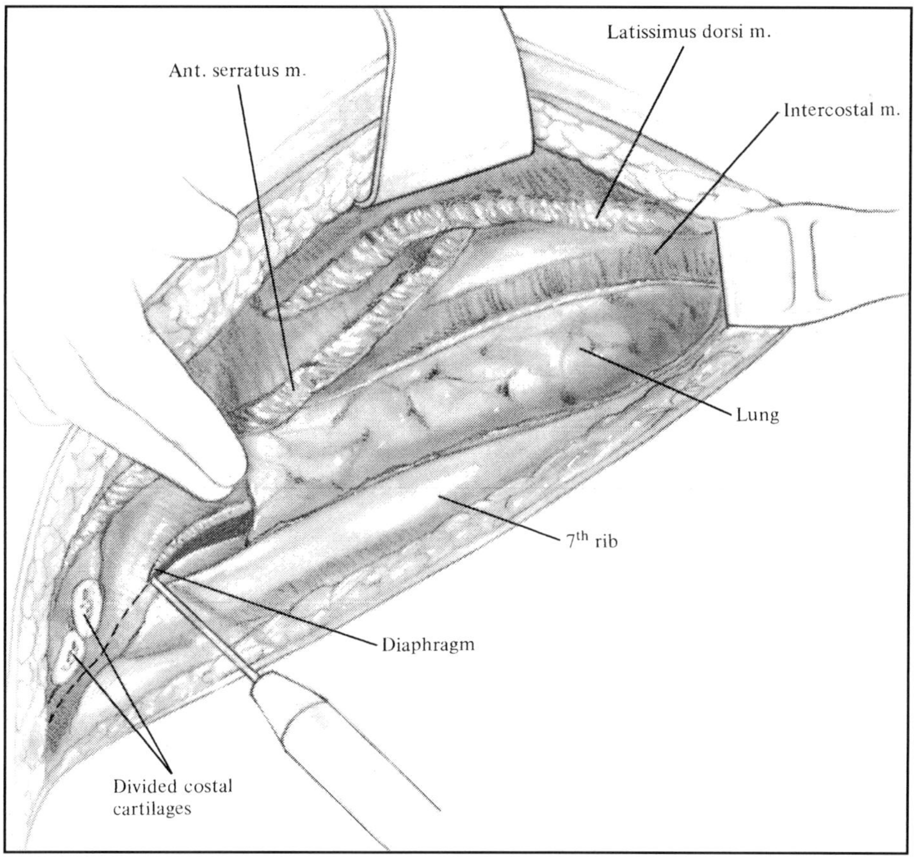
Latissimus dorsi m.
Ant. serratus m.
Intercostal m.
Lung
7th rib
Diaphragm
Divided costal
cartilages

Fig. 3-7

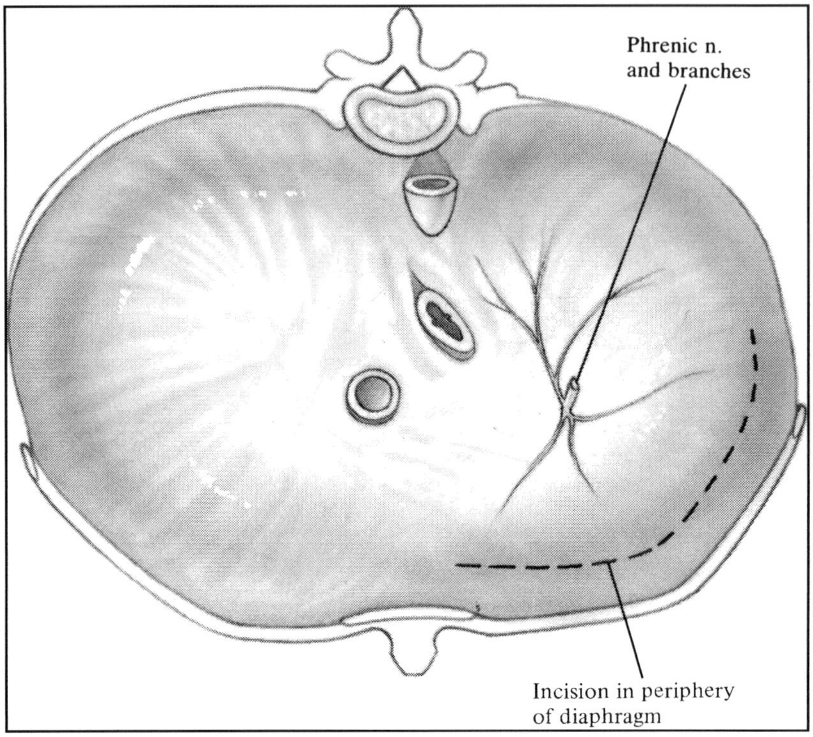

Fig. 3-8

finger and then with a latex drain **(Fig. 3–10)**. Divide the vagus nerves as they approach the esophagus from the hilus of the lung. Dissect the tumor and the attached vagus nerves away from the mediastinal structures. If the pleura of the right thoracic cavity or pericardium has been invaded by tumor, include it in the resection. Dissection of the esophagus should free this organ from the arch of the aorta down to the hiatus, including all the periesophageal areolar tissue. Generally, only two or three arterial branches of the descending aorta join the esophagus. They should be occluded by hemostatic clips and divided. Use an umbilical tape ligature or a 55/3.5 mm linear stapler to occlude the lumen of the proximal esophagus (above the tumor) to prevent cephalad migration of tumor cells **(Fig. 3–11)**. The esophagus may be divided at this time and reflected into the abdomen once hiatal mobilization is complete, or it may be delayed until the stomach is mobilized.

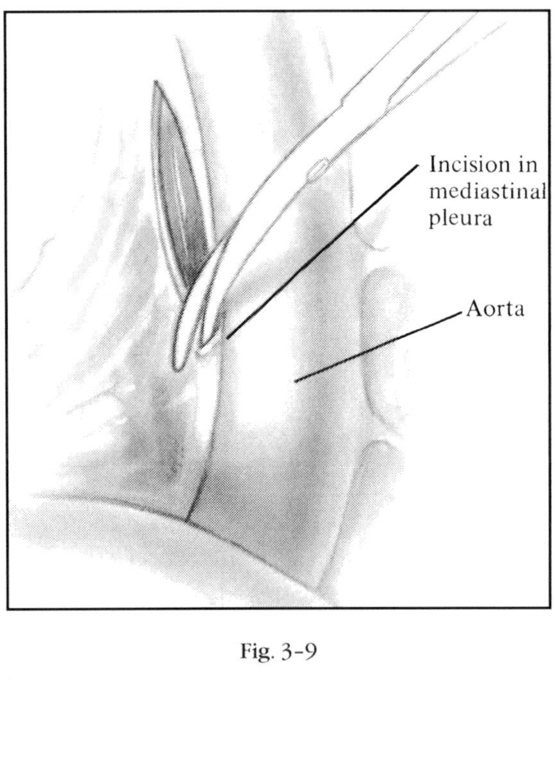

Fig. 3-9

Splenectomy

If the proximity of the carcinoma makes splenectomy necessary, retract the spleen medially and divide the lienophrenic ligament **(Fig. 3–12)**. Gently elevate the spleen and the tail of the pancreas from the retroperitoneal tissues by finger dissection. Divide the lienocolic ligament. Identify the splenic artery and vein on the posterior surface of the splenic hilus. Each should be divided and ligated with 2-0 silk. It may be convenient to remove the spleen as a separate specimen after dividing each of the short gastric vessels. Do this on the anterior aspect of the stomach to visualize the greater curvature accurately, thereby

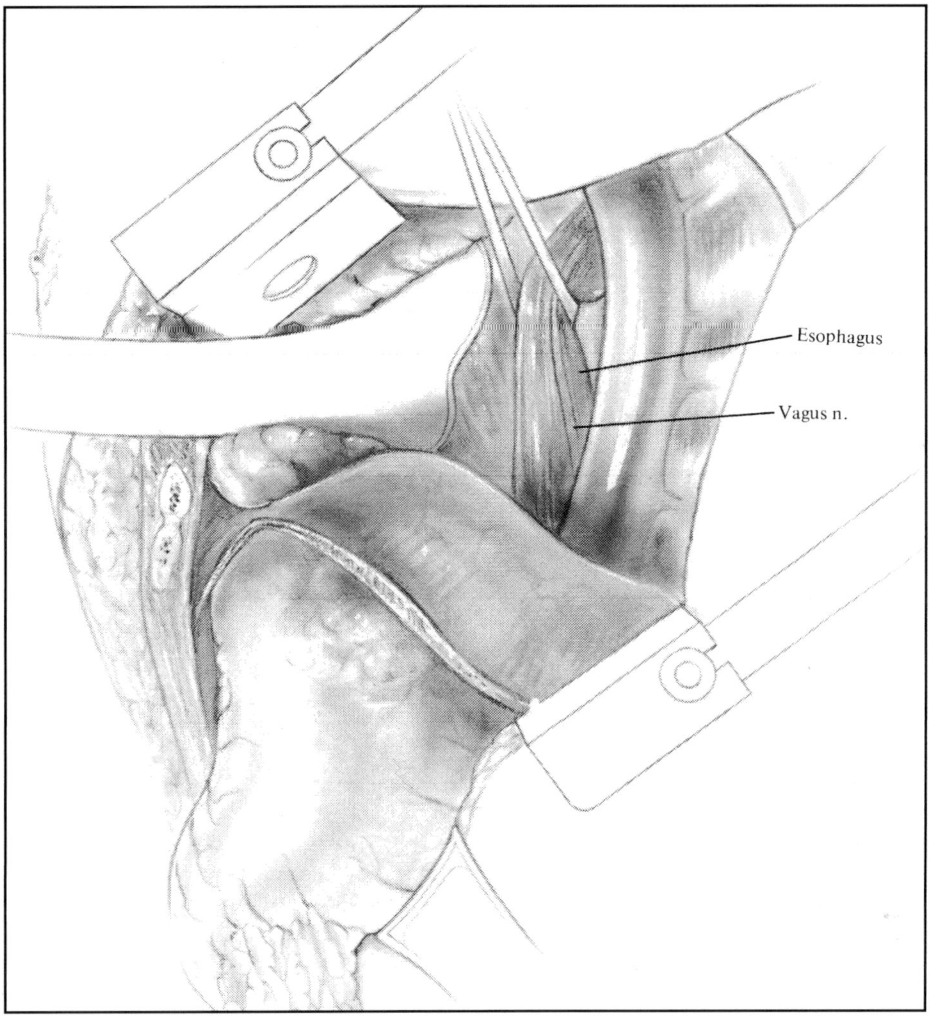

Fig. 3-10

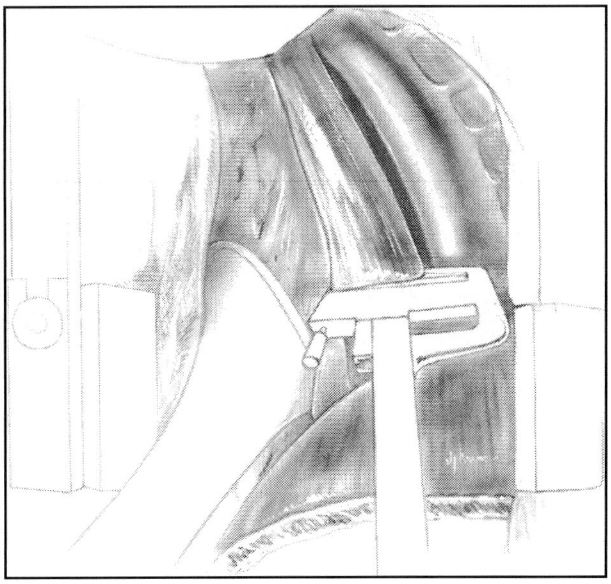

Fig. 3-11

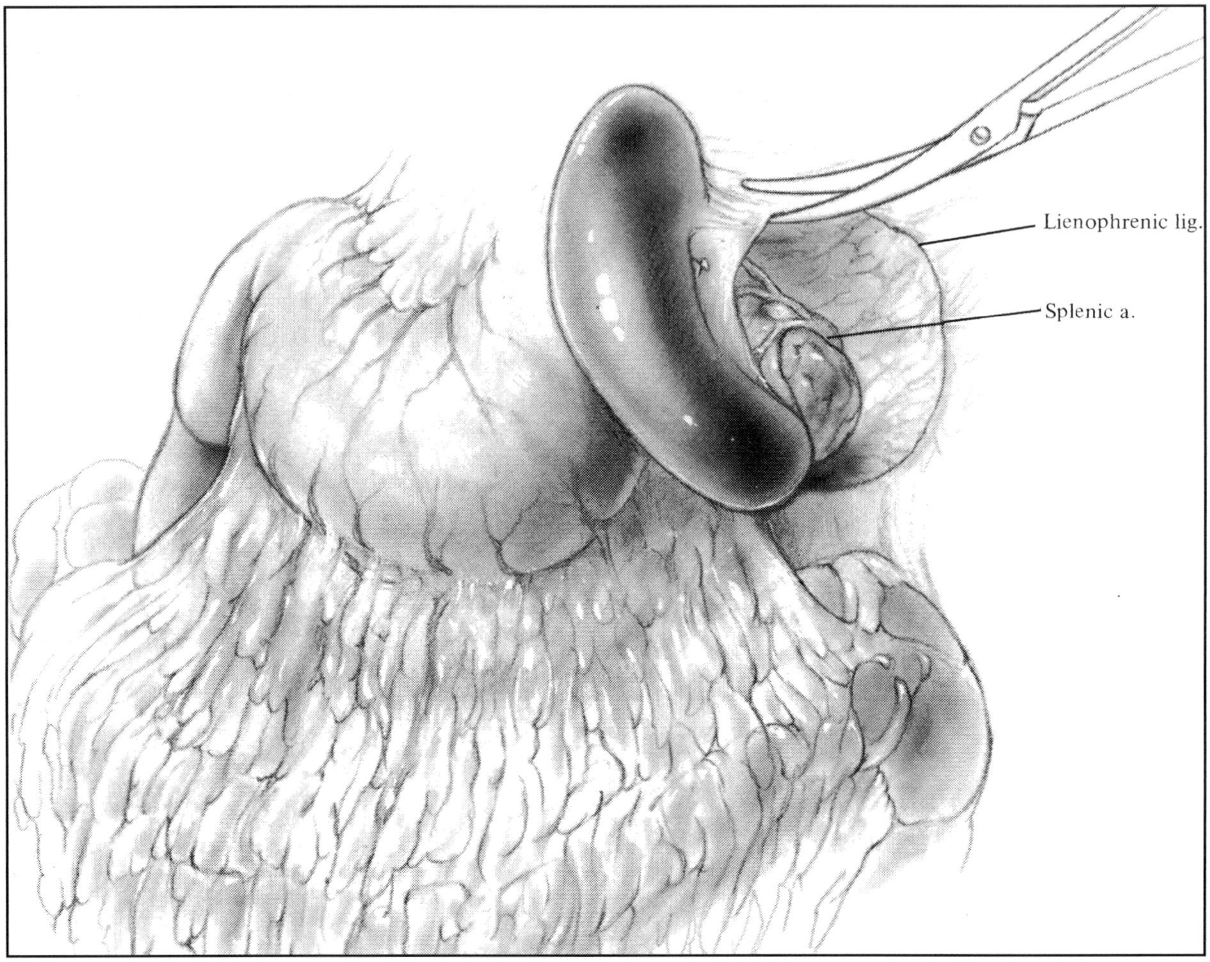

Fig. 3-12

avoiding any possibility of trauma to the stomach. If splenectomy is not necessary, enter the lesser sac through the avascular space above the left gastroepiploic vessels and individually control and divide the short gastric vessels.

Gastric Mobilization

The gastroepiploic arcade along the greater curvature of the stomach *must be preserved with compulsive attention to detail*, as the inadvertent occlusion of this vessel in a clamp or ligature results in ischemia of the gastric pouch and anastomotic leakage. Working from above down, divide the left gastroepiploic vessels and open the lesser sac to identify the gastroepiploic arcades from both front and back. Be sure always to *leave 3-5 cm of redundant omentum attached* to the vascular arcade. Identify the plane separating the colon mesentery from the gastroepiploic arcade. Continue the dissection to a point 6–8 cm cephalad to the pylorus **(Figs. 3–13a, 3–13b)**. The greater curvature now should be elevated. Complete posterior mobilization of the stomach by incising the avascular attachments that connect the back wall of the stomach to the posterior parietal peritoneum overlying the pancreas (gastropancreatic folds) and continue the dissection to the pylorus. Carefully preserve the subpyloric vessels (right gastroepiploic and right gastric).

Identify the celiac axis by palpating the origins of the splenic, hepatic, and left gastric arteries. Dissect lymphatic and areolar tissues away from the celiac axis toward the specimen. Skeletonize the coronary vein and divide and ligate it with 2-0 silk. Immediately cephalad to this structure is the left gastric artery, which should be doubly ligated with 2-0 silk and divided **(Figs. 3–14a, 3–14b)**. Incise the gastrohepatic ligament near its attachment to the liver **(Fig. 3–15)**. An accessory left hepatic artery generally can be found in the cephalad portion of

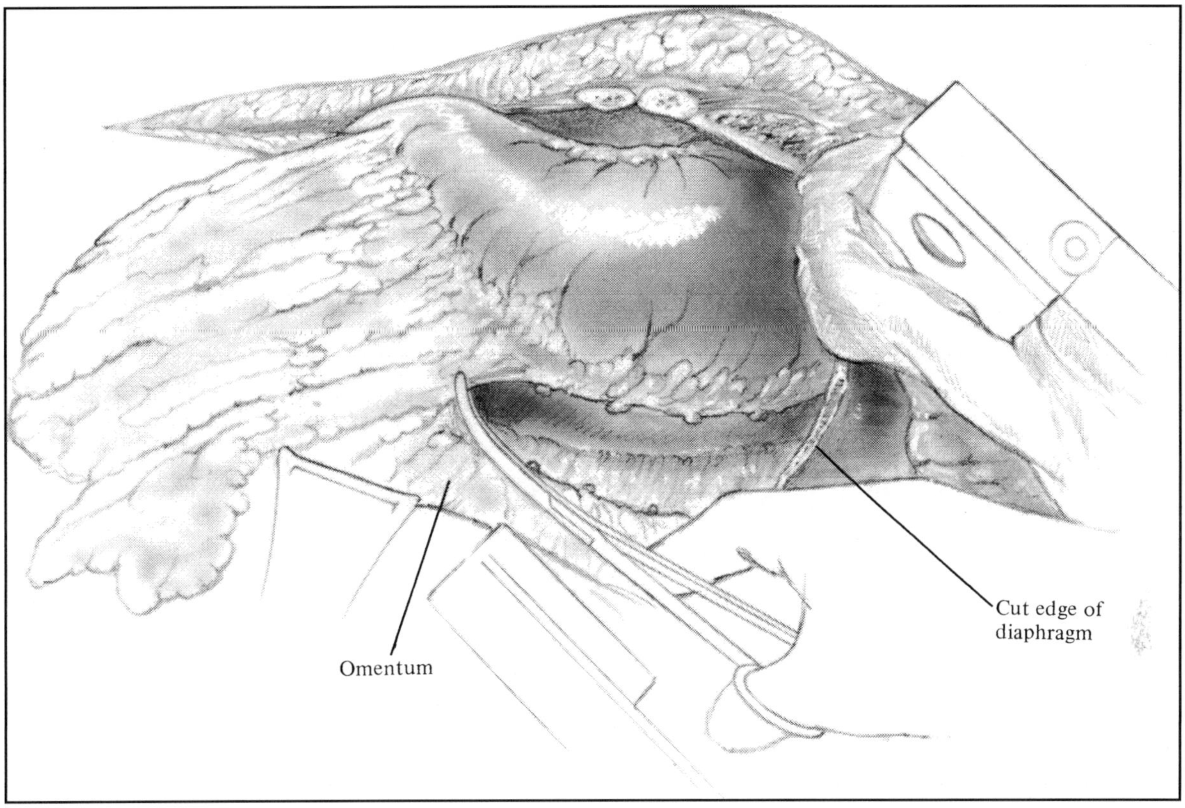

Fig. 3-13a

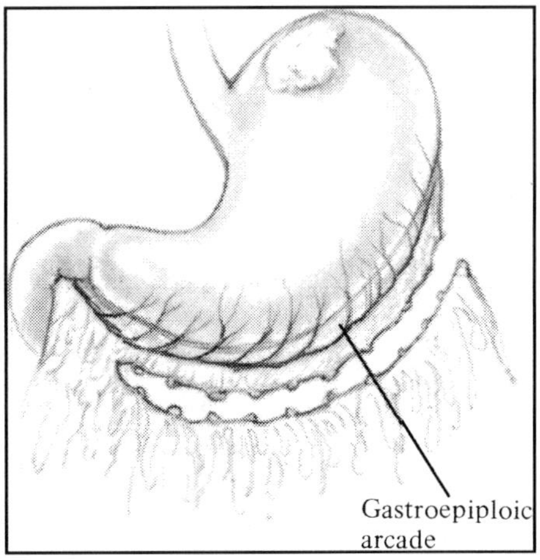

Fig. 3-13b

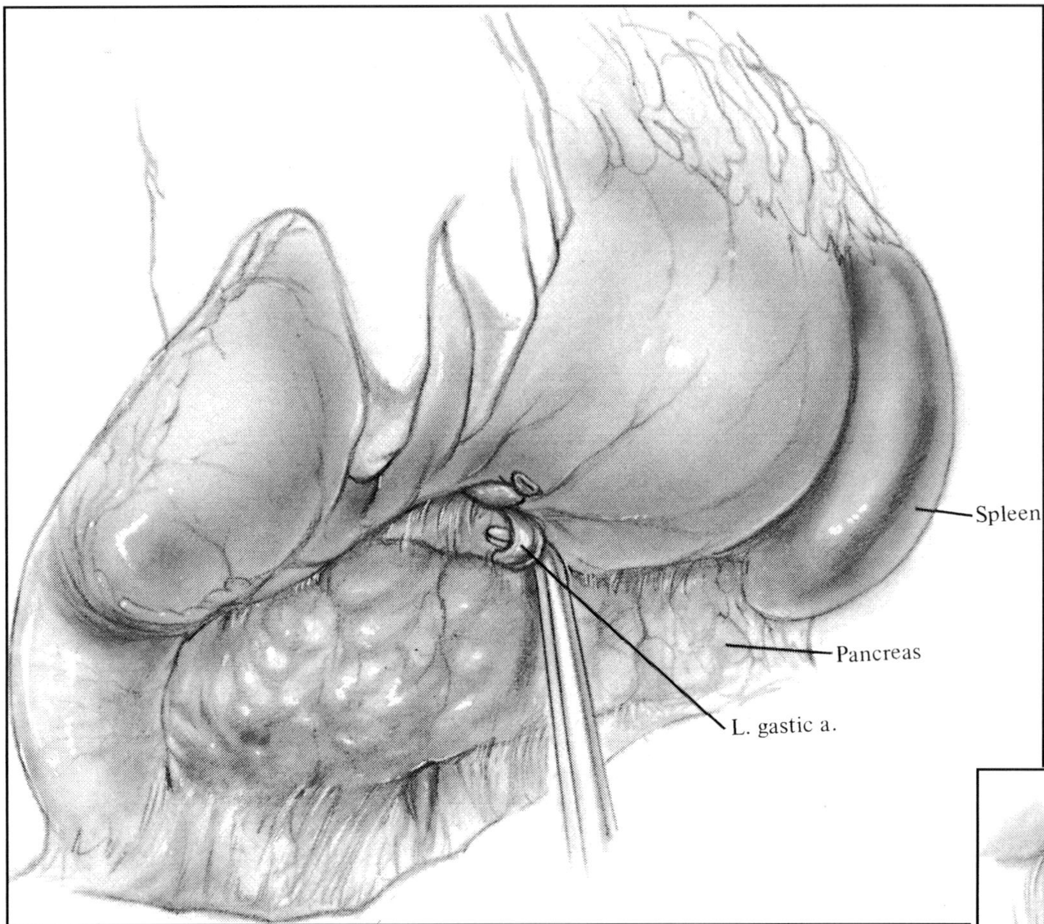

Fig. 3-14a

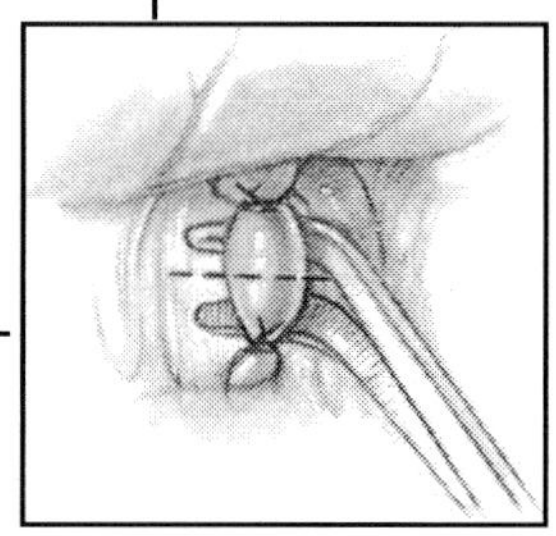

Fig. 3-14b

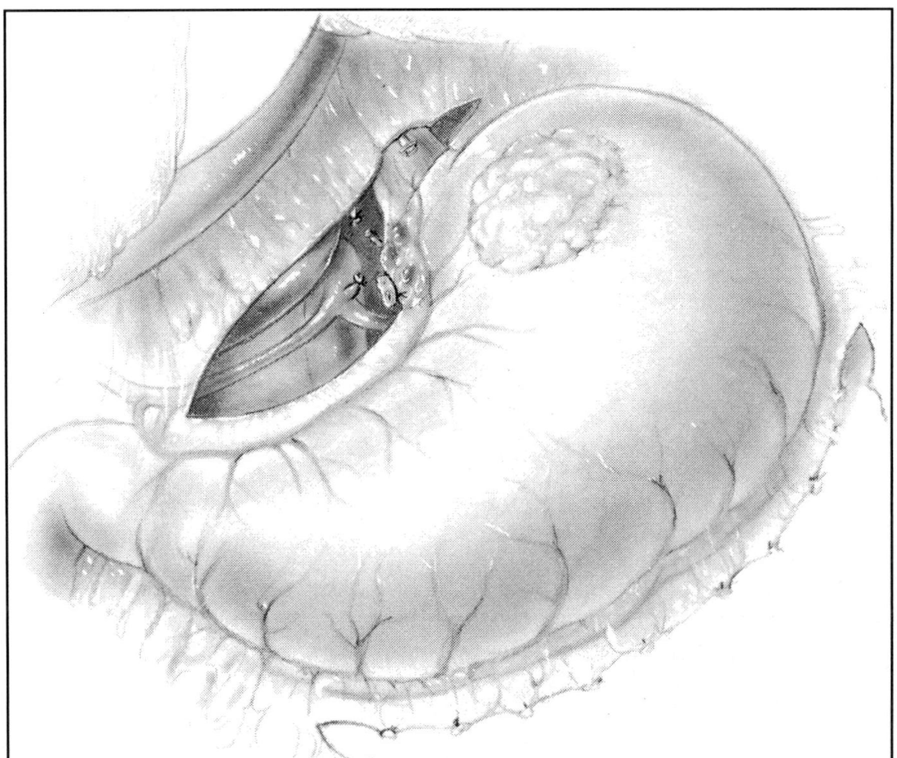

Fig. 3-15

the gastrohepatic ligament. Divide the artery and ligate it with 2-0 silk; then divide the remainder of the ligament and the peritoneum overlying the esophagus.

Hiatal Dissection

A gastrophrenic ligament attaches the posterior aspect of the gastric fundus to the posterior diaphragm. Divide the ligament using the left index finger as a guide. If tumor has encroached on the hiatus, leave crural musculature attached to the tumor and divide it from the surrounding diaphragm with electrocautery. This may require division and ligature of the inferior phrenic artery. Divide the vagus nerves just below the hiatus **(Fig. 3–16)** and divide the phrenoesophageal ligaments; this frees the esophagus and stomach from the arch of the aorta down to the duodenum.

Kocher Maneuver

To achieve maximum upward mobility of the gastric pouch, divide the avascular lateral duodenal ligament and pass a hand behind the duodenum and the head of the pancreas **(Figs. 3–17, 3–18)**. If necessary, continue this Kocher maneuver along the duodenum as far distally as the superior mesenteric vein (see Figs. 2-15, 2-16). Additional freedom of the mobilized stomach can be achieved by dividing the attachments of the greater omentum to the duodenum beyond the right gastroepiploic vessels.

Pyloromyotomy

Perform a pyloromyotomy as described in Chapter 2 (see Figs. 2-17 to 2-19).

Transection of Stomach and Esophagus

To treat a primary tumor of the lower esophagus, apply either a long linear cutting stapler or a 90mm linear stapler (loaded with 4.8mm staples) in an oblique fashion to remove the stump of the left gastric artery, the celiac lymph nodes on the lesser curvature of the stomach, and 5-6cm of the greater curvature.

To treat lesions of the proximal stomach, which is the operation illustrated in **Figures 3–19a**, and **3–19b**, apply the stapler so 5-6cm of normal stomach distal to the lesion is removed. *Ascertain that the nasogastric tube has been withdrawn*, and divide the stomach with a long linear cutting stapler or with two 90mm linear staplers applied in a parallel fashion.

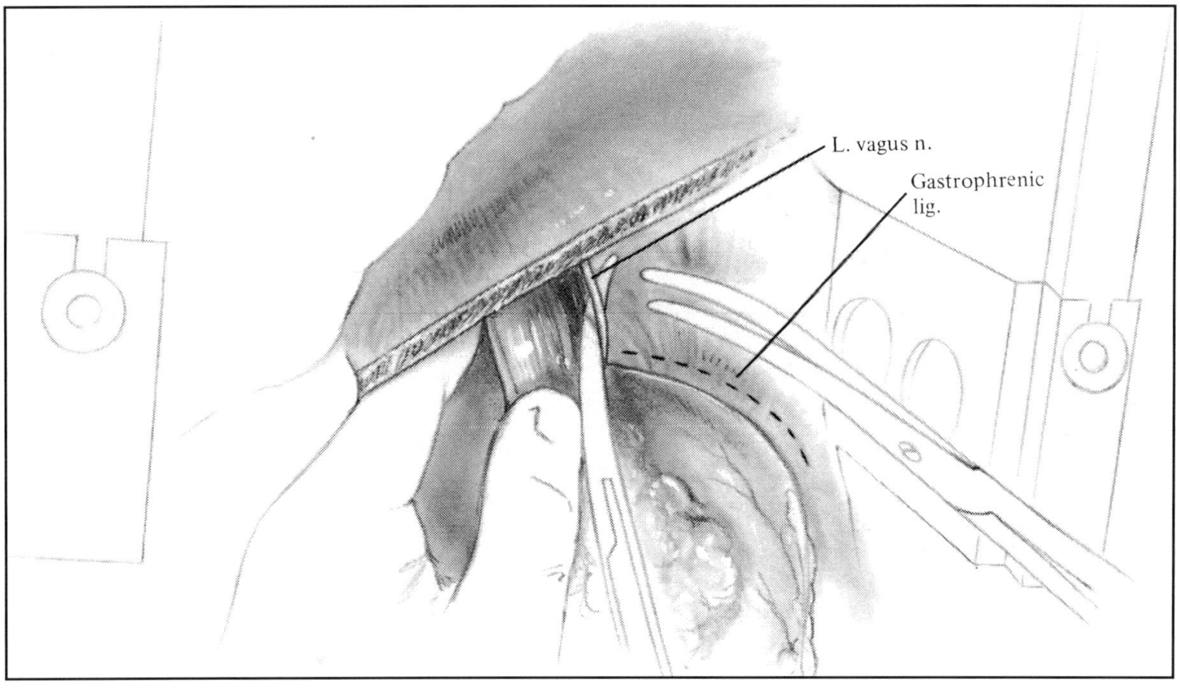

Fig. 3-16

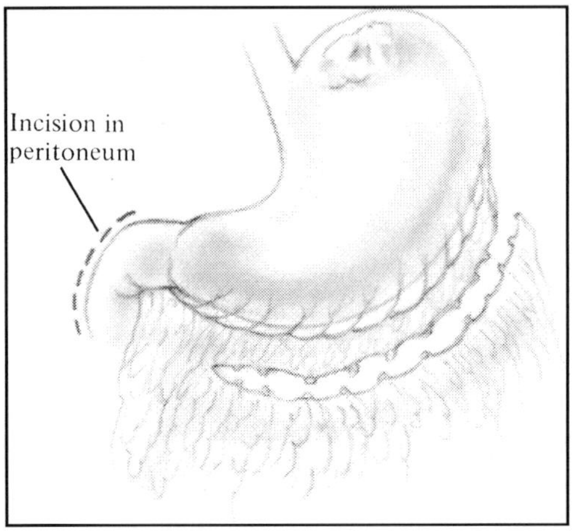

Fig. 3-17

Make an incision with the scalpel flush with the stapler attached to the residual gastric pouch. If two 90mm linear staplers are not available, the first stapler should be applied to the stomach, fired, and then reapplied 1cm lower on the gastric wall. The transection should be made flush with the stapler on the gastric pouch. Control individual bleeding vessels with electrocautery after removing the device. This staple line should be oversewn with fine inverting sutures. The gastric wall is of variable thickness, and we have seen isolated leakage from this staple line when it was not reinforced. If multiple applications of the cutting stapler were required, a running 4-0 polypropylene Lembert suture conveniently reinforces the staple line without excess inversion.

In a previous step the esophageal lumen proximal to the tumor was occluded with a row of staples

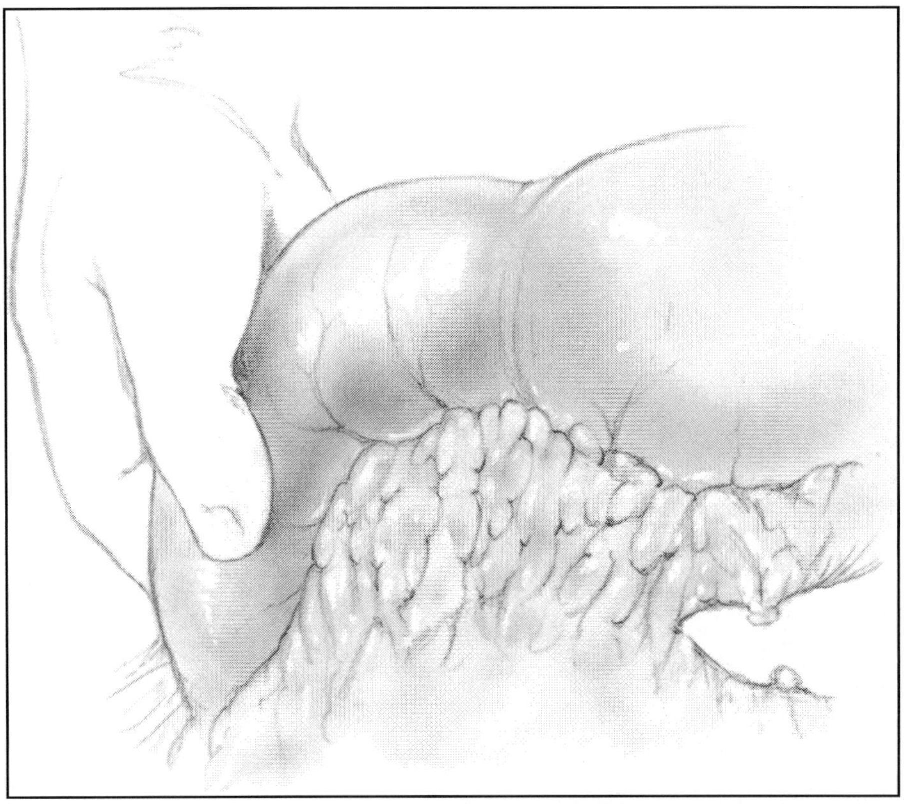

Fig. 3-18

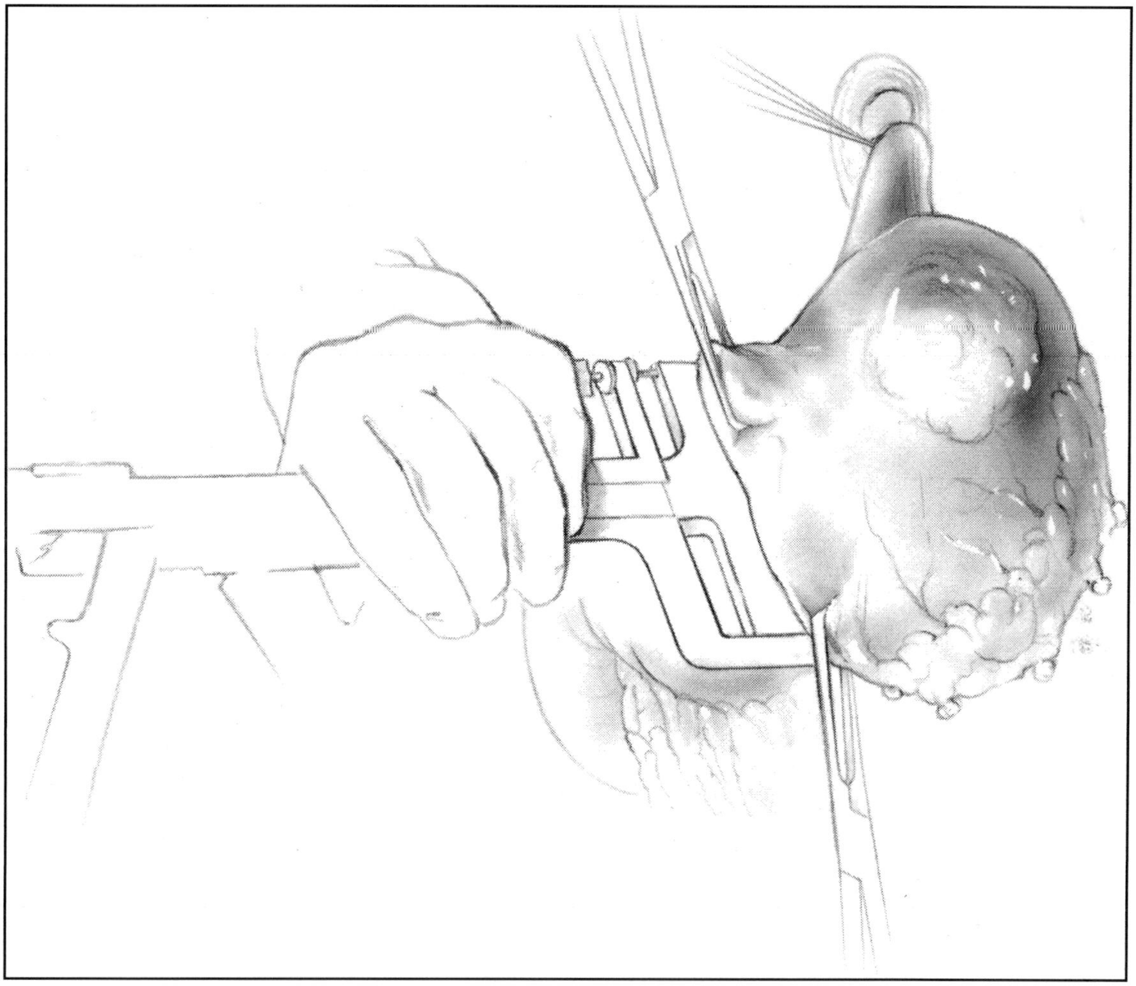

Fig. 3-19a

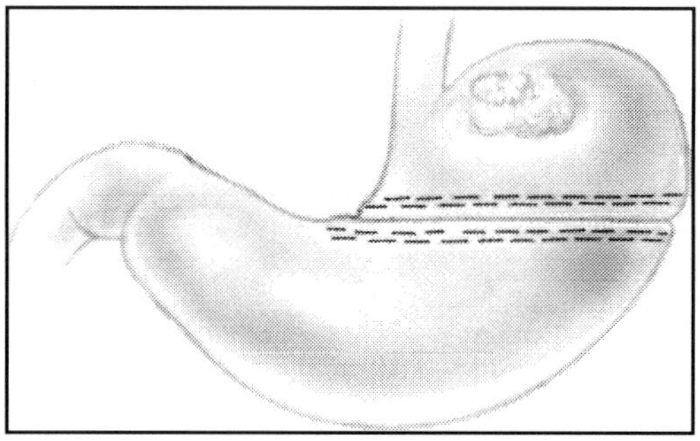

Fig. 3-19b

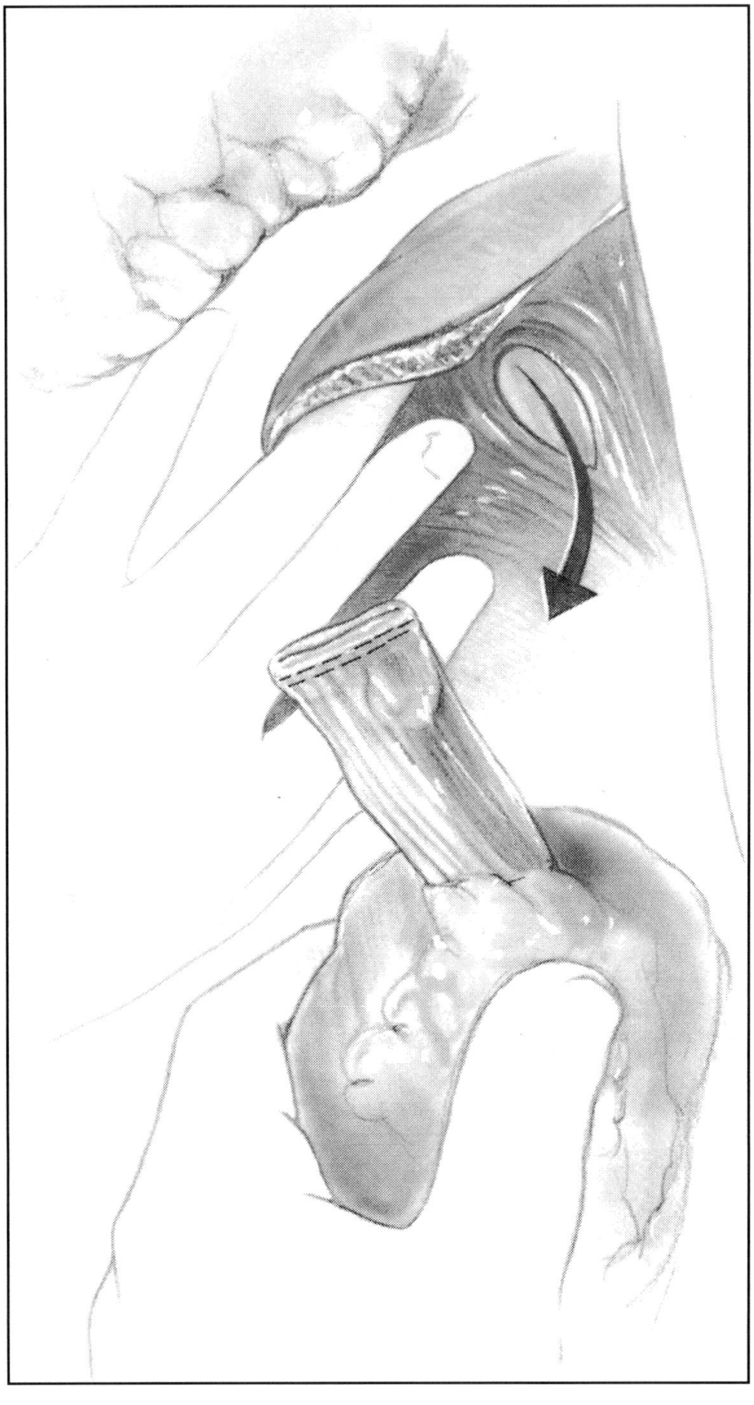

Fig. 3-20

(Fig. 3-11). If the esophagus has not yet been divided, transect it now 8-10 cm proximal to the tumor and remove the specimen **(Fig. 3–20)**. Submit the proximal and distal margins of the specimen to frozen section examination. Clean the lumen of the proximal esophagus with a suction device **(Fig. 3–21)**.

Enlargement of Hiatus

Enlarging the hiatus is rarely necessary if the crura have been skeletonized as described by division of the phrenoesophageal ligament. If the hiatus appears tight, make a transverse incision by electrocautery in the left branch of the crux **(Fig. 3–22)**. The incision

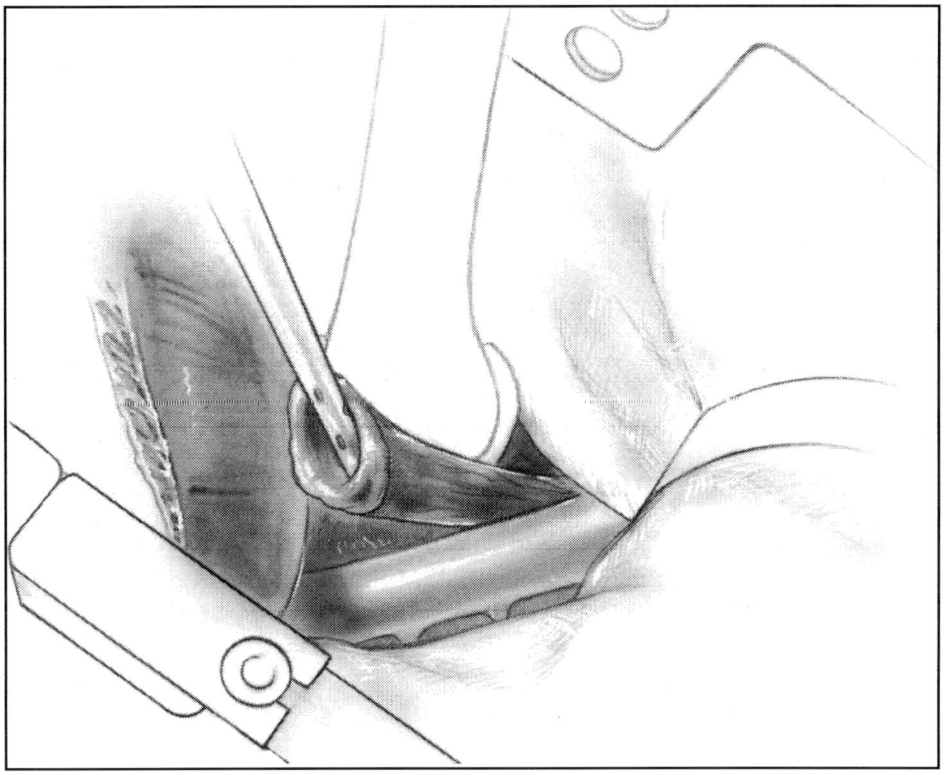

Fig. 3-21

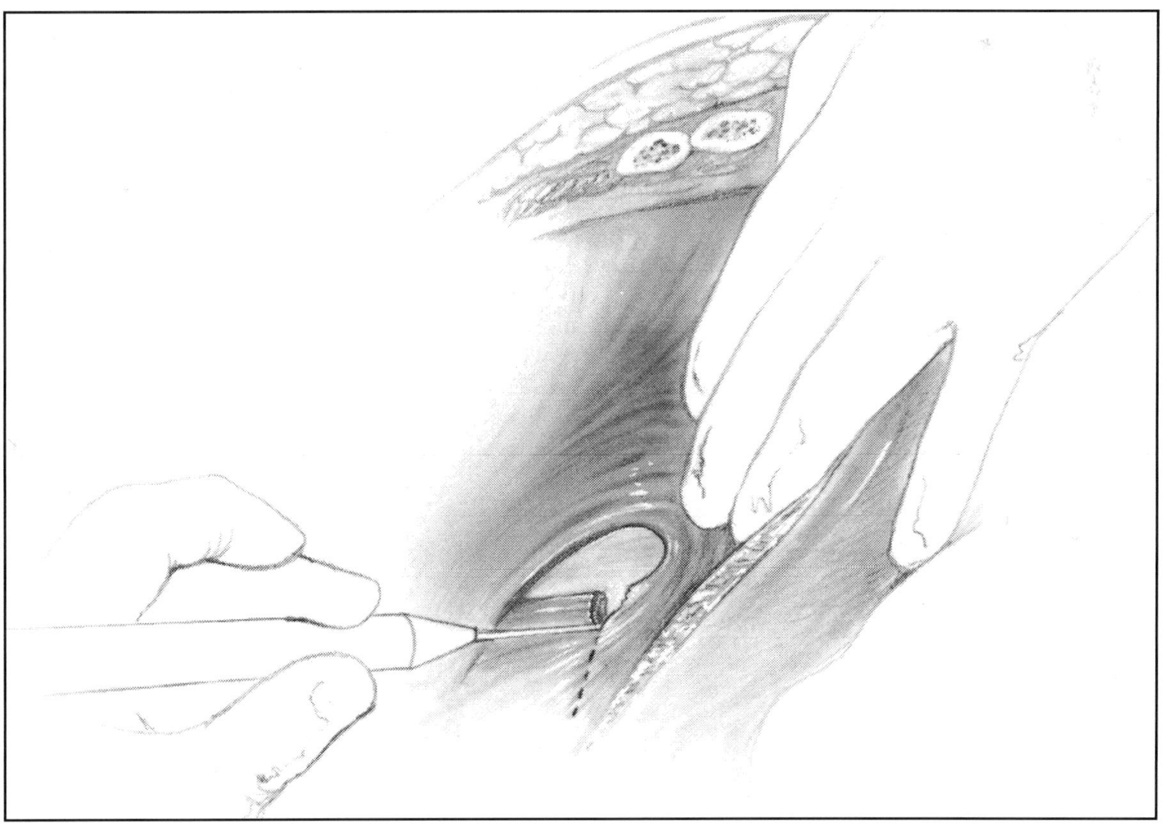

Fig. 3-22

should be of sufficient magnitude to allow the gastric pouch to pass into the mediastinum *without constriction* of its venous circulation.

Enlargement of Thoracic Incision If Supraaortic Anastomosis Is Necessary

A properly fashioned end-to-side esophagogastric anastomosis requires the presence of 6–8 cm of esophagus below the aortic arch. If there is not 6–8 cm of esophagus below the aortic arch, the surgeon should not hesitate to enlarge the thoracic incision so the esophagus can be passed behind the arch into a supraaortic position. This makes the anastomosis far simpler and safer to perform and requires only a few minutes to accomplish.

Move to a position on the left side of the patient. Extend the skin incision up from the tip of the scapula in a cephalad direction between the scapula and the spine. With electrocautery divide the rhomboid and trapezium muscles medial to the scapula. Retract the scapula in a cephalad direction and free the erector spinal muscle from the necks of the sixth and fifth ribs. Free a short (1 cm) segment of the sixth (and often of the fifth) rib of its surrounding periosteum and excise it **(Fig. 3–23)**. Divide and ligate or electrocoagulate the intercostal nerves with their accompanying vessels **(Fig. 3–24)**. Reinsert the Finochietto or other mechanical retractor **(Fig. 3–25)**. If the exposure is still inadequate, a segment of the fourth rib may also be excised, but this is rarely necessary.

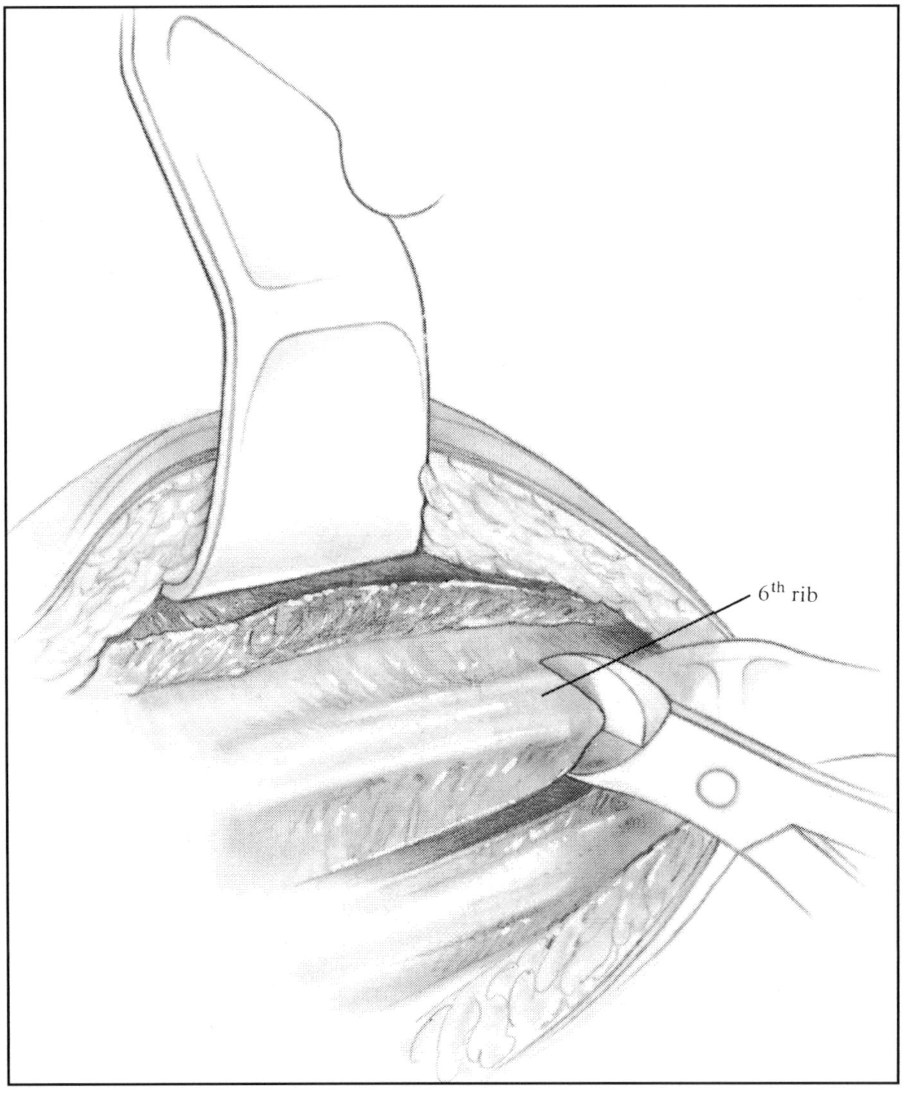

Fig. 3-23

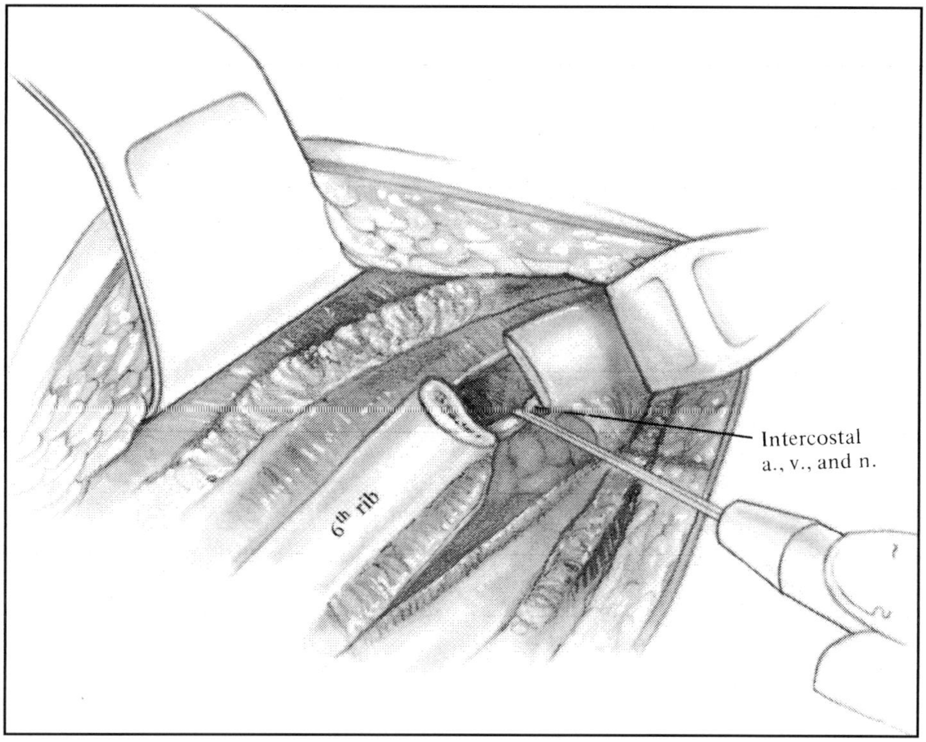

Fig. 3-24

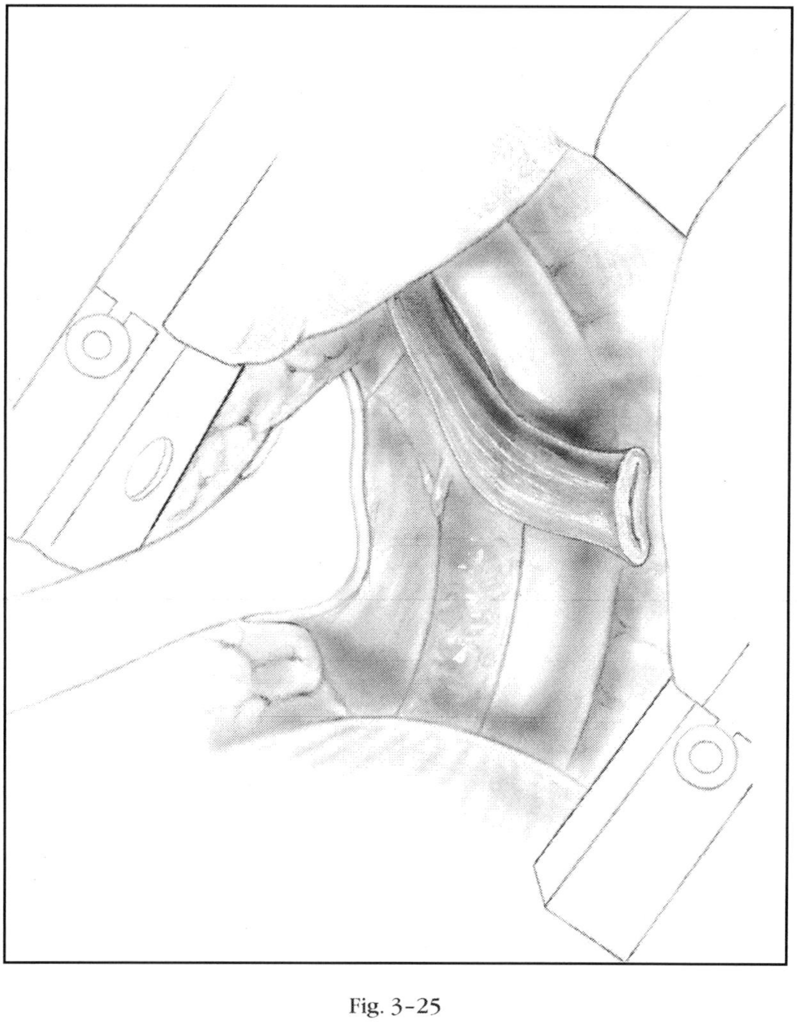

Fig. 3-25

Enter the space between the anterior wall of the esophagus and the aortic arch with the index finger **(Figs. 3–26a, 3–26b, 3–26c)**. There are no vascular attachments in this area. The index finger emerges cephalad to the aortic arch behind the mediastinal pleura. Incise the mediastinal pleura on the index finger, making a window extending along the anterior surface of the esophagus up to the thoracic inlet. Now dissect the esophagus free of all its attachments to the mediastinum in the vicinity of the aortic arch. Avoid damage to the left recurrent laryngeal nerve, the thoracic duct, and the left vagus nerve located medial to the esophagus above the aortic arch. One or two vessels may have to be divided between hemostatic clips.

Deliver the esophagus from behind the aortic arch up through the window in the pleura between the left carotid and subclavian arteries **(Fig. 3–27)**. If the space between the carotid and subclavian arteries is narrow, bring the esophagus out through a pleural incision lateral to the subclavian artery.

The esophagogastric anastomosis, as described below, should be constructed in a position lateral and anterior to the aortic arch. Exposure for the anastomosis in this location is excellent. Bring the esophagus down over the anterior wall of the stomach for a sutured anastomosis. An overlap of 6–7 cm is desirable. If the esophageal dissection has been carried out without undue trauma, the esophageal segment has an excellent blood supply even though its distal 10 cm has been liberated from its bed in the mediastinum. The anastomosis can readily be performed as high as the apex of the thorax by this method, and a level of resection comparable to that achieved by adding a cervical incision can often be used. Use of the circular stapling technique to perform the anastomosis high in the chest is an excellent alternative to sutured intrathoracic or cervical anastomosis. For this technique the stomach is placed in front of the esophagus for the end-to-side anastomosis.

Esophagogastric Anastomosis, Suture Technique

The technique for sutured esophagogastric anastomosis is described and illustrated in Chapter 2.

Esophagogastric Anastomosis, Stapling Technique (Surgical Legacy Technique)

In 1978 Chassin described a linear stapling technique for esophagogastric anastomosis. Although circular staplers are more commonly used currently, this method is still occasionally useful and applicable when other methods are difficult. It involves attaching the posterior aspect of the distal esophagus to the anterior wall of the stomach. It requires an overlap to enable 7–8 cm of the esophagus to lie freely over the front of the stomach. If a 7- to 8-cm overlap is not available, this stapling technique is contraindicated.

Make a stab wound, 1.5 cm long, on the anterior wall of the gastric pouch at a point 7–8 cm from the

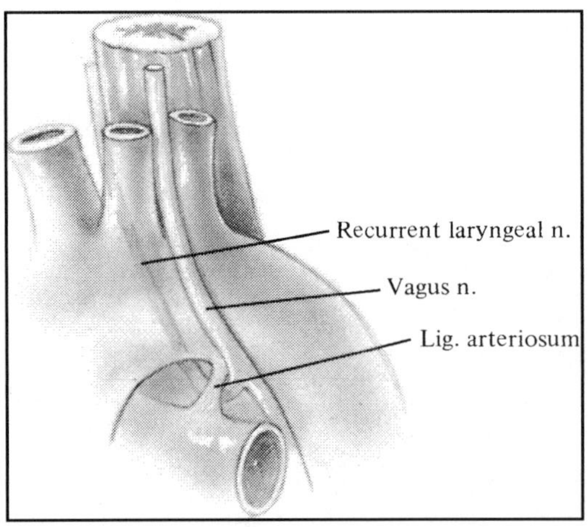

Fig. 3-26a

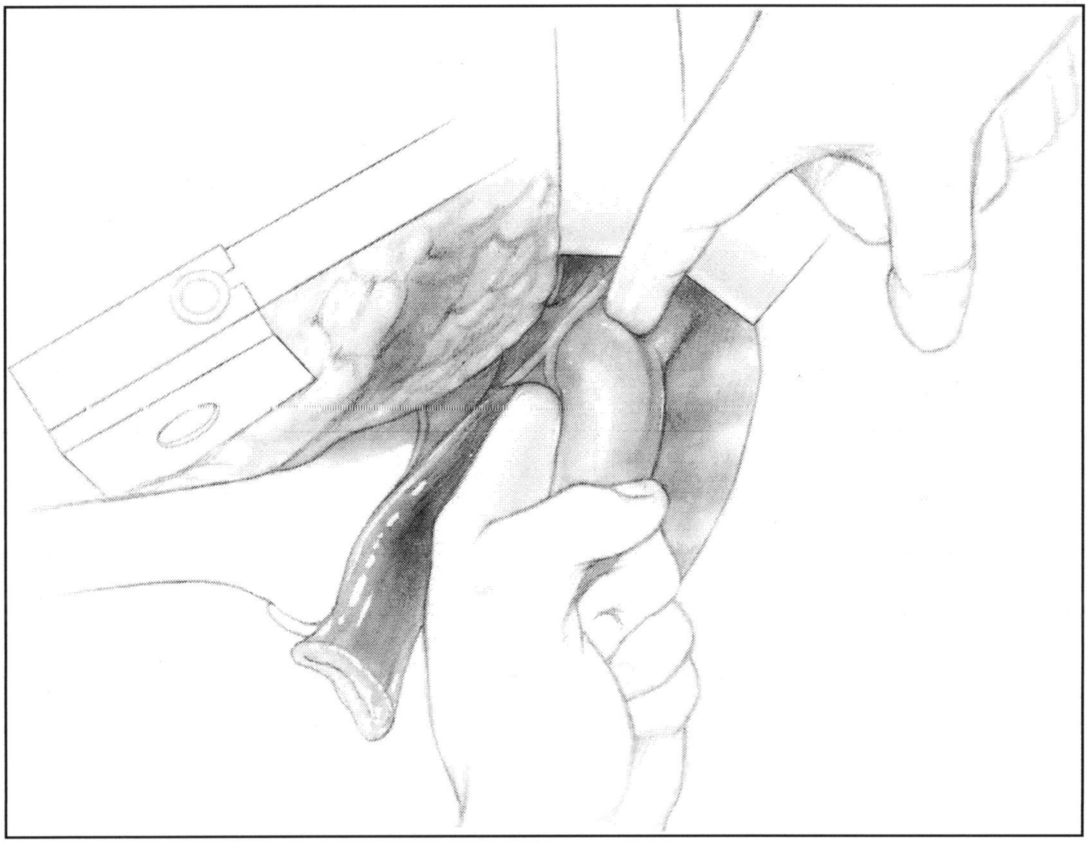

Fig. 3-26b

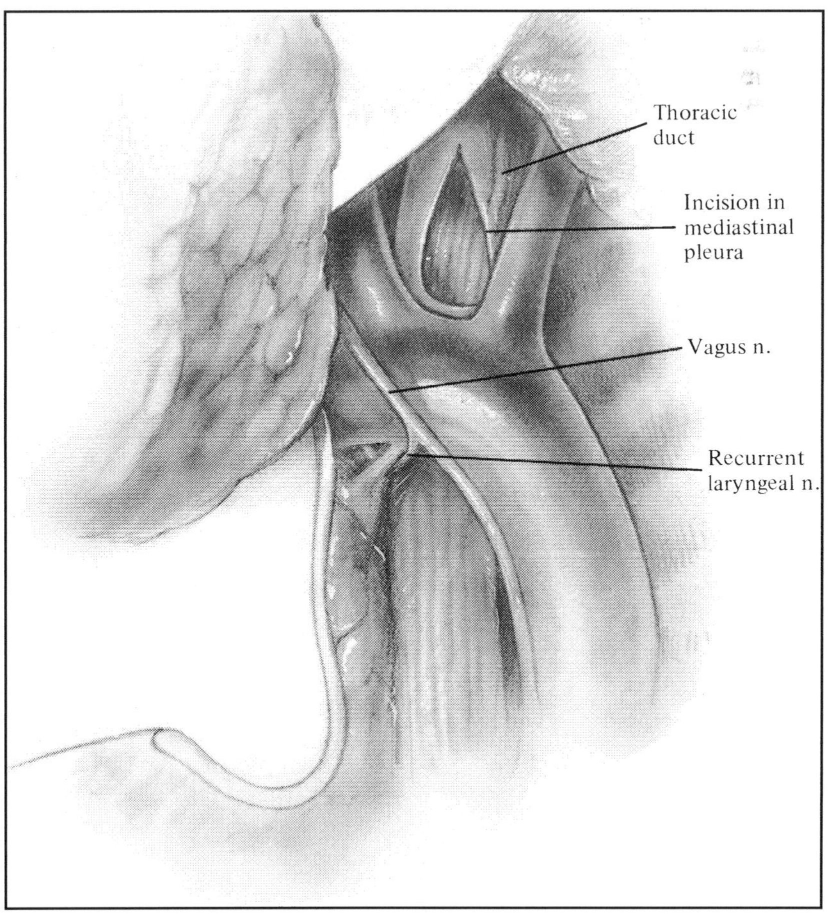

Fig. 3-26c

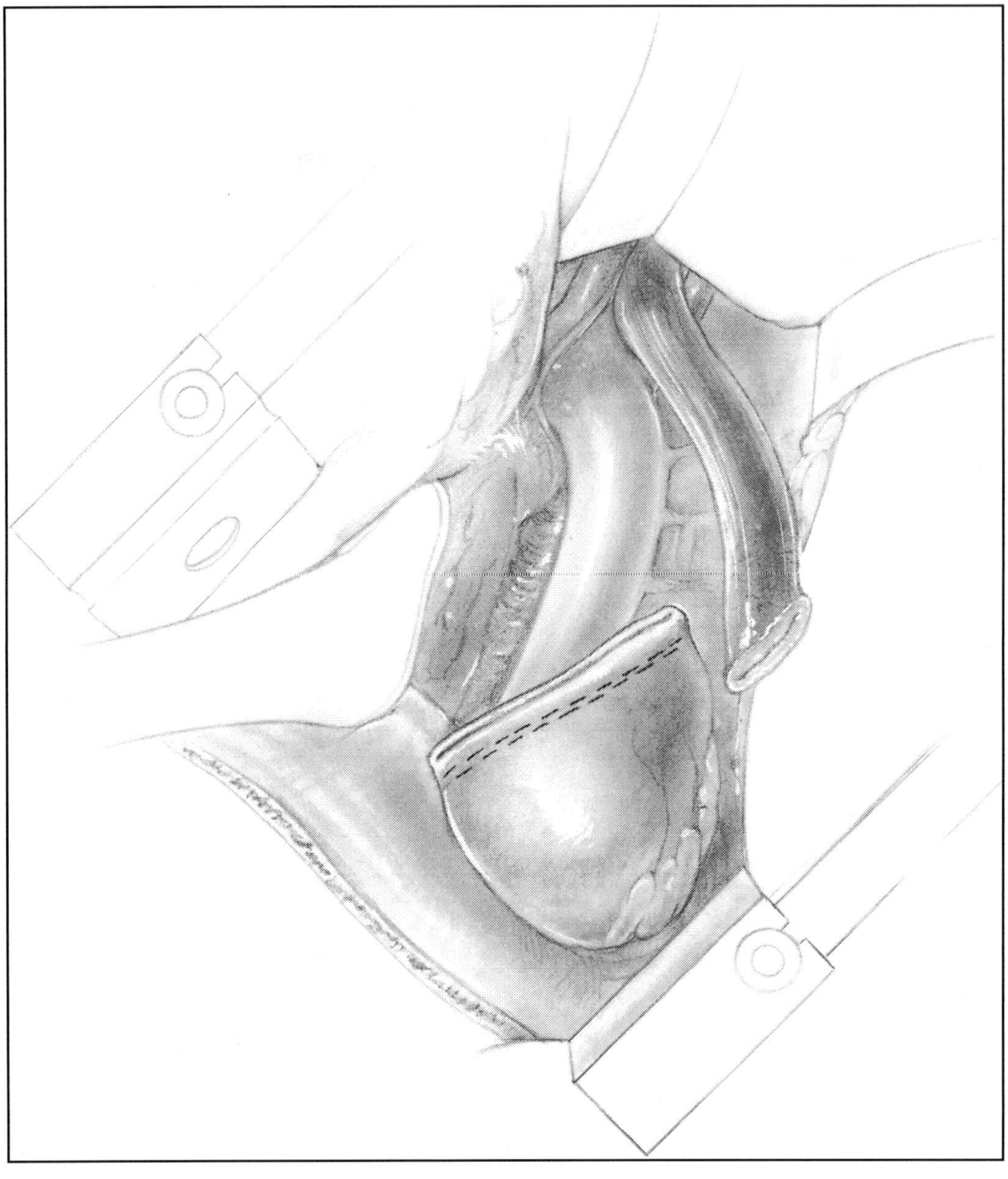

Fig. 3–27

cephalad margin of the stomach **(Fig. 3–28)**. Insert one fork of the cutting linear stapler through the stab wound into the stomach and the other fork into the open end of the overlying esophagus **(Fig. 3–29)**. Insert the stapling device to a depth of 3.5–4.0 cm. Fire and remove the stapling device. This step leaves both the end of the esophagus and a large opening in the stomach unclosed **(Fig. 3–30)**. The posterior layer of the anastomosis has already been accomplished by the stapling device. Complete the anastomosis in an everting fashion by triangulation with two applications of the 55 mm linear stapler. To facilitate this step, insert a 4-0 temporary guy suture through the full thickness of the anterior esophageal wall at its midpoint, carry the suture through the center of the remaining opening in the gastric wall **(Fig. 3–31)**, and tie the suture. Apply Allis clamps to approximate the everted walls of the esophagus and stomach. Apply the first Allis clamp just behind termination of the first staple line on the medial side. Hold the suture and the Allis clamps so the linear stapler can be applied just underneath the clamps and the suture **(Fig. 3–32)**. Tighten and fire the stapling device. Excise the esophageal and gastric tissues flush with the stapling device with Mayo scissors. Leave the guy suture intact.

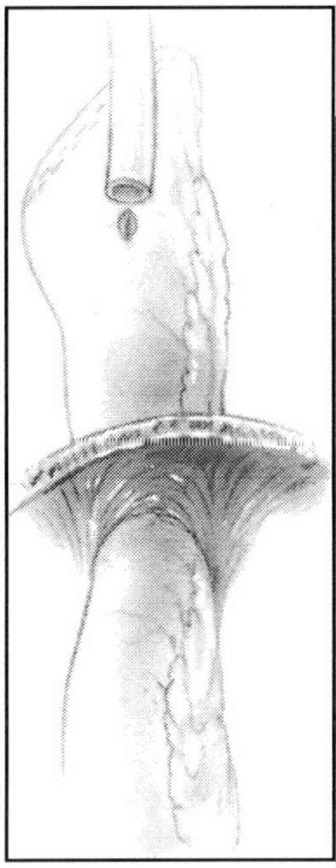

Fig. 3-28

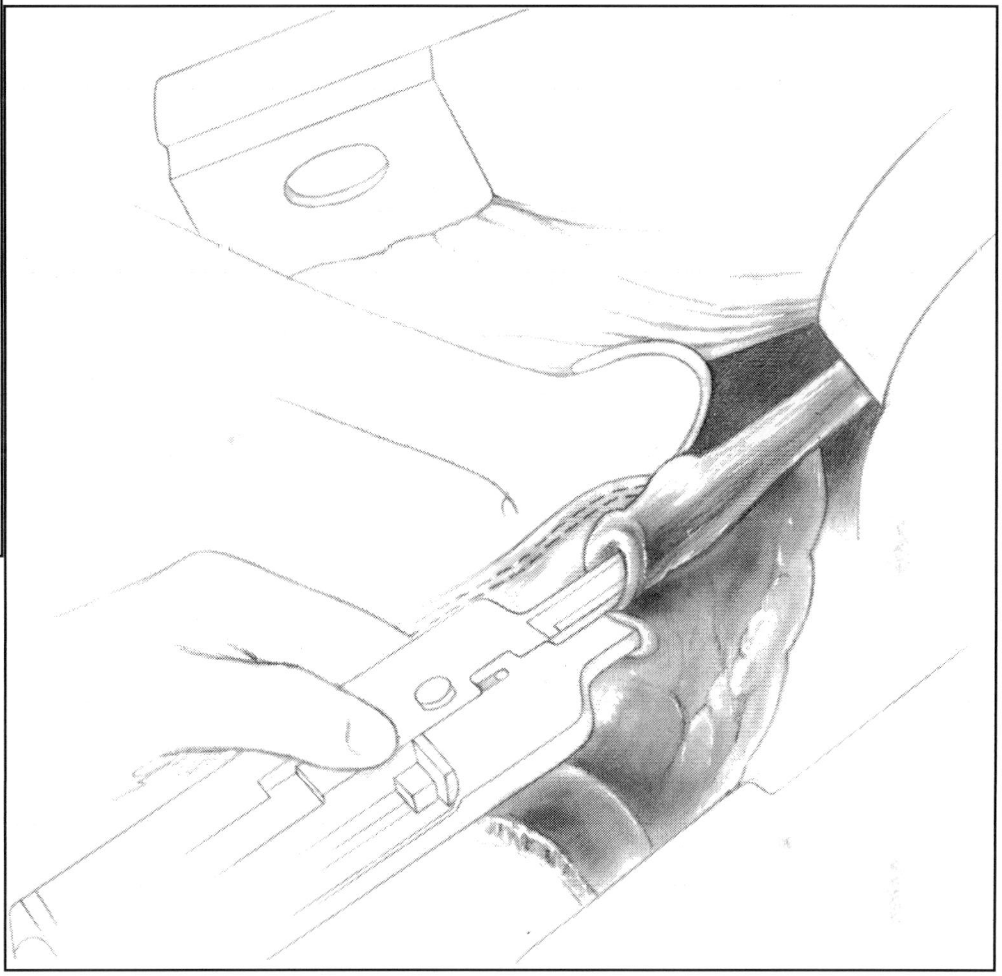

Fig. 3-29

Use an identical procedure to approximate the lateral side of the esophagogastric defect. Apply additional Allis clamps. Then place the 55 mm linear stapling device into position deep to the Allis clamps and the previously placed guy suture. Close and fire the stapler and remove the redundant tissue with Mayo scissors **(Fig. 3–33)**. It is essential that a small portion of the lateral termination of the stapled anastomosis be included in the final linear staple line. Include the guy suture also in this last application of the linear stapler. These measures eliminate any possibility of leaving a gap between the various staple lines. Test the integrity of the anastomosis by inserting a sterile solution of methylene blue through the nasogastric tube into the gastric pouch. The appearance of the completed stapled anastomosis is shown in **Figure 3–34**.

Whether a Nissen fundoplication is to be constructed following this anastomosis depends on the judgment of the surgeon and the availability of loose gastric wall. In some cases partial fundoplication can be done.

Esophagogastric Anastomosis Performed by Circular Stapling Technique

The circular stapling technique is especially suitable for patients in whom the lumen of the esophagus is large enough to admit a 28- or 31-mm circular stapling device. The esophageal lumen can be measured by attempting to insert sizers (which come in 25, 28, and 31 mm sizes). It is dangerous to stretch the esophagus with these sizers, because it can result in one or more longitudinal tears of the mucosa and submucosa. Gentle dilatation with a Foley catheter balloon is the safest way to achieve lumen of adequate size for

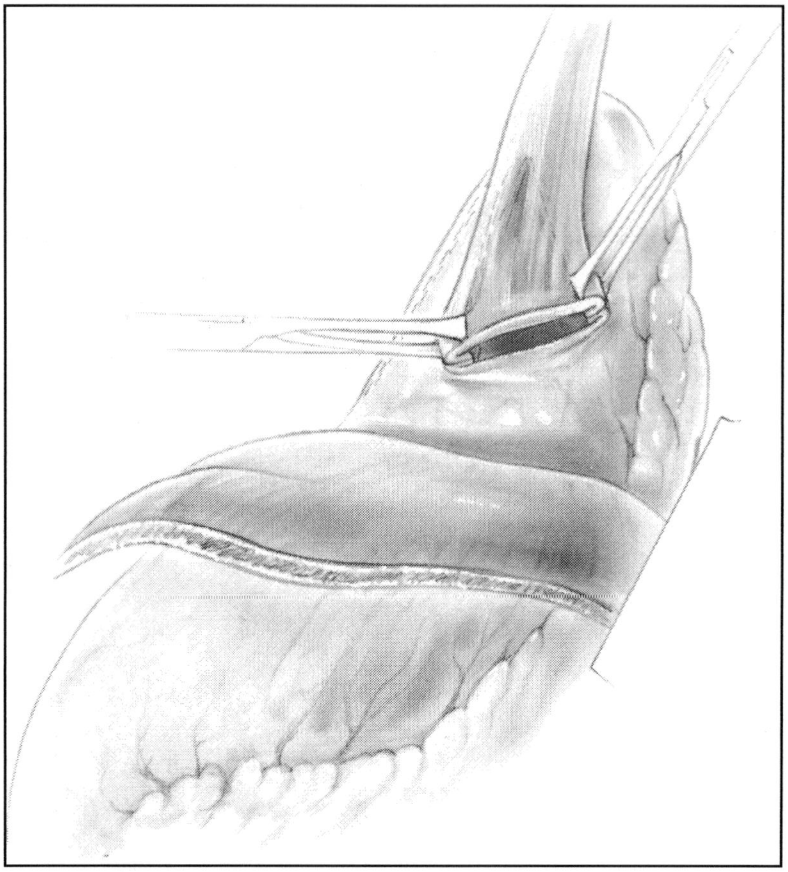

Fig. 3-30

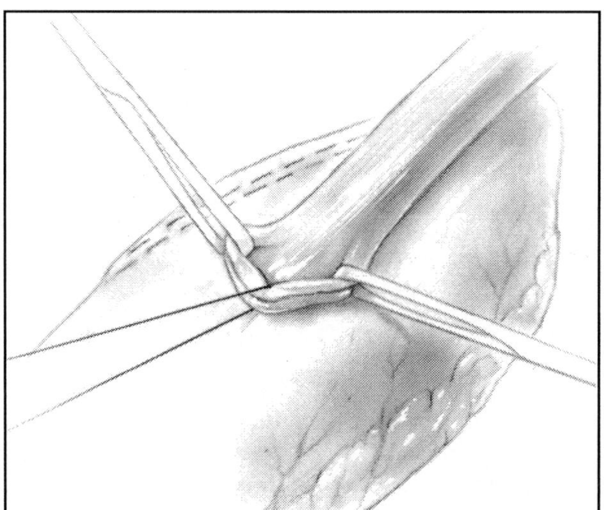

Fig. 3-31

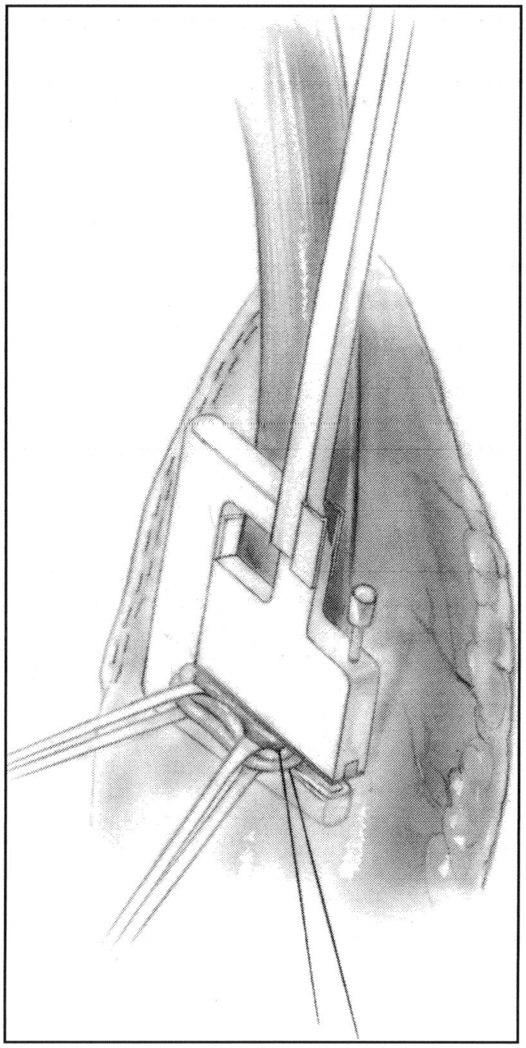

Fig. 3-32

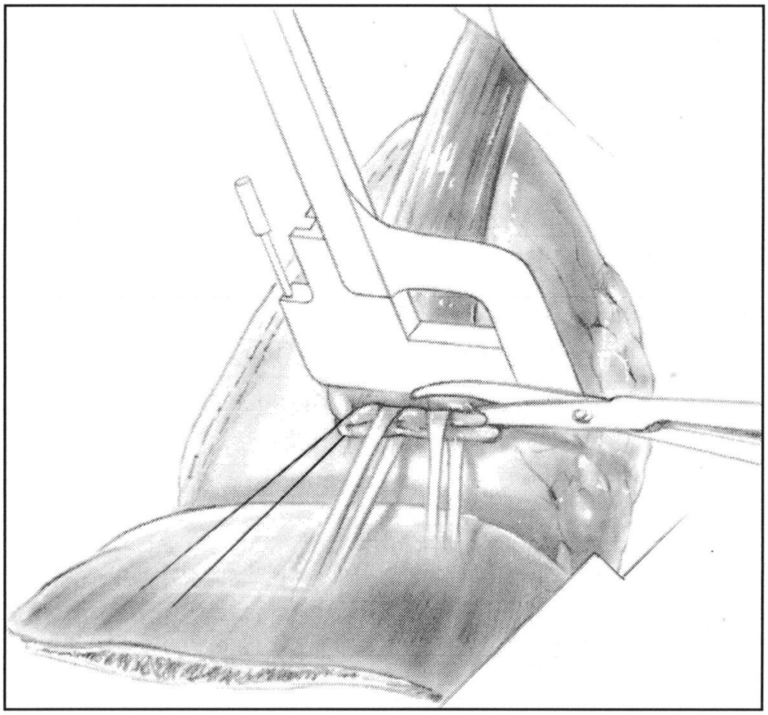

Fig. 3-33

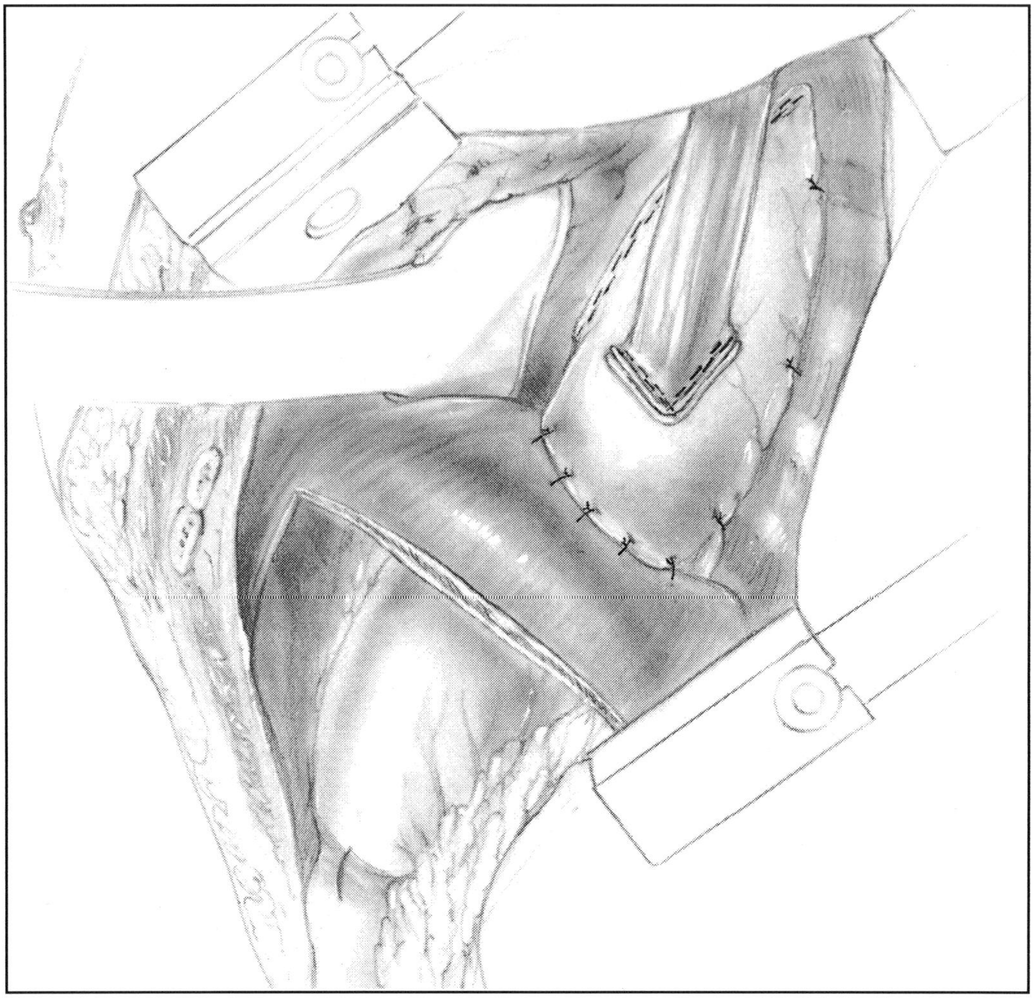

Fig. 3-34

anastomosis. Use a 16F Foley catheter with a 5 cc balloon attached to a 20 cc syringe filled with saline. Insert the Foley catheter well above the site for anastomosis and inflate the balloon in 2.5 cc increments. Withdraw the inflated balloon slowly after each inflation. A 28 mm circular staple can almost always be inserted with ease (use the largest size that can be inserted easily). Place four long Allis clamps or guy sutures equidistant around the circumference of the esophagus to maintain a wide lumen and minimize difficulty with insertion of the stapler head.

If a tear is detected, resect an additional segment of the esophagus to remove the laceration. If the tear is not detected and a stapled anastomosis is constructed, postoperative leakage is a potentially dangerous complication.

Next, insert the 25 mm sizer and then the 28 mm sizer. If the 28 mm sizer passes easily, the circular stapling technique is a good one. If only the 25 mm sizer can be inserted, there is danger of postoperative stenosis when this size staple cartridge is used. Although this type of stenosis frequently responds well to postoperative dilatation, we prefer to utilize the alternative technique described above (Fig. 3-28 to 3-34), which corrects for the narrow esophagus without requiring postoperative dilatation. Use a purse-string suture to tighten the esophagus around the shaft of the stapler. After inserting a 28- or 31-mm sizer, place one or two purse-string sutures of 0 or 2-0 Prolene, making certain to include the mucosa and the muscularis in each bite.

The anastomosis can be done to the anterior or posterior wall of the stomach. We generally prefer to use the posterior wall if the anastomosis is high in the chest, as it allows an easy anterior hemifundoplication.

Make a 3 cm linear incision somewhere in the antrum of the gastric pouch utilizing electrocautery. Through this opening in the anterior wall of the

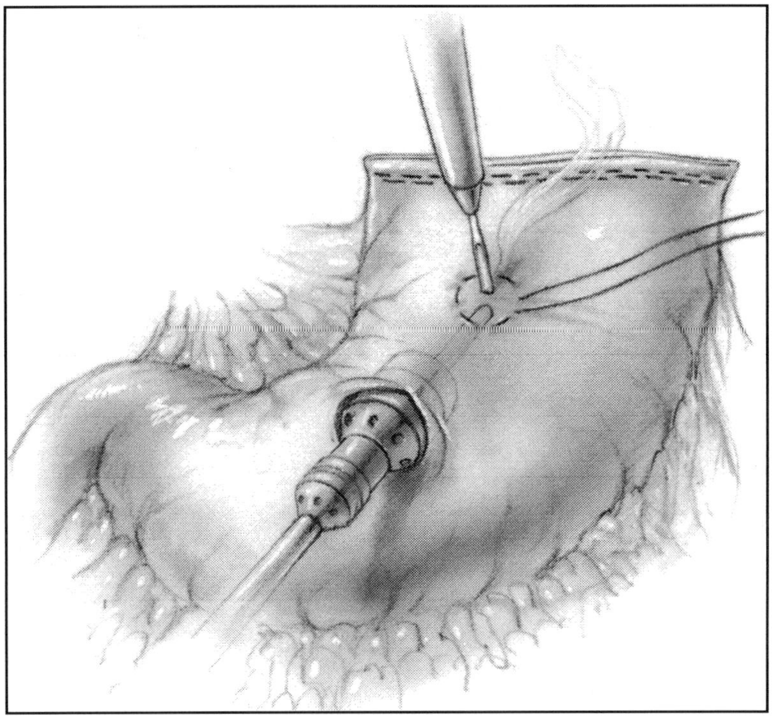

Fig. 3–35

gastric pouch, insert the cartridge of a circular stapling device after having removed the anvil.

Then choose a point 5–6 cm from the proximal cut end of the gastric pouch and use the spike of the stapler to puncture it. Advance the shaft as far as it will go and then insert a small purse-string suture of 2-0 Prolene around the shaft. Alternatively, place the purse-string suture first; then make a stab wound in the middle of it **(Fig. 3–35)** and permit the shaft of the circular stapler to emerge from the stab wound. Tie the purse-string suture around the shaft. Remove the spike. Gently insert the anvil of the device into the open end of the esophagus. Draw the esophagus down over the anvil. When this has been accomplished, tie the purse-string suture around the instrument's shaft, fixing the esophagus in position **(Fig. 3–36)**. Ensure that there is no axial rotation of the stomach. Now attach the anvil to the shaft of the device and approximate the anvil to the cartridge of the circular stapling device by turning the wing-nut in a clockwise direction to the indicated tightness. Be certain that the purse-string suture fits snugly around the shaft and that it does not catch on grooves in the shaft. After this has been accomplished, fire the stapling device.

Now rotate the wing-nut the appropriate number of turns in a counterclockwise direction, gently disengage the anvil from the newly created anastomosis,

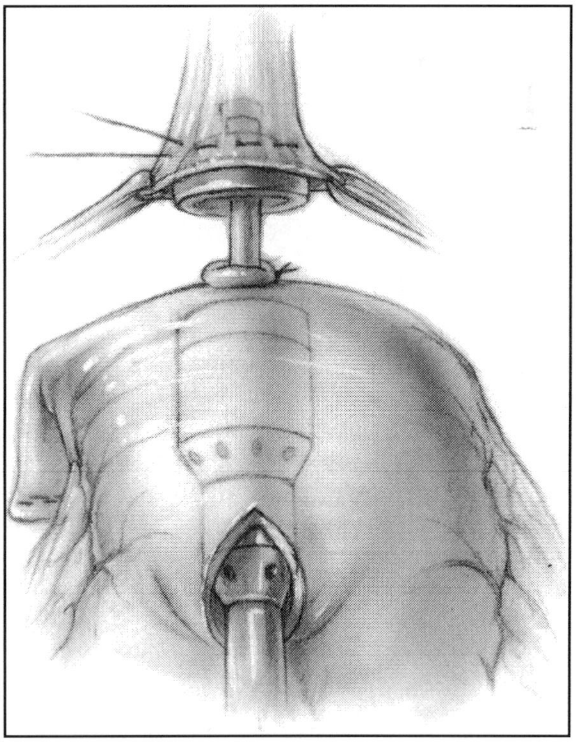

Fig. 3–36

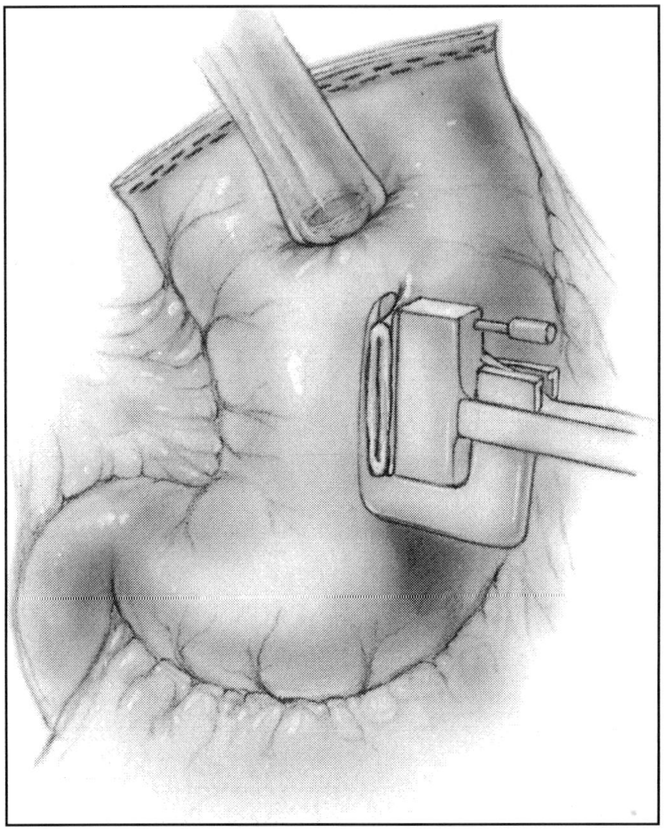

Fig. 3–37

and remove the entire device from the gastric pouch. Carefully inspect the newly constructed circular anastomosis between the open end of the esophagus and the gastric pouch to see that all the staples have fired and that the anastomosis is intact. Confirm this by inserting the index finger through the previously made gastrotomy incision and pass the finger into the esophagus, confirming the presence of an open lumen. Now apply Allis clamps to the gastrotomy incision on the anterior wall of the gastric pouch. Apply a linear stapling device for thick tissue (4.8mm) and fire. Excise any redundant gastric tissue, remove the stapler, and lightly electrocoagulate bleeding vessels. Carefully inspect the staple line to be sure all of the staples have closed. Many surgeons oversew the gastrotomy incision with a layer of continuous or interrupted Lembert sutures of a nonabsorbable nature, although this step may not be essential if 4.8mm staples are used **(Fig. 3–37)**. Do not convert the linear gastrotomy to a transverse closure as you would for a pyloroplasty because it increases tension on the suture line.

Muehreke and Donnelly reported four leaks from stapled gastrotomies in 195 patients undergoing esophageal resection using circular stapling instruments. A possible explanation for failure of the stapled gastrotomy closure to heal properly is the use of a 3.5mm staple. In a stomach of normal thickness, using a small staple can produce a line of necrosis. We prefer that a 4.8mm staple be used when closing the stomach. These authors found that there was a reduction in the leak rate from their gastrotomy closures if they oversewed the gastrotomy staple line with a continuous noninverting layer of 3-0 Mersilene. We have used a 4-0 polypropylene running, inverting seromuscular suture to cover the staple line and have seen leaks only when this step was omitted.

Stabilizing the Gastric Pouch

To prevent any gravity-induced tension on the anastomosis, the apex of the gastric pouch should be sutured to the mediastinal pleura or the prevertebral fascia with 2-0 or 3-0 nonabsorbable sutures. The gastric pouch should then be fixed to the enlarged diaphragmatic hiatus with interrupted 2-0 or 3-0 nonabsorbable sutures, which attach the gastric wall to the margins of the hiatus (Fig. 3–34). These sutures should be 2cm apart and should not penetrate the gastric mucosa lest they induce a gastropleural fistula.

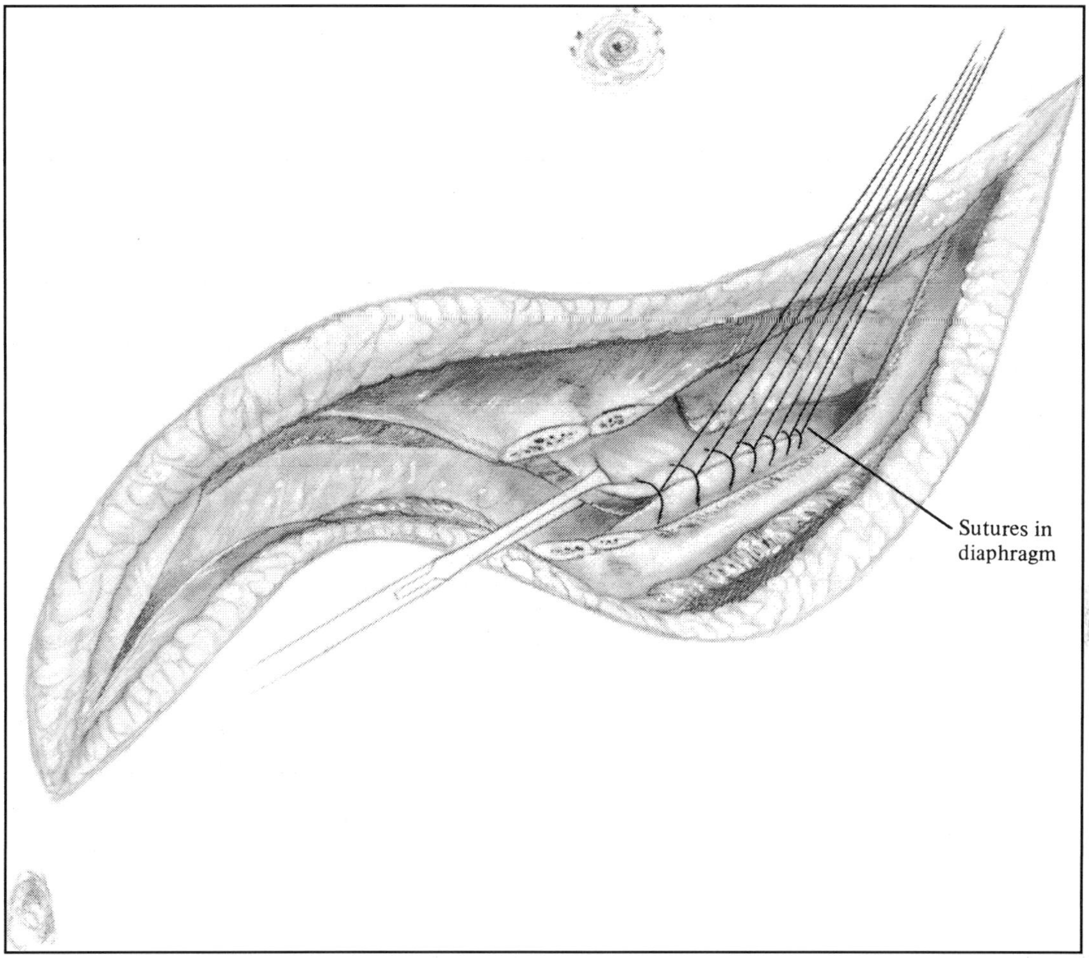

Fig. 3-38

Consider performing a jejunostomy for immediate postoperative enteral alimentation.

Closure

Irrigate the thoracic and abdominal cavities and close the incision in the diaphragm with interrupted sutures of 2-0 Tevdek or a running suture of 0 monofilament **(Fig. 3–38)**. In either case, take fairly large (1 cm) bites, as dehiscence of this suture line can have serious consequences, such as herniation of small intestine into the chest. Do not try to complete this closure until the costal margin has been approximated to avoid tearing the diaphragm.

Excise approximately 1 cm of cartilage from the costal margin to improve apposition **(Fig. 3–39)**. Close the incision in the costal margin with one or two sutures of monofilament stainless steel wire **(Fig. 3–40)**. Either 2-0 or no. 5 wire may be used. Insert four or five pericostal sutures of no. 1 PDS to approximate the ribs **(Fig. 3–41)**. Bring a 30F chest

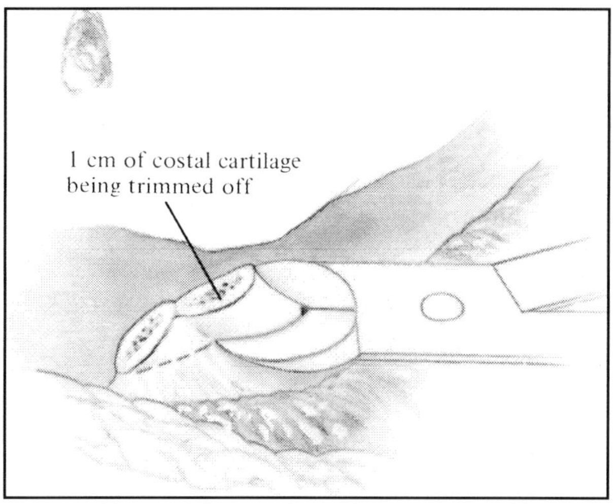

Fig. 3-39

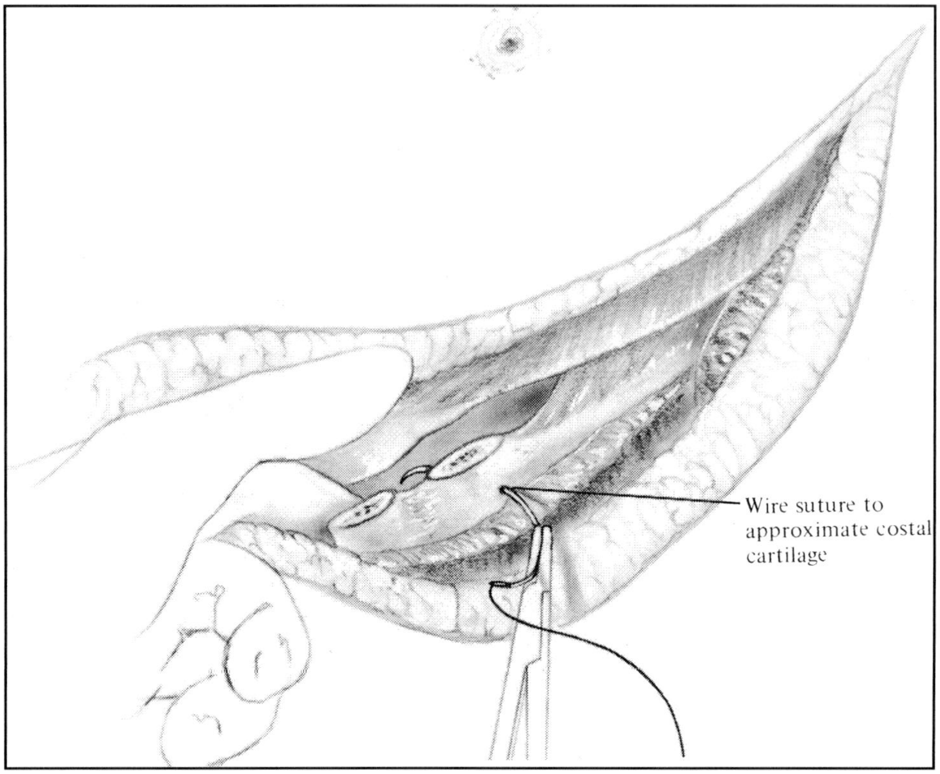

Fig. 3-40

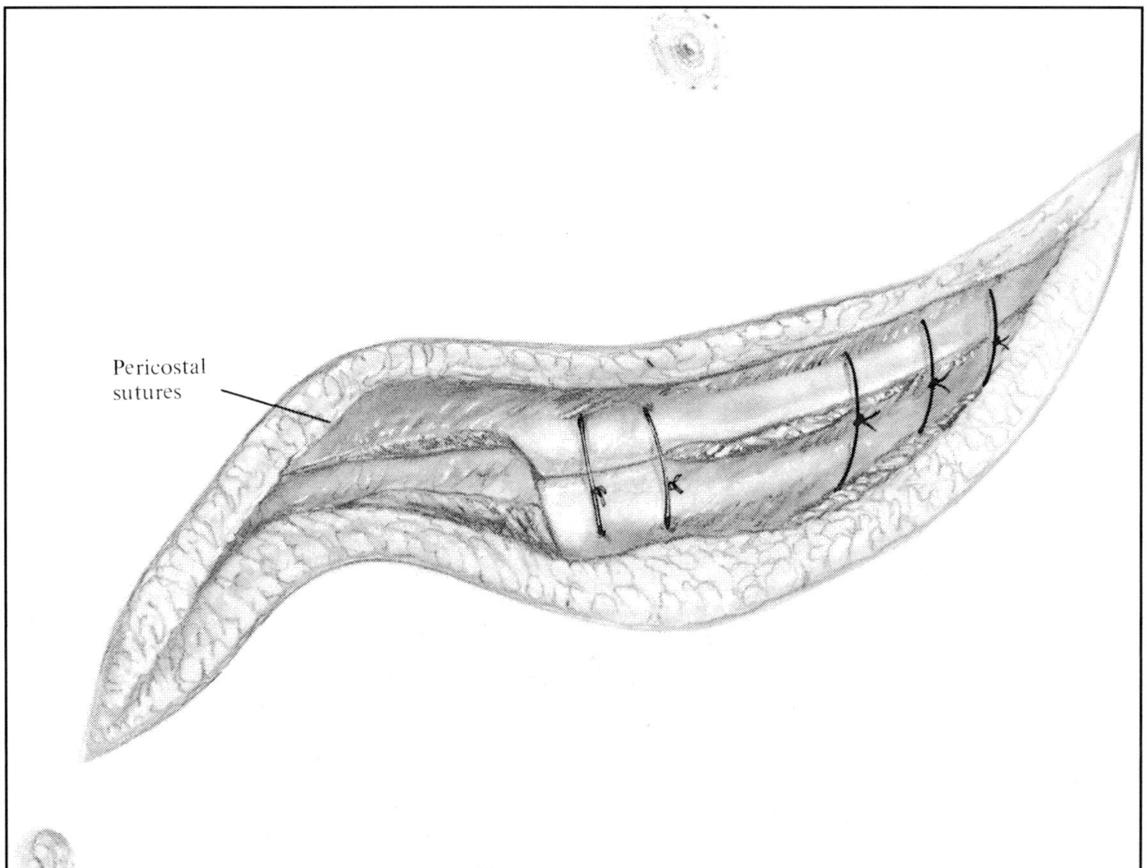

Fig. 3-41

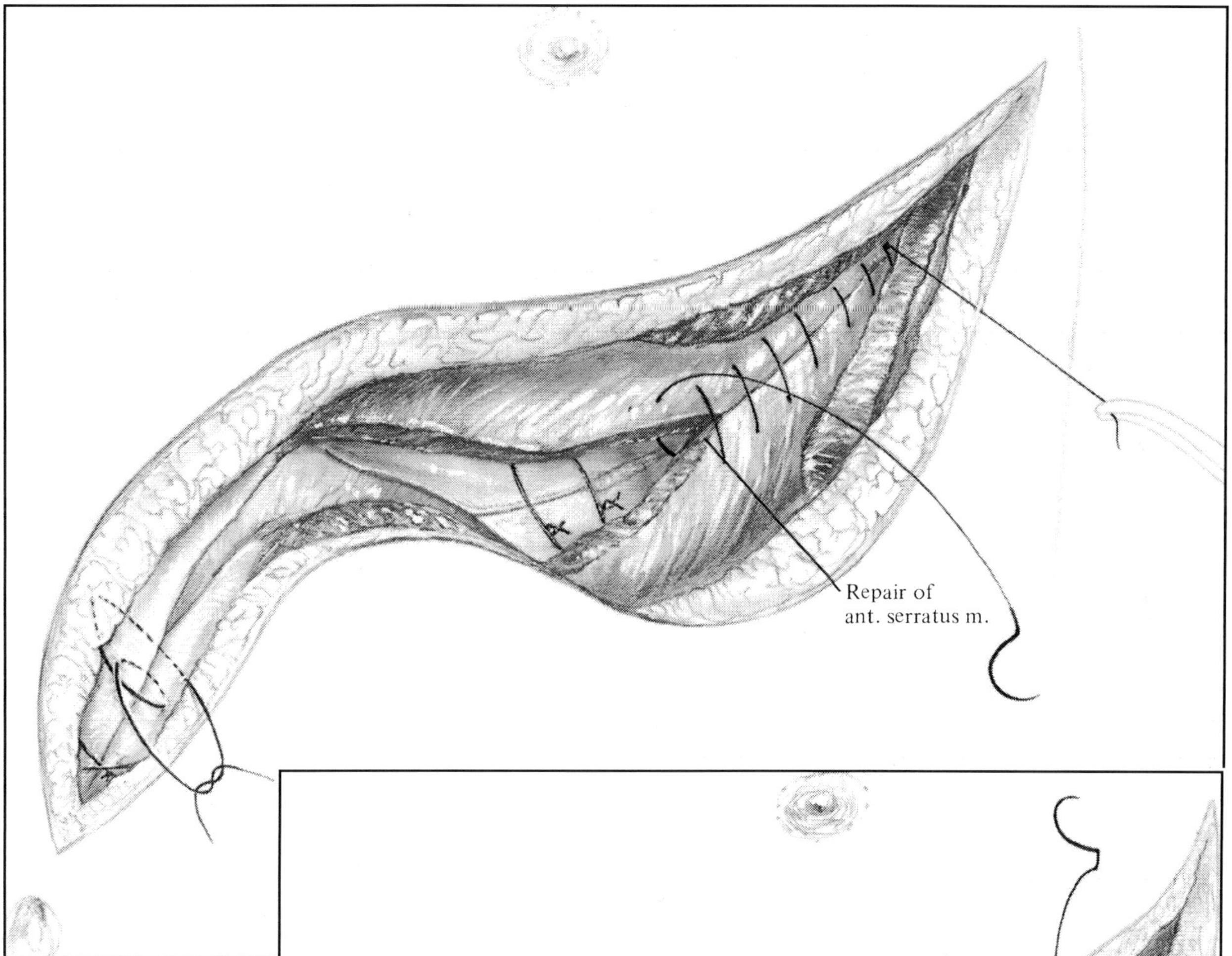

Fig. 3-42

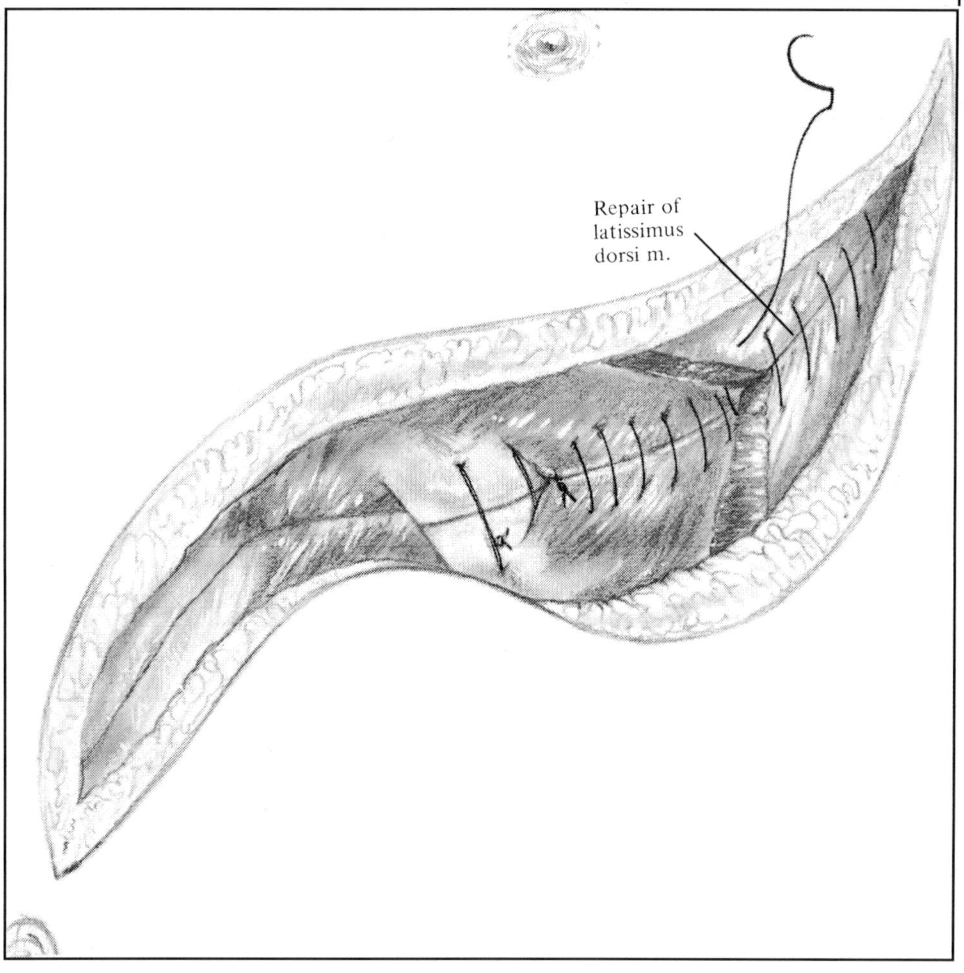

Fig. 3-43

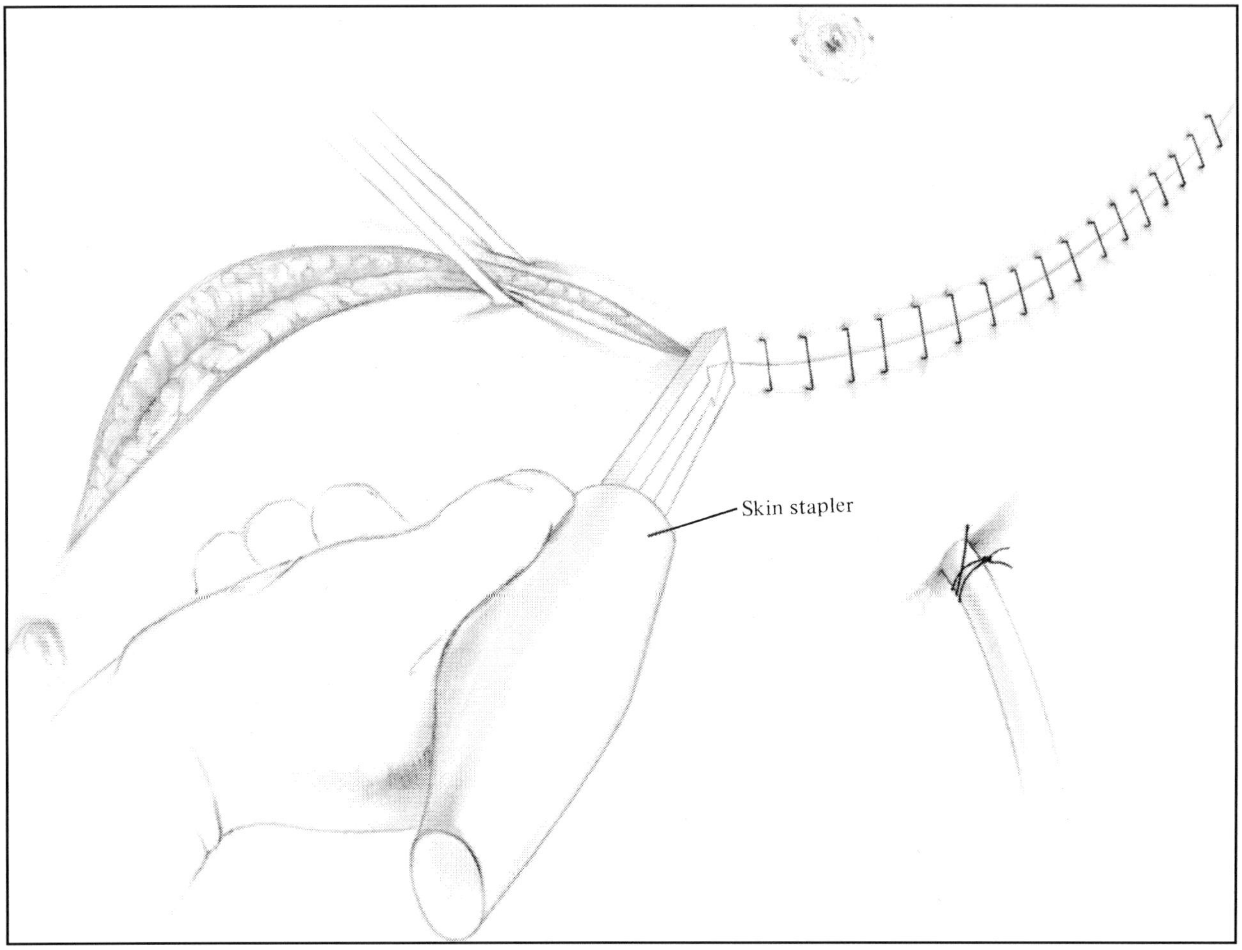

Fig. 3–44

tube through the ninth intercostal space in the anterior axillary line and carry it up to the level of the anastomosis. Place it under direct vision. If it does not sit comfortably, suture it to the parietal pleura posterior to the aorta using fine absorbable sutures. Inflate the lung to eliminate any atelectatic patches. If a significant number of air leaks from the lung are noted, pass a second chest catheter anterior to the lung up to the apex of the thorax. Tie the pericostal sutures and the final diaphragm sutures and close the muscles in two layers with a continuous 2-0 or 0 PG atraumatic synthetic absorbable suture in each **(Figs. 3–42, 3–43)**.

Close the abdominal portion of the incision with interrupted no. 1 PDS Smead-Jones sutures. The diaphragm is continuous with the endoabdominal fascia, and separate closure of this layer to meet the diaphragmatic closure facilitates closure of both diaphragm and abdominal wall. Use staples or a subcuticular suture to close the skin **(Fig. 3–44)**. No drains should be needed in the abdominal cavity.

POSTOPERATIVE CARE

See Chapter 2.

COMPLICATIONS

See Chapter 2.

REFERENCES

Chassin JL. Esophagogastrectomy: data favoring end-to-side anastomosis. Ann Surg 1978;188:22.

Chassin JL. Stapling technic for esophagogastrostomy after esophagogastric resection. Am J Surg 1978;136:399.

Ellis FH, Heatley GJ, Krasna MJ, Williamson WA, Balogh K. Esophagogastrectomy for carcinoma of the esophagus and cardia: a comparison of findings and results after standard resection in three consecutive eight-year intervals with improved staging criteria. J Thorac Cardiovasc Surg 1997;113:836.

Fisher RD, Brawley RK, Kieffer RF. Esophagogastrostomy in the treatment of carcinoma of the distal two-thirds of the esophagus. Ann Thorac Surg 1972;14:658.

Humphrey EW. Stapling techniques in esophageal replacement. Surg Clin North Am 1984;64:499.

Krasna MJ. Advances in the staging of esophageal carcinoma. Chest 1998;113:107S.

Muehrcke DD, Donnelly RJ. Complications after esophagogastrectomy using stapling instruments. Ann Thorac Surg 1989;48:257.

Skandalakis JE, Ellis H. Embryologic and anatomic basis of esophageal surgery. Surg Clin North Am 2000; 80:85.

Steichen FM. Varieties of stapled anastomoses of the esophagus. Surg Clin North Am 1984;64:481.

4 Transhiatal Esophagectomy

INDICATIONS

Carcinoma of the esophagus

Esophageal stricture

PREOPERATIVE PREPARATION

See Chapter 2.

Prepare for possible massive blood loss during the blunt phase of the thoracic dissection.

Prepare a single-lumen endotracheal tube, not cut short.

Consider hemodynamic monitoring.

PITFALLS AND DANGER POINTS

Excessive bleeding

Laceration of membranous trachea

Injury to spleen

Hypotension during mediastinal dissection due to compression of the heart

Trauma to thoracic duct; chylothorax

Traction injury or laceration of the recurrent laryngeal nerve

Bowel herniation through a too large diaphragmatic hiatus

Undetected pneumothorax

Ischemia or trauma to tip of gastric tube in the neck inducing necrosis and sepsis

Anastomotic leak

Inadvertent laceration of right gastroepiploic artery

OPERATIVE STRATEGY

Although a large portion of this operation is accomplished by blunt dissection, there are five areas where dissection must be performed with consummate delicacy to avoid devastating complications.

1. *Membranous trachea.* A small linear laceration of the membranous trachea can be repaired by suturing. However, if a patch of the membranous trachea is avulsed while dissecting an esophageal cancer that has invaded the trachea, adequate repair may be impossible. In the absence of a malignancy in the area of the trachea, dissection of the esophagus away from the trachea should not be difficult if carried out in a gentle manner.

2. *Right gastroepiploic artery.* While dissecting the omentum away from the gastroepiploic artery, continually keep in mind that this vessel constitutes the major blood supply to the tip of the gastric tube to be constructed. In many areas this vessel is covered by omental fat so its exact location is not obvious to the naked eye. Consequently, when dividing the omentum, leave a few centimeters of omentum attached to the artery, as inadvertent division of this vessel makes the stomach useless as an esophaeal substitute.

3. *Gastric tip.* Be aware that the gastroepiploic artery does not continue to the tip of the gastric tube. Beyond the termination of this artery the blood supply to the gastric tip consists of intramural circulation. Although this circulation is *normally* adequate to sustain the healing process of the gastroesophageal anastomosis in the neck, *unnecessary trauma* to this area can threaten this precarious anastomosis. Consequently, be aware throughout the operation that this tissue must be protected from rough handling. Even inserting a suture between the gastric tip and the prevertebral fascia in the neck has been reported to have caused focal necrosis of the stomach and a gastric fistula with vertebral osteomyelitis. If an anchoring stitch is considered necessary, use 5-0 PG suture material, do not place the suture too deeply, and do not tie a tight knot.

4. *Recurrent laryngeal nerve.* Aside from hoarseness, damage to the left recurrent laryngeal nerve during the cervical dissection can also result in swallowing difficulty and aspiration. Use the assistant's

index finger rather than a rigid instrument to retract the trachea and the thyroid gland.

5. *Azygos vein*. Laceration or avulsion of the azygos vein results in massive hemorrhage that in most cases requires right thoracotomy for control. Avoid this by careful preoperative staging and careful dissection at the point where the azygous vein crosses the esophagus.

OPERATIVE TECHNIQUE

Place the patient in a supine position on the operating table and insert bilateral intravenous catheters and one intraarterial catheter, which permits continuous monitoring of the patient's blood pressure. Both arms are padded and aligned alongside the body. If a central venous pressure or a Swan-Ganz catheter is to be used, insert it into the right internal jugular vein, as the left side of the neck is preserved for the esophagogastric anastomosis. Request that the anesthesiologist use a standard endotracheal tube of standard length that has not been shortened. If the membranous trachea is inadvertently lacerated, the anesthesiologist can then advance the tip of the endotracheal tube into the left main bronchus. After the balloon is inflated, this maneuver enables the anesthesiologist to control the patient's respiration while repair of the laceration is attempted. Place a small blanket roll under the upper thorax to keep the neck extended.

Turn the head to the right. Attach a self-retaining Thompson, Omni, or similar retractor to the operating table for later use.

Abdomen

Make a midline incision from the xyphoid to a point a few centimeters distal to the umbilicus, and enter the abdominal cavity. Check the stomach carefully to ascertain that it is indeed suitable for the development of a gastric tube that reaches up into the neck. Check the celiac lymph nodes for metastases. Liberate the left lobe of the liver by incising the triangular ligament. Expose the spleen and divide any adhesions that involve the capsule of the spleen, so the short gastric and left gastroepiploic vessels are easily identified. Insert the Weinberg blade of the Thompson retractor underneath the sternum and retract the liver in a cephalad direction, exposing the esophageal hiatus. Thereupon free the lower esophagus and divide the gastrophrenic ligament as described in Figures 2-7 to 2-11. Encircle the esophagus with the index finger and then with a 2 cm wide Penrose drain. Divide the right and left vagus nerves. Apply caudad traction to the esophagus via the Penrose drain and free up the lower esophagus by blunt dissection. If the tumor can be reached by digital palpation, ascertain that it is not fixed to the aorta or vertebral column. If it is fixed, transhiatal esophagectomy without thoracotomy is contraindicated. If not, expose the gastric cardia and then carefully divide and ligate each of the short gastric vessels as well as the left gastroepiploic artery.

Divide the greater omentum serially between Kelly clamps leaving 3-5 cm of omentum attached to the right gastroepiploic arcade to avoid injury to the gastroepiploic artery. Remember that this vessel will be the main blood supply to the gastric conduit (see Figs. 2-12a,b).

Elevate the greater curvature of the stomach in a cephalad direction and identify the origin of the left gastric artery. Divide and ligate it as described in Figure 2-13 and then perform an extensive Kocher maneuver (see Figs. 2-14 to 2-16). Perform a pyloromyotomy (see Figs. 2-17 to 2-19). Cover the abdominal incision with sterile towels and start the neck operation.

Cervical Dissection

Expose and mobilize the cervical esophagus as described in Chapter 2. Encircle the esophagus with a Penrose drain and apply cephalad traction. Use the index finger with the volar aspect of the fingers facing the esophagus to dissect the esophagus away gently from the overlying trachea and the posterior prevertebral fascia. With this dissection, the index finger can reach down almost to the carina of the trachea.

Transhiatal Dissection

Wear a headlamp for this phase of the operation. Adjust the Thompson retractor to elevate the sternum and liver. Enlarge the hiatal opening by incising the diaphragm with electrocautery in an anterior direction through the middle of the central tendon, dividing and ligating the transverse phrenic vein during this step. Dissect the central tendon away from the pericardium. If necessary, insert a flat malleable retractor behind the heart and elevate gently. Push the right and left diaphragmatic plurae laterally to improve exposure. Palpate the esophagus and the tumor. Determine that they are flexible and mobile, and that there are no points of tumor invasion that would make resection without thoracotomy inadvisable. Before embarking on further dissection, pass a 28F Argyle Saratoga suction catheter into the neck incision and then down into the lower mediastinum to facilitate evacuation of blood from the surgical field.

Despite the limited exposure allowed by the transhiatal approach, the transhiatal esophagectomy is neither a blind nor a crude operation. Dissection of the esophagus from the diaphragm to the arch of the aorta is performed under direct vision. Exposure can be enhanced by inserting long, narrow retractors along the lateral aspects of the hiatal aperture. Many of the vascular attachments to the esophagus can be divided and occluded by hemostatic clips or ligatures. When dissecting the esophagus in the mediastinum, make no special effort to excise any pleura or lymph nodes. The strategy of the operation is to separate the surrounding anatomy from the esophageal tube as efficiently as possible. When dissecting the esophagus along its posterior surface, keep the hand flat against the vertebral column. Orringer et al. stated that entry into one or both pleural cavities occurs in 75% of patients during this operation. After the esophagus has been removed from the mediastinum, and before the stomach is brought into the chest, examine the pleura visually and by palpation. If a tear has occurred, insert an appropriate chest tube to prevent a postoperative tension pneumothorax.

After the lower esophagus has been mobilized, insert a small sponge on a long sponge-holder ("sponge on a stick") along the prevertebral fascia in the neck behind the esophagus while the other hand is placed behind the esophagus in the mediastinum **(Fig. 4–1)**. When the sponge-stick meets the hand, the posterior dissection of the esophagus has been completed. Try not to compress the heart unduly with the hand in the prevertebral space. Remind the anesthesiologist to monitor the arterial pressure carefully during this dissection. Now remove the sponge-stick from the neck. With the assistant exerting traction in a caudal direction on the Penrose drain encircling the esophagogastric junction, place the hand, palm down, on the anterior surface of the esophagus and with finger dissection free the esophagus from overlying pericardium and carina. With the other hand insert one or two fingers, volar surface down, over the anterior face of the esophagus in the neck while cephalad traction is being applied to the Penrose drain encircling the cervical esophagus. Working with both hands simultaneously, disrupt the filmy attachments between the esophagus and the membranous trachea-left main stem bronchus. After this has been accomplished, there remain lateral attachments to be disrupted before the esophagus is freed. Again retract the upper esophagus in a cephalad direction and separate the esophagus from these attachments until the upper 8 cm of thoracic esophagus is freed circumferentially. Now insert the hand into the hiatus and slide upward along the anterior esophagus behind the trachea until the circumferentially freed upper esophagus is contacted. Trap the esophagus against the vertebral column between the index and middle fingers. Then with a down-ward raking motion, avulse the lateral attachments until the esophagus has been completely mobilized.

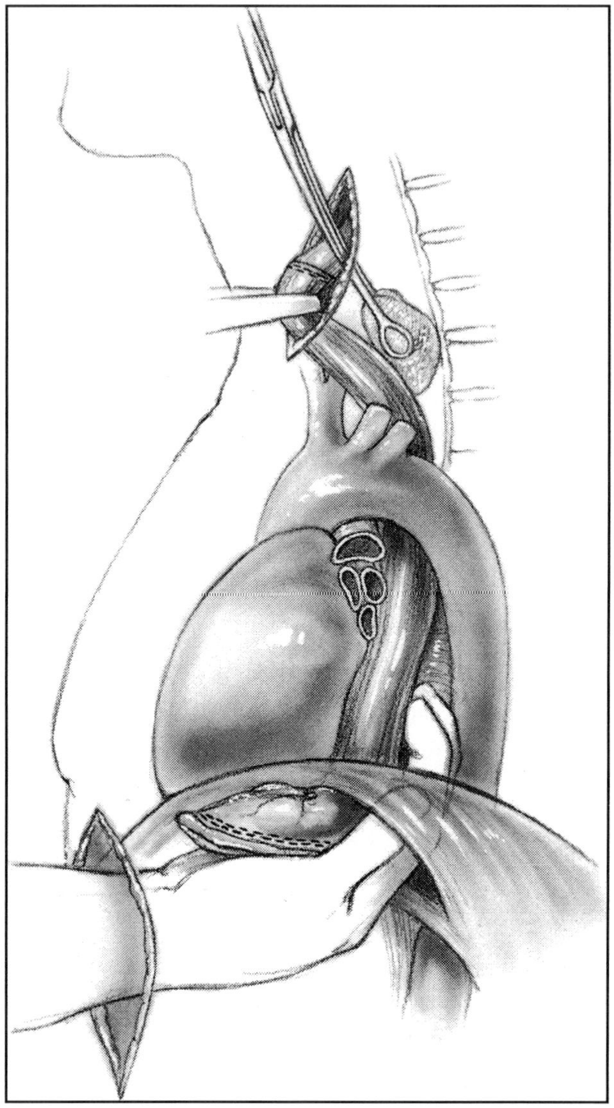

Fig. 4-1

Deliver 7–8 cm of thoracic esophagus into the neck and transect the esophagus with a linear cutting surgical stapler. This maneuver provides a few centimeters of extra esophagus, allowing the option of selecting the best length when the anastomosis is performed.

Suture a long 2 cm wide Penrose drain to the distal end of the divided esophagus. Apply a hemostat to the proximal end of the drain in the neck. Draw the thoracic esophagus down into the abdomen. Then cut

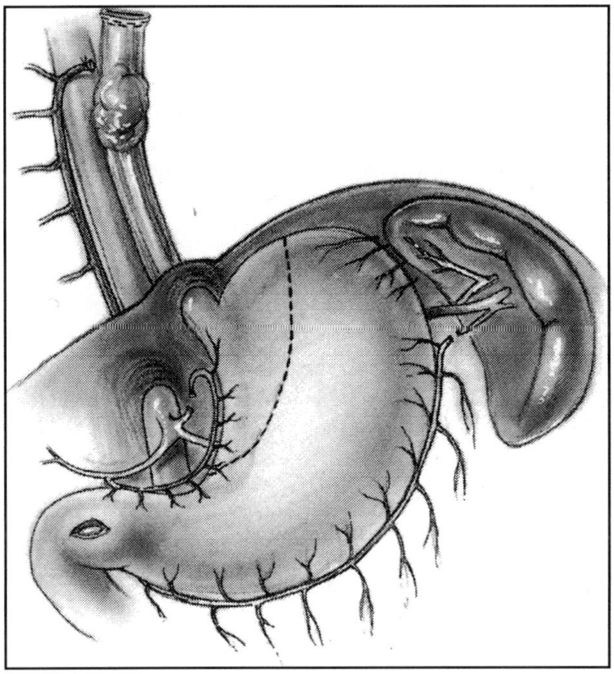

Fig. 4-2

application of the stapler a small portion of the previous staple line must be included. Now invert the entire staple line by means of a continuous 4-0 Prolene Lembert suture. Remove the identifying hemostat from the previously positioned Penrose drain that was brought down from the neck into the mediastinum. Suture this Penrose drain to the most cephalad point of the gastric cardia using 3-0 silk the drain and apply a hemostat to the proximal cut end in the abdomen. This drain with its two identifying hemostats is later used to draw the stomach up through the posterior mediastinum into the neck.

Insert two narrow retractors into the mediastinum and retract laterally. Inspect the mediastinum for any laceration of the pleura. If a laceration is encountered, insert a 32F chest tube into the chest cavity on the side of the laceration, in the mid-axillary line. Then insert moist gauze packing into the mediastinum to help achieve hemostasis while the stomach is being prepared.

Exteriorize the stomach and attached esophagus by spreading it out along the patient's anterior chest wall. Because the blood supply to the lesser curvature subsequent to ligation of the left gastric artery is poor (Akiyama), the lesser curvature is excised, converting the stomach into a tubular structure **(Fig. 4–2)**. Manually stretch the proximal tip of the cardia in a cephalad direction. Observe the esophagogastric junction and note where the second or third branch down of the left gastric artery enters the lesser curvature. At this point, apply the linear cutting stapler and aim it in a cephalad direction toward the cardia. While continuing to apply cephalad traction on the cardia, fire the stapler. Sequentially reapply and fire the stapler until the lesser curvature has been amputated, leaving about 6–8 cm width of cardia intact at the gastric tip **(Fig. 4–3)**. Remember that with each

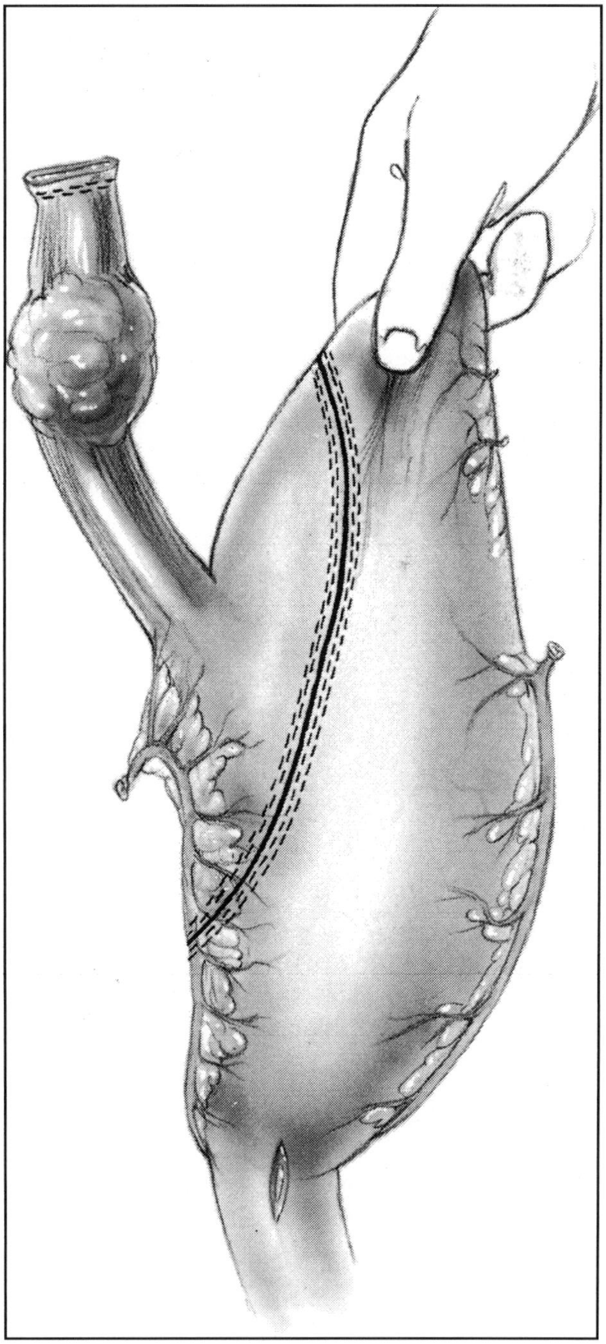

Fig. 4-3

sutures. Leave a 4- to 5-cm tail on the medial suture to identify the lesser curvature side of the gastric tube. Place gentle cephalad traction on the proximal end of the Penrose drain that remains in the cervical incision while using the right hand to maneuver the gastric tip gently through the hiatus and into the posterior mediastinum until the stomach has been manipulated into the neck. To avoid the possibility of gastric torsion, be certain that the staple line along the lesser curvature is located to the patient's right and the greater curvature to the patient's left. The long-tailed suture at the junction of the Penrose drain and the gastric cardia identify the medial aspect of the gastric tube. Confirm the absence of torsion by inserting the right hand through the hiatus and palpating the anterior surface of the stomach up to the aortic arch and with the left hand from the cervical approach. With both hands, deliver the gastric tip up to the apex of the cervical incision. Insert several sutures of 5-0 Vicryl to attach the gastric fundus to the fascia of the longus colli muscles on both sides of the neck. Do not take deep bites of stomach or tie the sutures so tight that necrosis of the gastric wall occurs.

Return to the abdomen and close the incision in the diaphragm with interrupted 2-0 silk sutures but do not constrict the newly formed hiatus to the point where it obstructs venous return from the gastric tube. Leave about three fingers' space between the diaphragm and the stomach. Then insert enough interrupted 3-0 silk sutures between the muscle surrounding the hiatus and the stomach to prevent the possibility of bowel herniating through the newly formed diaphragmatic hiatus. Cover the pyloromyotomy with omentum. Perform a feeding needle catheter jejunostomy in the proximal jejunum. Close the abdominal incision and then return to the neck to perform the esophagogastric anastomosis.

To avoid any tension whatsoever on the anastomosis, divide the cervical esophagus at a point where it can easily reach the clavicle. When dividing the esophagus, cut the anterior flap of esophagus so it is at least 1 cm longer than the posterior flap, as illustrated in Figure 2–24. This maneuver converts the anastomotic suture line into an ellipse instead of a circle and should result in a larger stoma. Now reflect the esophagus in a cephalad position above the cervical incision. The uppermost gastric cardia has already been sutured to the neck muscles as high as is comfortable in the cervical incision. Using Babcock forceps, gently elevate the anterior wall of the stomach from behind the clavicle to a more superficial and superior location in the neck. The anastomosis between the end of the esophagus and the anterior wall of the stomach should be located 3–5 cm down from the apex of the gastric tube and above the level of the clavicle. Bring the esophagus back into the neck so it rests on the anterior wall of the gastric tube. Make an incision in the anterior wall of the gastric tube in a vertical direction, the length being appropriate to the diameter of the elliptical esophageal orifice, which is approximately 2.5 cm.

Be certain that the esophagus and stomach are positioned such that there is no tension on the suture line. Using 4-0 PG or PDS insert the first stitch in the mucosa 4 mm from the cut end. This stitch passes through the muscle layer of the esophagus and then enters the cephalad margin of the gastric incision 4 mm above the incision, entering the lumen of the stomach. When tying these sutures, make the knot just tight enough to afford approximation, not strangulation. Place the second stitch through the left lateral wall of the esophagus into the lumen, again catching at least 4 mm of mucosa, and bring the stitch into the stomach and out the center of the left lateral wall of the stomach. Do not tie this stitch; rather, clamp it in a hemostat and place the third stitch in the same fashion in the right lateral margin of the esophagus and stomach. Ask the assistant to apply hemostats to stitches 2 and 3 and then to apply lateral traction to separate the two stitches. This maneuver lines up the esophagus and stomach so closing the posterior layer is simple. Insert interrupted sutures about 4 mm apart from each other. When the knots are tied the mucosa will automatically have been inverted into the lumen. Cut the tails of all the sutures in the posterior anastomosis but retain the hemostats on stitches 2 and 3. Maintain lateral traction on these two stitches and begin the anterior anastomosis by inserting the first stitch at 12 o'clock at the midpoint of the inferior esophagus. Bring this stitch into the lumen of the stomach and bring it out of the stomach at 6 o'clock. Apply a hemostat to this stitch, which serves as an anchor. Now close the anterior layer by inserting Lembert sutures and then invert the tissues as the knots are being tied. These knots remain outside the lumen **(Fig. 4–4)**. We frequently use the technique of successive bisection. After the anastomosis is completed, ask the anesthesiologist to pass a nasogastric tube and guide it through the anastomosis into the gastric pouch.

Closure

Close the cervical incision in layers with interrupted 4-0 PG after inserting a 1.5 cm latex drain to a point near the anastomosis. Consider a needle catheter jejunostomy. Close the abdominal cavity without drainage using the modified Smead-Jones

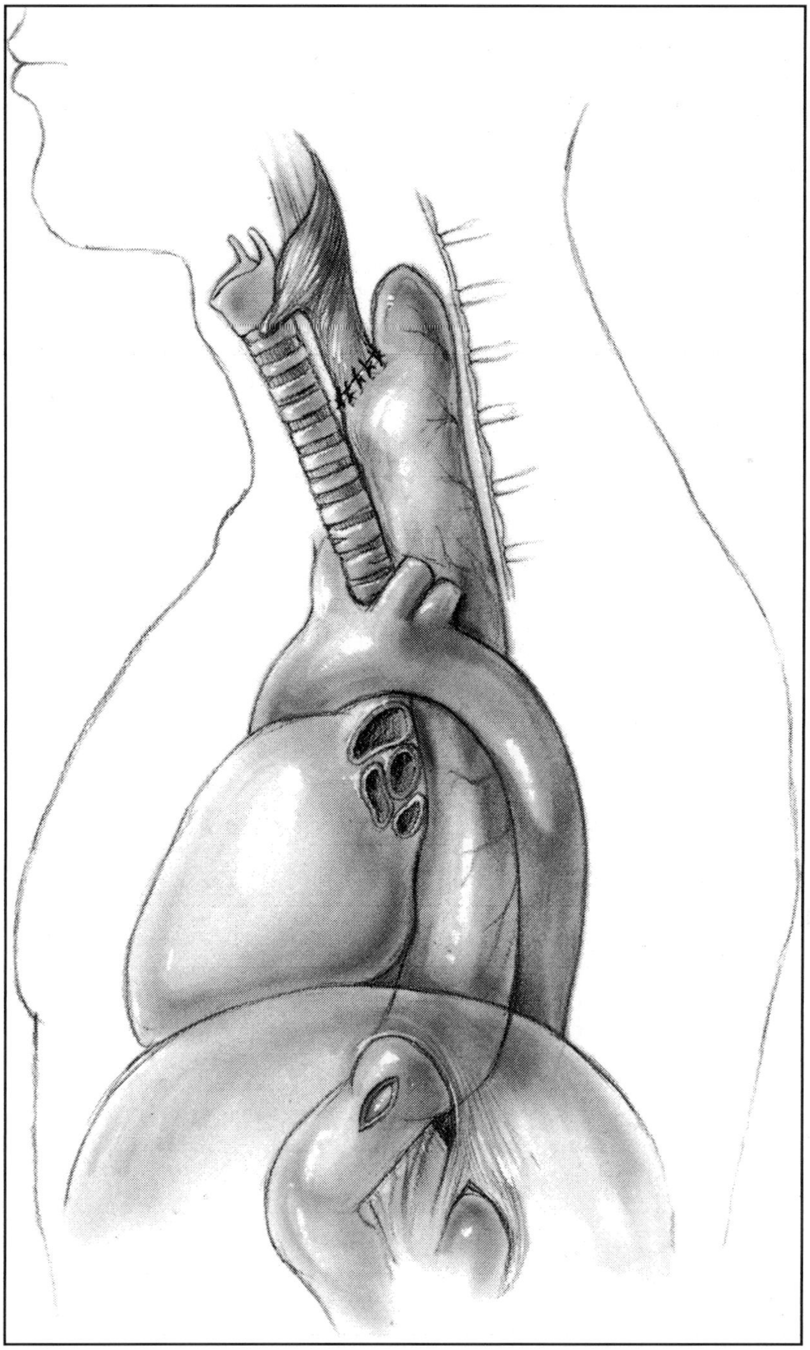

Fig. 4-4

closure and no. 1 PDS sutures. Close the skin with interrupted fine nylon, subcuticular continuous 4-0 PG, or staples.

POSTOPERATIVE CARE

Continue nasogastric suction for 4-5 days. Maintain the chest catheter on some type of underwater drainage for 4-5 days or until the volume of drainage becomes insignificant. Leave the cervical drain in place 7-10 days.

COMPLICATIONS

Anastomotic leak. This is seen especially in cases of anastomoses involving the cervical esophagus.

Stricture of the cervical anastomosis. This occurs especially after leaks.

Intestinal obstruction. Obstruction is due to adhesions.

Trauma to recurrent laryngeal nerve. The nerve is traumatized during dissection of the cervical esophagus.

Pneumothorax and intraoperative or postoperative hemorrhage. Insert a large drainage tube into the right or left hemithorax (or both) if a pneumothorax has been produced by the transhiatal dissection. Inspection of the mediastinum reveals most gaps in the mediastinal pleura.

Chylothorax. Chylothorax may follow transhiatal esophagectomy. It should be suspected whenever the chest tube drainage exceeds 800 ml per day after the third postoperative day. The diagnosis can be confirmed by administering cream via the jejunostomy catheter and observing an opalescent tinge to the pleural drainage. Early recognition, exploration, and transthoracic ligation may hasten resolution when compared with traditional conservative management.

Leaking thoracic duct. To identify the leaking thoracic duct at reoperation, Orringer et al. injected cream into the jejunostomy feeding tube at a rate of 60–90 ml/hr for 4–6 hours prior to reoperation for duct ligation. A limited fifth-interspace posterolateral thoracotomy under one-lung anesthesia was the approach these authors employed for the reoperation.

REFERENCES

Akiyama H. Surgery for carcinoma for the esophagus. Curr Probl Surg 1980;17:56.

Bolton JS, Fuhrman GM, Richardson WS. Esophageal resection for cancer. Surg Clin North Am 1998;78:773.

Chu KM, Law SY, Fok M, Wong J. A prospective randomized comparison of transhiatal and transthoracic resection for lower-third esophageal carcinoma. Am J Surg 1997;21:320.

Gluch L, Smith RC, Bambach CP, Brown AR. Comparison of outcomes following transhiatal or Ivor Lewis esophagectomy for esophageal carcinoma. World J Surg 1999;23:271.

Orringer MB, Stirling MC. Cervical esophagogastric anastomosis for benign disease: functional results. J Thorac Cardiovasc Surg 1988;96:887.

Orringer MB, Bluett M, Deeb GM. Aggressive treatment of chylothorax complicating transhiatal esophagectomy without thoracotomy. Surgery 1988;104:720.

Orringer MB, Marshall B, Iannettoni MD. Eliminating the cervical esophagogastric anastomotic leak with a side-to-side stapled anastomosis. J Thorac Cardiovasc Surg 2000;119:277.

Orringer MB, Marshall B, Iannettoni MD. Transhiatal esophagectomy: clinical experience and refinements. Ann Surg 1999;230:392.

Pinotti HW, Cecconello I, De Oliveira MA. Transhiatal esophagectomy for esophageal cancer. Semin Surg Oncol 1997;13:253.

Rindani R, Martin CJ, Cox MR. Transhiatal versus Ivor-Lewis oesophagectomy: is there a difference? Aust NZ J Surg 1999;69:187.

Stark SP, Romberg MS, Pierce GE, et al. Transhiatal versus transthoracic esophagectomy for adenocarcinoma of the distal esophagus and cardia. Am J Surg 1996;172:478.

Swanstrom LL, Hansen P. Laparoscopic total esophagectomy. Arch Surg 1997;132:943.

5 Operations to Replace or Bypass the Esophagus

Colon or Jejunum Interposition

INDICATIONS

Esophageal stricture or perforation

PREOPERATIVE PREPARATION

Nutritional rehabilitation, if needed

Perioperative antibiotics

Preoperative assessment of colon or jejunum by contrast studies, colonoscopy, and arteriography (if necessary)

Routine bowel preparation

OPERATIVE STRATEGY

Resect the damaged esophagus and replace it with a conduit whenever possible. When this is not feasible, a bypass leaving the damaged esophagus in situ is occasionally warranted. Patients who have an irreversible stricture due to peptic esophagitis require esophageal resection. Esophagectomy is also performed on patients who have undergone failed operations for neuromotor esophageal disorders or who have had diversion-exclusion operations (see Chapter 14) for esophageal perforations or anastomotic leakage. Orringer and Orringer (1983) did not open the chest in most of these patients but instead performed transhiatal esophagectomy from the abdominal and cervical approaches.

The colon is a versatile conduit that is applicable to most situations unless the patient has had a previous colon resection. Sufficient length can be obtained to perform a cervical anastomosis if necessary. Jejunum provides a better size match than colon but is considerably more difficult to use owing to the small size of the vessels. It has been used for cervical reconstructions using microsurgical free flap techniques.

The conduit must be carefully developed to preserve the blood supply, positioned in an isoperistaltic fashion without kinking or twisting, and the gastrointestinal continuity restored. These complex operations require thorough preoperative planning and must be individualized.

OPERATIVE TECHNIQUE

Incision and Resection of Esophagus

The choice of incision is determined by whether, and how much, esophagus is to be resected. Transhiatal esophagectomy is an option that obviates the need for a thoracic incision (see Chapter 4).

We prefer a sixth interspace left thoracoabdominal incision for most of these esophagectomies (see Figs. 3-3 to 3-8). Close the gastroesophageal junction in an area relatively free of disease using a 55- or 90-mm linear stapler on the stomach side. Close the esophageal end with another application of the stapling device. Dissect the esophagus out of the mediastinum. If the esophagus is markedly fibrotic, this dissection may require a scalpel. After the esophagus has been freed to the arch of the aorta, dissect the esophagus from underneath the arch of the aorta, as illustrated in Figure 3-26. Temporarily leave the esophagus in its bed until the colon has been liberated.

Long Segment Colon Interposition: Colon Dissection

The initial step for preparing a long colon segment is to liberate the hepatic flexure and the transverse and descending colon. If necessary, extend the thoracoabdominal incision below the umbilicus. Dissect the omentum away from the transverse colon and its mesentery.

With this accomplished, inspect the blood supply of the left and transverse colon. Preserving the left colic artery in most cases permits transection of the middle colic vessels close to the point of origin and yields a segment of colon that could include a good portion of the descending colon as well as the entire transverse colon if it should be necessary. We have not encountered any cases where the "marginal artery" did not continue unimpeded from the left colon around to the transverse colon. However, verify this by careful palpation of the marginal artery and transillumination of the mesentery. Apply bulldog vascular clamps along the marginal artery at the points selected for division and check the adequacy of the pulse in the vessels being retained to supply the transplanted segment.

To ensure a vigorous blood supply to the proximal portion of the transverse colon, with sufficient length to reach the cervical region, ligate and divide the middle colic artery at a point well proximal to its bifurcation (along line At rather than line B in **Figure 5–1a**). This allows the blood flow from the left colic artery to enter the left branch of the middle colic artery and to continue along the right branch to nourish the right portion of the transverse colon. For this reason it is critical that this division and ligature of the middle colic artery and vein be done with great care.

Estimating the Length of Colon Required to Reach the Neck

After the omentum has been dissected off the colon and after both the left and right colon segments have been freed from the posterior abdominal wall, grasp the splenic flexure at the point of termination of the left colic artery and draw this segment of colon in a cephalad direction toward the sternum. Then measure the distance from this point (point X in **Fig. 5–1b**) on the sternum to the neck. This distance approximates the amount of colon required going in a proximal direction from the termination of the left colic artery. Add about 4–5 cm to the estimate and insert a marking stitch in the right transverse colon at this point. In most cases the point marked is at the right of the middle colic vessels, indicating that division of the origin of the middle colic artery and vein is required.

Transect the colon at the proximal margin of the segment selected for transplantation. Restore continuity to the colon by performing a stapled anastomosis. Close the proximal (right) margin of the colon transplant (temporarily) with a 55 mm linear stapler and leave the distal end of the colon segment open.

Cologastrostomy

Elevate the stomach with its attached omentum away from the pancreas. Divide the avascular attachments between the peritoneum overlying the pancreas and the back wall of the stomach. Also incise the avascular portion of the gastrohepatic omentum; then draw the colon transplant with its mesentery in an isoperistaltic direction through the retrogastric plane and through the opening in the gastrohepatic omentum. Be certain not to twist the mesentery. Verify that the colon does indeed reach the cervical esophagus without tension.

Prepare to anastomose the open end of the distal colon transplant to a point on the stomach approximately one-third the distance down from the fundus to the pylorus. The anastomosis may be made on the anterior or posterior side of the stomach. As illustrated in **Figure 5–2**, make a 1.5 cm vertical incision in the stomach about one-third of the way down from the fundus; then insert the cutting linear stapler—one fork in the stab wound of the stomach and one in the open lumen of the colon—to a depth of 3 cm and lock it **(Fig. 5–3)**. Fire the stapler and remove it. Inspect the staple line for bleeding. Then apply Allis clamps to the left and right terminations of this staple line. Place a guy suture through the midpoint of the stab wound of the stomach as illustrated in **Figure 5–4**. Close the remaining defect by two applications of the 55 mm linear stapler. First, apply the stapler just deep to the Allis clamp and the guy suture to close the left half of the gap. After firing the stapling device **(Fig. 5–5)**, excise the surplus tissue but preserve the guy suture. Lightly electrocoagulate the everted mucosa and remove the stapling device. Then reapply the stapler in similar fashion to close the remaining defect. Be sure to place the stapler deep to the Allis clamp and the guy suture. After firing the stapling device, cut away the surplus tissue and lightly electrocoagulate the mucosa. This creates a fairly large anastomosis between the stomach and colon, as illustrated in **Figure 5–6**.

DeMeester et al. pointed out that it is possible to divide the descending colon as it comes behind the stomach without simultaneously dividing the marginal artery of the descending colon. If the marginal artery is not divided, it provides an added avenue of blood flow to the colon that has been transplanted into the neck. By carefully transecting the colon behind the stomach and then dividing and ligating the end branches of the marginal artery close to the colon for a distance of about 4 cm, sufficient colon will have been liberated that a cologastric anastomosis can be constructed to the posterior wall of the stomach, and the distal segment of descending colon can be anastomosed to the remaining hepatic flexure. If the anastomosis is made at the junction between the upper third and the lower two-thirds of the stomach, it seems not to matter whether the cologastrostomy is constructed on the posterior wall or the anterior wall of the stomach. However, if one wishes to preserve the marginal artery of the descending colon, it is necessary to place the cologastrostomy on

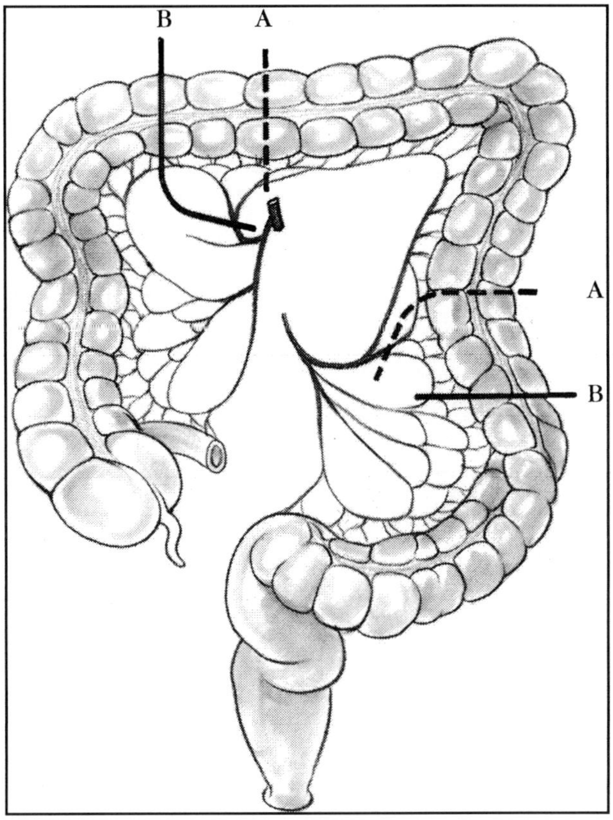

Fig. 5-1a

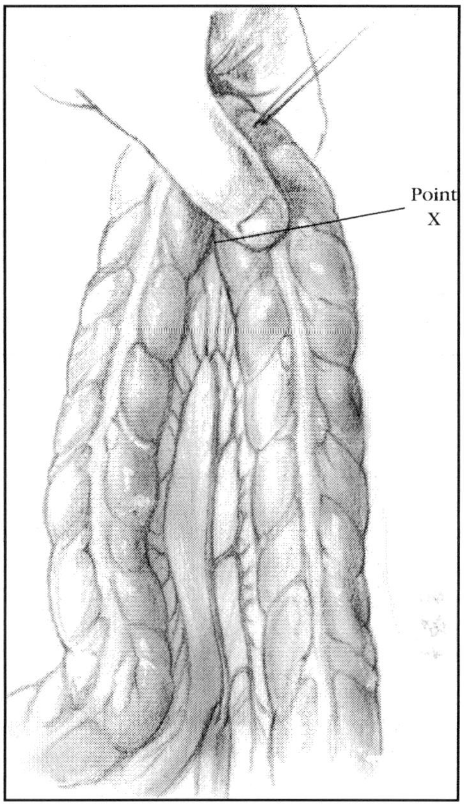

Fig. 5-1b

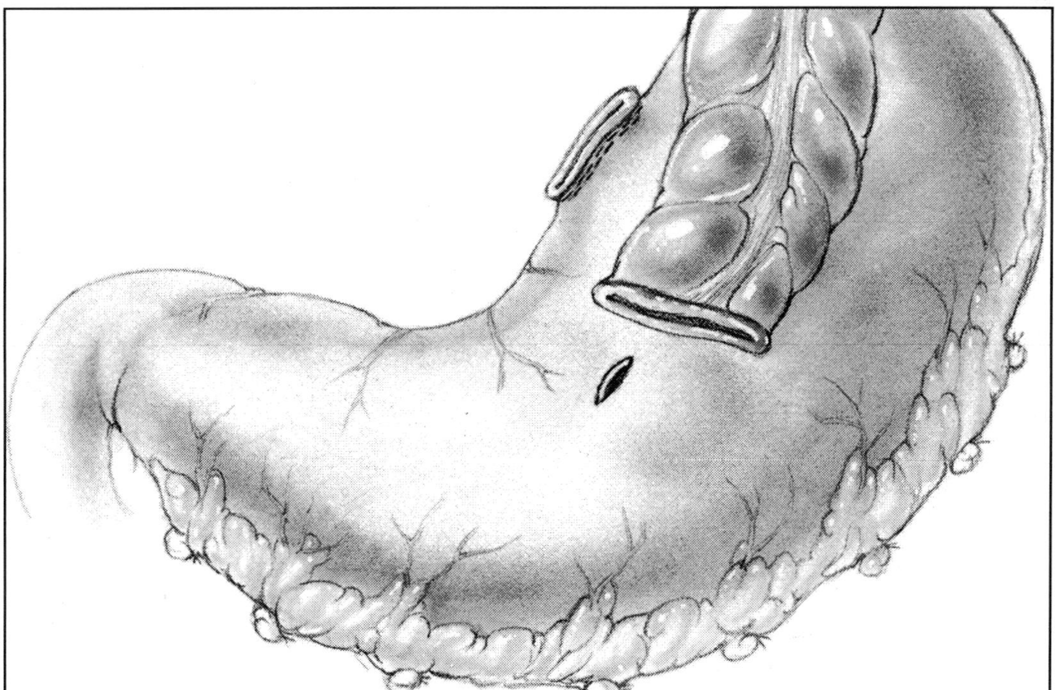

Fig. 5-2

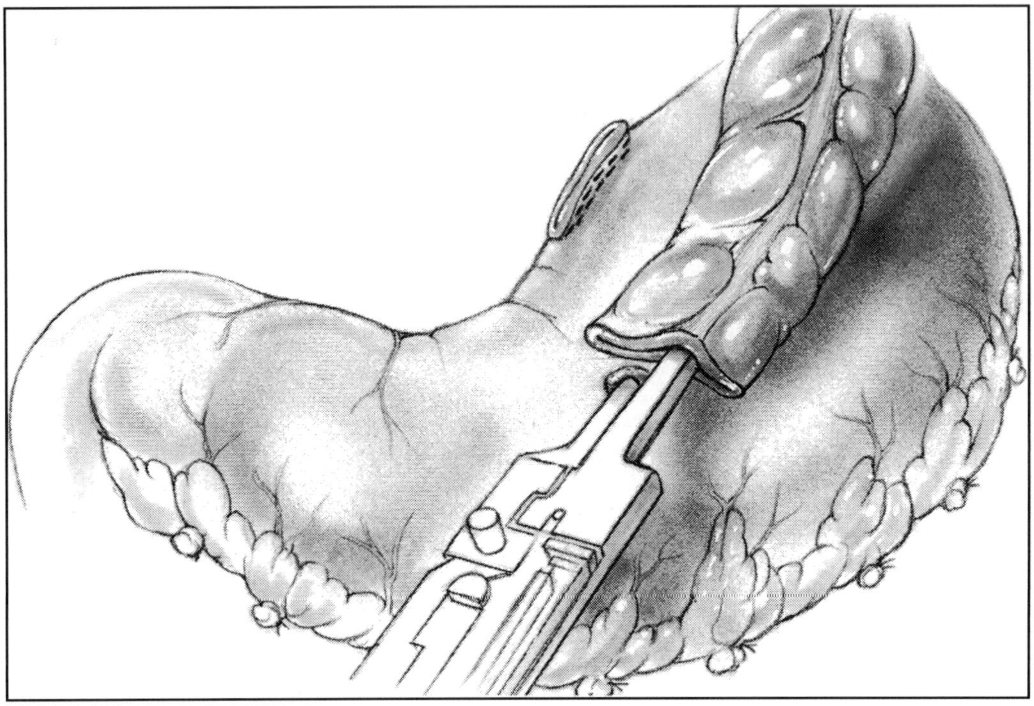

Fig. 5-3

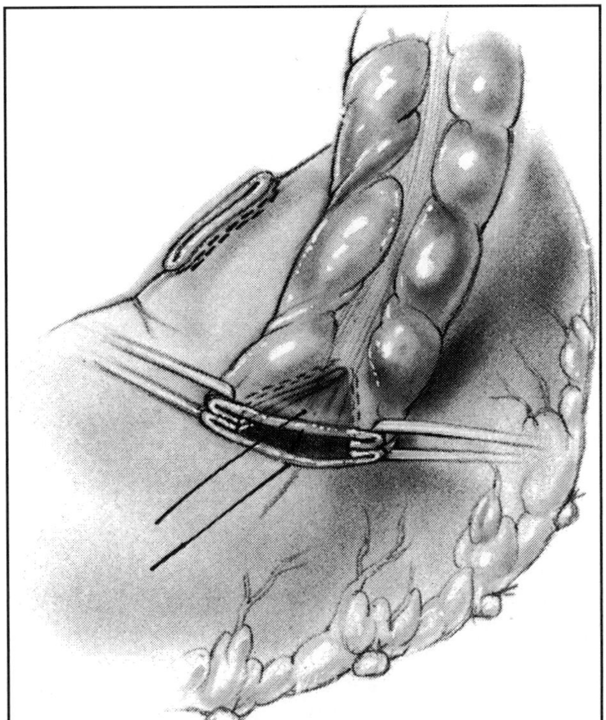

Fig. 5-4

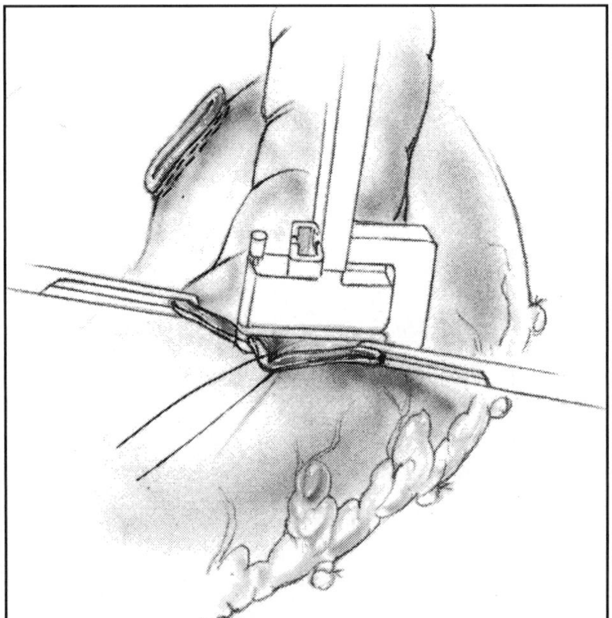

Fig. 5-5

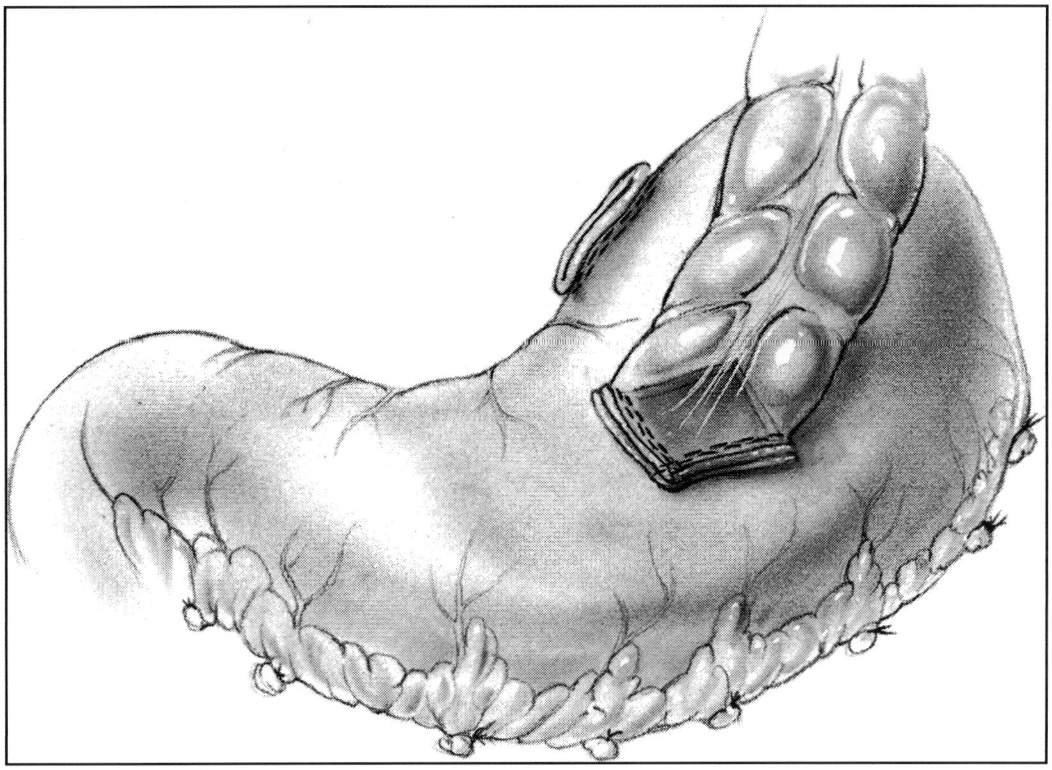

Fig. 5-6

the posterior wall of the stomach **(Fig. 5–7a)**. The posterior cologastric anastomosis may be constructed by suturing (as illustrated here) or by stapling (as described in Figs. 5-3 to 5-6). In this manner the colocolostomy can also be performed close by, preserving the marginal artery **(Fig. 5–7b)**.

Pyloromyotomy

In most conditions for which a thoracic esophagectomy is being performed, the vagus nerves are destroyed, which impairs gastric emptying to a fairly severe degree in about 20% of cases. To prevent this complication, a pyloromyotomy may be performed by the technique illustrated in Figures 2-17 to 2-19.

Advancing the Colon Segment to the Neck

Be certain to enlarge the diaphragmatic hiatus (see Fig. 2-20) sufficiently that the veins in the colon mesentery are not compressed by the muscles of the hiatus. The most direct route to the neck follows the course of the original esophageal bed in the posterior mediastinum. Place several studies between the proximal end of the colon transplant and the distal end of the esophagus; then draw the colon up into the neck by withdrawing the esophagus into the neck. This brings the colon into the posterior mediastinum behind the arch of the aorta and into the neck posterior to the trachea. If there is no constriction in the chest along this route, the sternum and clavicle at the root of the neck are also not likely to compress the colon. On the other hand, if a substernal tunnel is selected for passing the colon up to the neck, it is generally necessary to resect the head of one clavicle and a 2 cm width of adjacent sternal manubrium to be certain there is no obstruction at that point.

A good alternative method for transporting the colon up to the neck is to pass a 36F rubber catheter from the neck down into the abdominal cavity. Obtain a sterile plastic sheath such as a laser drape and suture the end of this plastic cylinder to the termination of the rubber catheter. Insert the proximal end of the colon into this plastic sheath and suture it lightly to the red rubber catheter. By withdrawing the catheter through the thoracic cavity into the neck, the colon with its delicate blood supply can be delivered into the neck without trauma.

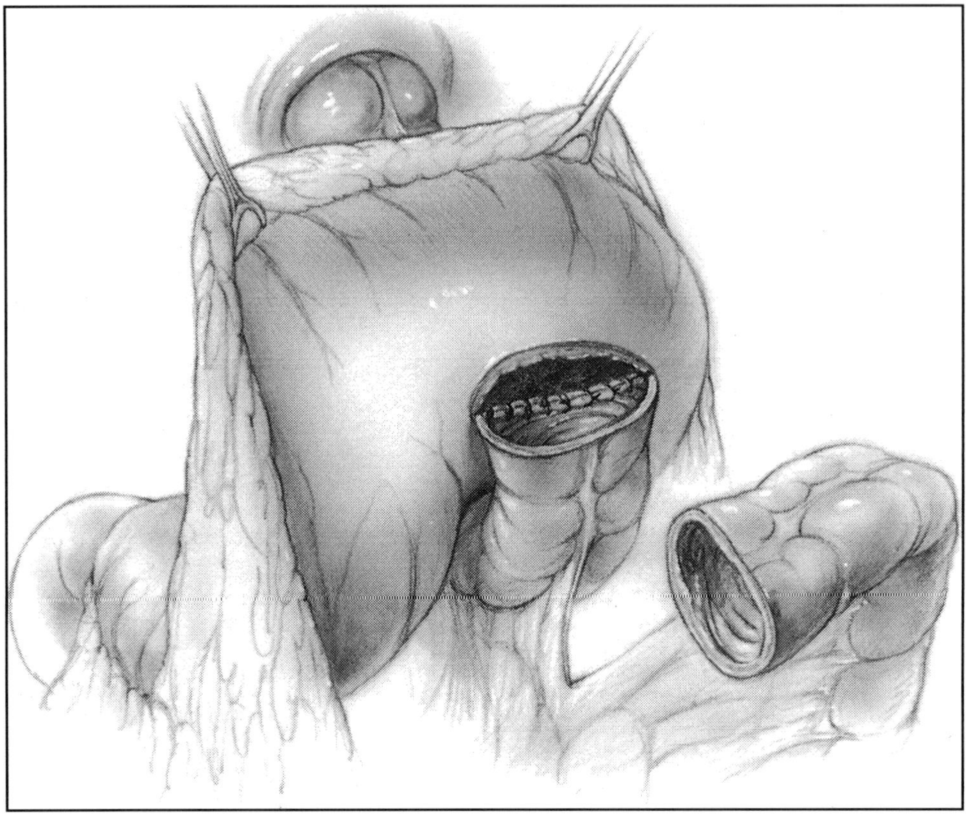

Fig. 5-7a

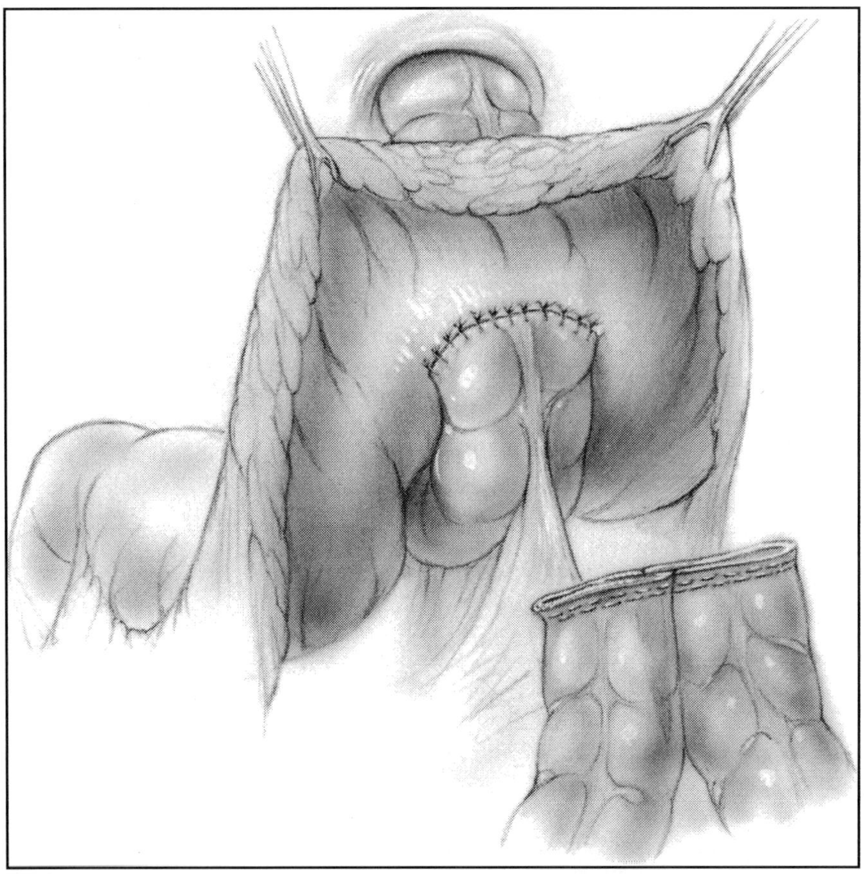

Fig. 5-7b

Verify that the tube of colon from the neck to the abdominal cavity lies in a straight line and there is no surplus of colon in the chest. Leaving redundant colon in the thorax may produce a functional obstruction to the passage of food. Then suture the colon to the muscle of the diaphragmatic hiatus with interrupted sutures of atraumatic 4-0 Tevdek at intervals of about 2 cm around half the circumference of the colon. This helps maintain a direct passageway from the neck into the abdomen. Be sure not to pass the needle deep to the submucosa of the colon, as colonic leaks have been reported to result from this error.

Dissecting the Cervical Esophagus

Change the position of the patient's left hand, which is suspended from the ether screen. Bring the left hand laterally and place it along the left side of the patient. Turn the head slightly to the right and make an incision along the anterior border of the left sternomastoid muscle; continue the dissection as described in Figures 2-27 to 2-30. Be careful not to damage the left or the right recurrent laryngeal nerve. After dissecting the esophagus free down into the superior mediastinum, extract the thoracic esophagus by applying gentle traction in the neck. In this way the thoracic esophagus and the attached colon interposition segment may be drawn gently into the neck. Divide the distal cervical esophagus and remove the thoracic esophagus. Inspect the end of the colon. There should be a good pulse in the marginal artery. Cyanosis indicates venous obstruction, which must be corrected. Draw the closed stapled end of the colon transplant to a point about 6–7 cm above the cut end of the esophagus and, taking care not to penetrate the lumen of the colon, suture the colon to the prevertebral fascia with several interrupted 4-0 silk sutures.

Esophagocolonic Anastomosis

Perform an end-to-side esophagocolonic anastomosis at a point about 4 cm below the proximal end of the colon using a technique similar to that described in Figures 2-22 to 2-26 and by using interrupted 4-0 silk Cushing sutures for the outer layer and 5-0 PG or PDS for the mucosal layer. Before closing the anterior portion of the anastomosis, ask the anesthesiologist to pass a nasogastric tube into the esophagus and guide this tube through the anastomosis into the colon.

Retrosternal Passage of Colon Transplant

When the posterior mediastinum is not a suitable pathway for the colon or if the esophagus has not been removed, make a retrosternal tunnel to pass the colon up to the neck. If the left lobe of the liver is large or if it appears to be exerting pressure on the posterior aspect of the colon transplant, liberate the left lobe by dividing the triangular ligament. This permits the left lobe to fall in a posterior direction and thereby relieves this pressure. If the xiphoid process curves posteriorly and impinges on the colon, resect the xiphoid.

Enter the plane just posterior to the periosteum of the sternum. Start the dissection with Metzenbaum scissors; then insert one or two fingers of the right hand. Finally, pass the entire hand just deep to the sternum up to the suprasternal notch. This is generally an avascular plane. Orient the colon segment so the mesentery enters from the patient's left side. Resect the medial 3–4 cm of clavicle using a Gigli saw. Then rongeur away about 2 cm of adjacent sternal manubrium to be certain the aperture at the root of the neck is sufficiently large to avoid any venous obstruction in the mesentery. Pass a long sponge-holder into the retrosternal tunnel from the neck down into the abdomen and suture the proximal end of the colon segment to the tip of the sponge-holder. Gently pass the colon into the substernal tunnel while simultaneously drawing the sutures in a cephalad direction.

There may be fewer symptoms after resection of the clavicular head if it is performed on the side opposite the dominant hand. Once it has been ascertained that the circulation to the colon segment is good, perform the esophagocolonic anastomosis as above. The final appearance of the colon interposition is depicted in **Figures 5–8** and **5–9**.

Closure

Close the cervical incision in layers with interrupted 4-0 PG sutures. Insert one or two drains in the general vicinity of the anastomosis and leave them in place 7–10 days. Close the skin in the usual fashion. Close the thoracoabdominal incision as illustrated in Figures 3-35 to 3-41.

Colon Interposition, Short Segment

In rare cases of benign peptic stricture of the lower esophagus, it is impossible to dilate the stricture, even in the operating room, without rupturing the esophagus. If there is no significant amount of disease above the level of the inferior pulmonary ligament, resect the diseased esophagus down to the esophagogastric junction and replace the missing esophagus with a short isoperistaltic segment of colon to extend from the divided esophagus to a point about one-

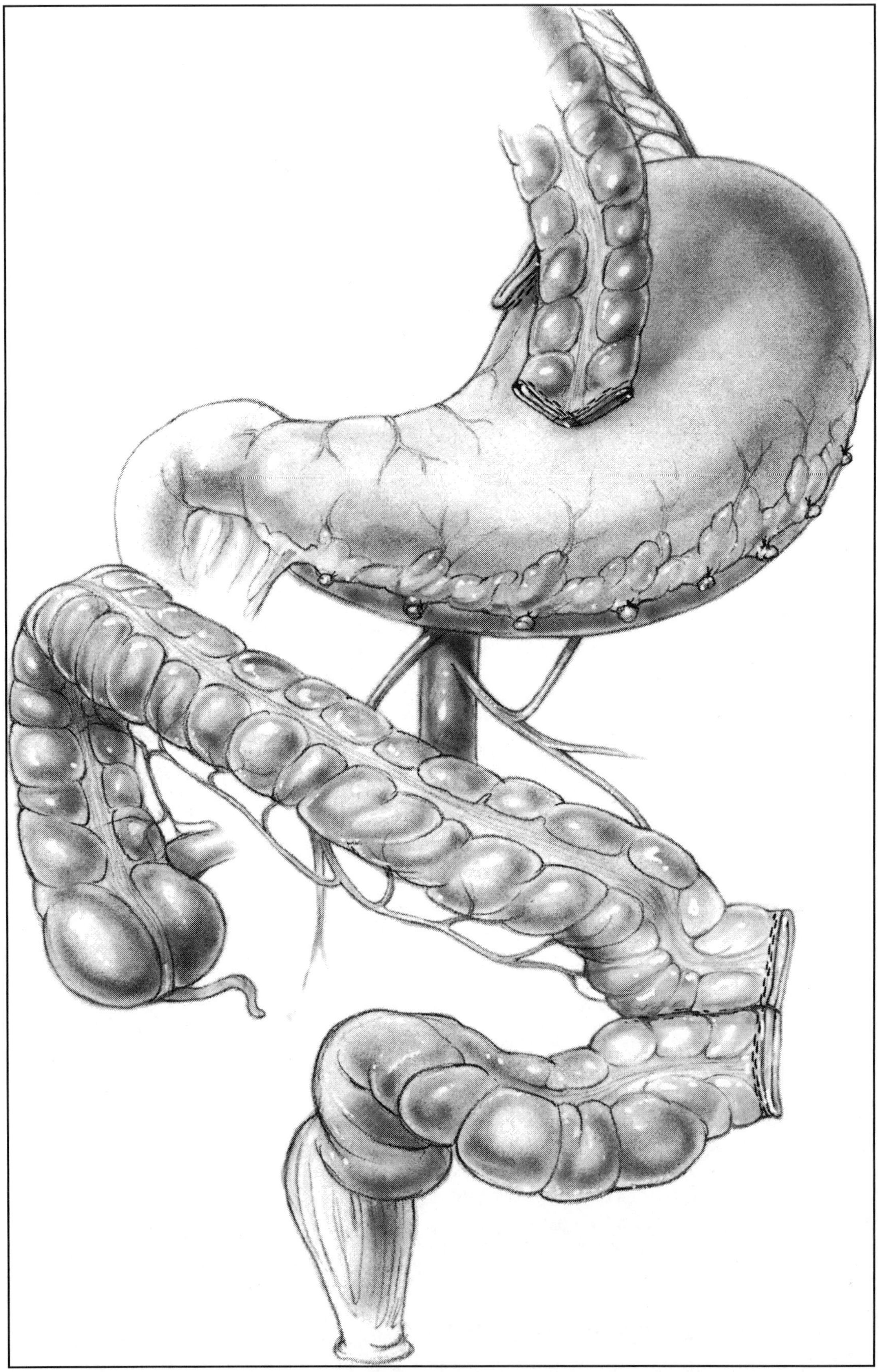

Fig. 5-8

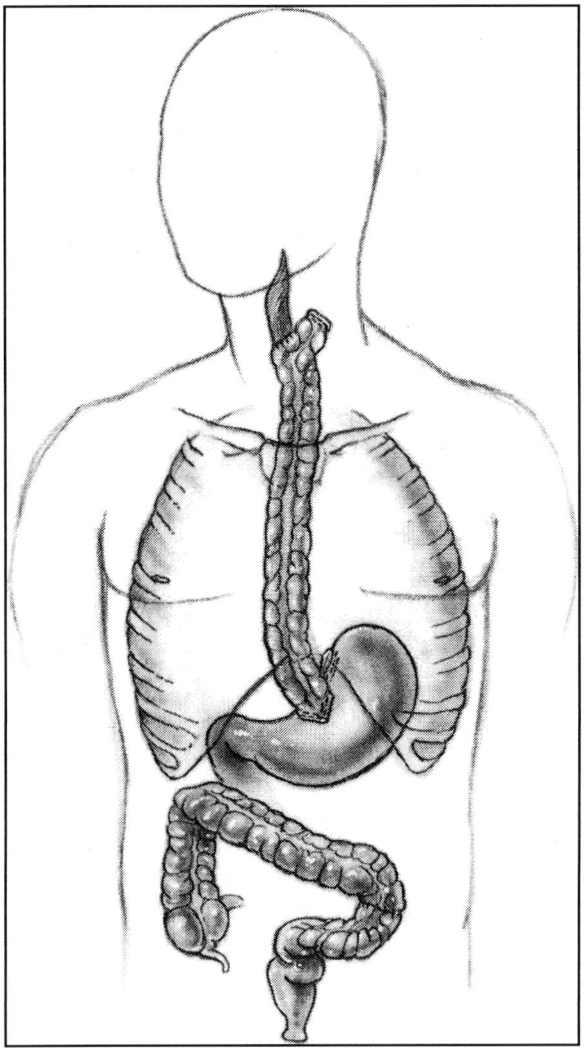

Fig. 5-9

third the distance between the fundus and the pylorus of the stomach. For a short segment operation it is not necessary to divide the middle colic artery, and only the distal portion of the transverse colon and the splenic flexure need be employed. Otherwise, the operation is much the same as described above. The cologastric anastomosis is identical. The esophagocolonic anastomosis may be sutured in an end-to-end fashion, an end-to-side fashion, or even by a stapling technique. The latter involves inserting a proper circular stapling cartridge (generally 28 or 25 mm) into the open proximal end of the colonic segment. The anastomosis is made between the end of the esophagus and the side of the colon by the usual circular stapling technique. Then, after disengaging the instrument, explore the anastomosis visually and manually with a finger through the open end of the colon. If the exploration appears satisfactory, close the opening in the colon about 1 cm away from the circular stapled anastomosis using a 55/3.5 mm linear stapler. Excise the redundant tissue and remove the stapler.

Jejunum Interposition

Incision and Mobilization

Although Polk advocated mobilizing the esophagogastric junction through an upper midline abdominal incision, we prefer the left sixth interspace thoracoabdominal incision with a vertical midline abdominal component. This is because the jejunal interposition operation is performed primarily in patients who have had multiple failed previous operations for reflux esophagitis. The Collis-Nissen gastroplasty combined with dilatation of the esophageal stricture suffices in most patients. This leaves a few of the most advanced cases that require a colon (short-segment) or jejunum interposition.

The combined thoracoabdominal incision provides superb exposure and makes this operation as safe as possible. It should be emphasized that creating a jejunal segment is much more difficult than the short-segment colon interposition. When performing the thoracoabdominal incision, incise the diaphragm with electrocautery in a circumferential fashion, as depicted in Figure 3-8.

Dissect the left lobe of the liver carefully away from the anterior wall of the stomach; in doing so, approach the dissection from the lesser curvature aspect of the stomach. At the same time, incise the gastrohepatic omentum by proceeding up toward the hiatus. This may require division of the accessory left hepatic artery, provided it has not been done at a previous operation (see Fig. 8-4). It may also be difficult to free the upper stomach from its posterior attachments to the pancreas. Careful dissection with good exposure from the thoracoabdominal incision should make it possible to preserve the spleen from irreparable injury. At the conclusion of this dissection, the upper portion of the stomach and lower esophagus should be free. Freeing the esophagus in the upper abdomen may be expedited by first dissecting the esophagus out of its bed in the lower mediastinum.

Resection of Diseased Esophagus

After the esophagus has been freed from its fibrotic attachments in the mediastinum and upper stomach, select a point near the esophagogastric junction for resection. If the upper stomach has been perforated during this dissection and the perforation can be included in the specimen, do so. If the upper stomach is not excessively thickened, apply a 55 or 90 mm linear stapling device with 4.8 mm staples and fire it. Transect the esophagogastric junction just above the stapling device. Lightly electrocoagulate the everted mucosa and remove the stapler. Deliver the transected esophagus into the chest and select the point of transection on the esophagus above the stricture. A mild degree of mucosal inflammation in the esophagus is acceptable at the point of transection. Remove the specimen.

If the point of division of the esophagus is not higher than the inferior pulmonary vein, jejunal interposition is a good method for establishing continuity. If the esophagus must be transected at a higher level, use a short segment of colon for the interposition or remove the remainder of the thoracic esophagus and reestablish continuity by means of a long-segment colon interposition from the neck to the stomach or by bringing the stomach up into the neck for this purpose, as described below. The graft of jejunum may be lengthened safely if its circulation can be boosted by creating microvascular anastomoses from a thoracic artery and vein to the upper end of the graft.

Mobilizing the Jejunum Graft

Because the vascular anatomy of the proximal jejunum varies somewhat from patient to patient, it is necessary to individualize the dissection according to the conditions encountered. First, try to stretch the proximal jejunum in a cephalad direction to determine where the greatest mobility is located. Be certain to leave intact at least the first major jejunal artery to the proximal jejunum. The average length of the jejunal segment to be transplanted varies between 12 and 20 cm, and the pedicle should consist of at least one major arcade vessel with careful preservation of the veins. Most jejunal grafts fail not because of poor arterial circulation but because the veins have been injured or compressed at some point. Try to preserve a vascular pedicle containing two arcade vessels with their veins intact. When dividing an arcade vessel, be sure to place the point of transection sufficiently proximal to a bifurcation so the continuity of the "marginal" artery and vein is not interrupted. Divide and temporarily close the jejunum proximally and distally with a linear cutting stapler, preserving a segment measuring 15–20 cm for interposition.

Make an incision in the transverse mesocolon through its avascular portion just to the left of the middle colic vessels. Carefully pass the jejunal graft together with its vascular pedicle through this incision into the previously dissected lesser sac behind the stomach. Be absolutely certain the incision in the mesentery does not constrict the veins of the vascular pedicle. Also be careful not to twist the pedicle. Pass the proximal portion of the jejunal segment through the hiatus into the chest. Be certain that the hiatus is large enough that it does not compress the veins in the vascular pedicle.

Esophagojejunostomy

Establish an end-to-side esophagojejunal anastomosis on the antimesenteric border of the jejunum beginning about 1 cm distal to the staple line on the proximal closed end of the jejunal segment. A similar technique is using 4-0 atraumatic interrupted silk Cushing or Lembert sutures for the outer layer and interrupted or continuous 5-0 Vicryl for the mucosal layer may be employed. Pass the nasogastric tube through this anastomosis down to the lower end of the jejunal graft. It is also possible to perform a stapled esophagojejunostomy if necessary.

Jejunogastrostomy

Place the jejunogastric anastomosis 5–7 cm below the proximal margin of the stomach in an area of stomach that is relatively free of fibrosis and that permits the vascular pedicle to be free of tension. This may be done by the same suture technique as mentioned above, but if there is sufficient length of jejunum it may also be performed by a stapled anastomosis similar to that described in Figures 5–2 to 5–6. The appearance of the completed anastomosis is shown in **Figure 5–10**.

Jejunojejunostomy

Reestablish the continuity of the jejunum by creating a functional end-to-end anastomosis using the stapling technique. Then carefully resuture the defect in the jejunal mesentery without compressing the vascular pedicle jejunal graft.

Use interrupted 4-0 Tevdek sutures to approximate the diaphragmatic hiatus to the seromuscular wall of the jejunum to avoid herniation of bowel through the hiatus. Be certain not to compress the vascular pedicle.

Gastrostomy; Pyloromyotomy

Although the nasogastric tube has been passed through the jejunal graft into the stomach to maintain the position of the graft, there is a risk that the nasogastric tube may be inadvertently removed before the patient's gastrointestinal tract has resumed function. For this reason, perform a Stamm gastrostomy, and remove the nasogastric tube.

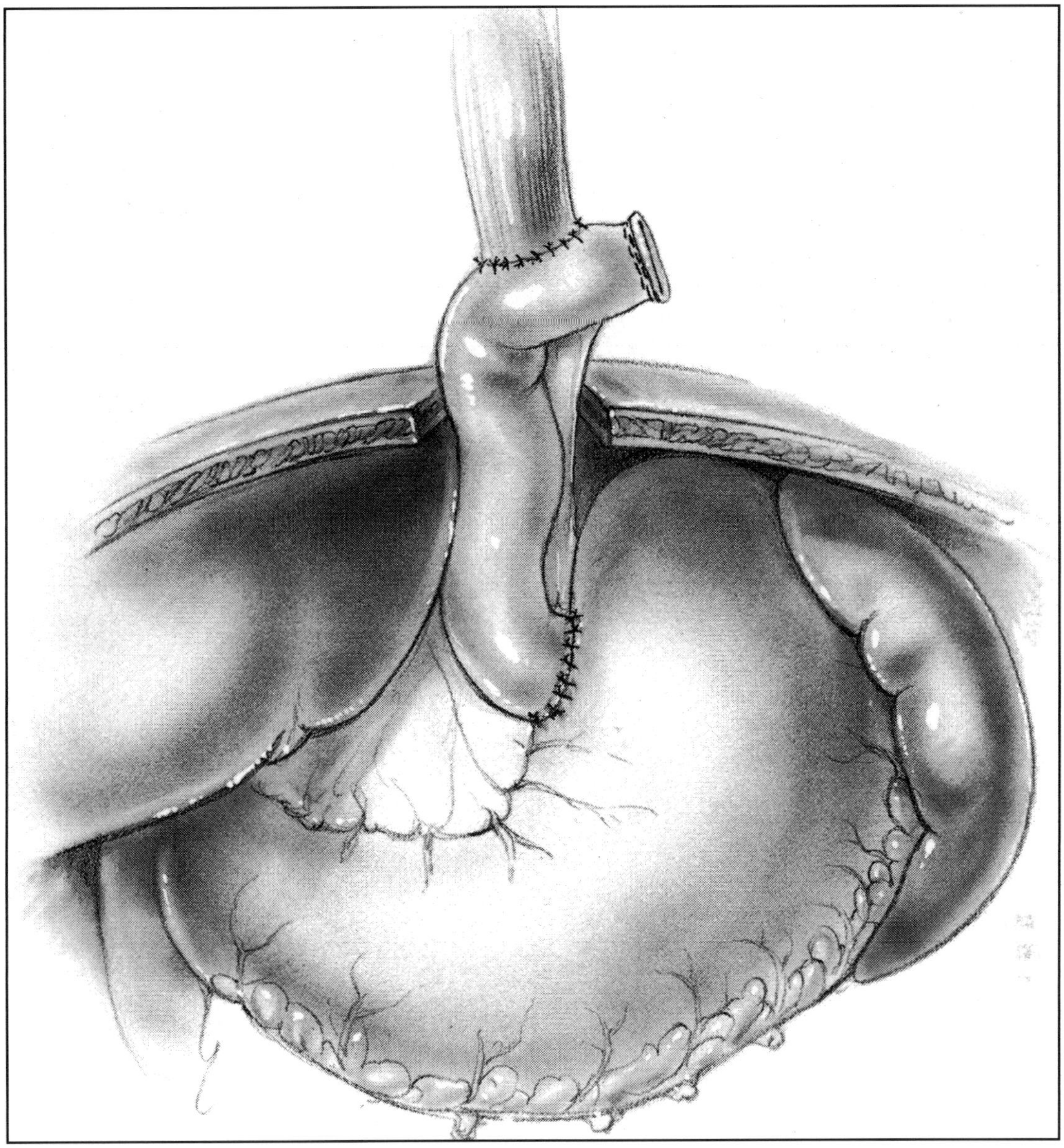

Fig. 5-10

Most surgeons advocate performing a pyloromyotomy or pyloroplasty during this type of operation because it is assumed that the vagus nerves have been interrupted during the course of dissecting a heavily scarred esophagus out of the mediastinum. Polk stated that this step may not be necessary.

Closure

Repair the diaphragm and close the thoracoabdominal incision as illustrated in Figures 3-38 to 3-44 after inserting a chest tube. No abdominal drains are utilized.

REFERENCES

Belsey R. Reconstruction of the esophagus with the left colon. J Thorac Cardiovasc Surg 1965;49:33.

Curet-Scott M, Ferguson MK, Little AG, et al. Colon interposition of benign esophageal disease. Surgery 1987; 102:568.

DeMeester TR, Johansson K-E, Franze I, et al. Indications, surgical technique, and long-term functional results of colon interposition and bypass. Ann Surg 1988;208:460.

Furst H, Hartl WH, Lohe F, Schildberg FW. Colon interposition for esophageal replacement: an alternative technique based on the use of the right colon. Ann Surg 2000;231:173.

Loinaz C, Altorki NK. Pitfalls and complications of colon interposition. Chest Surg Clin North Am 1997;7:533.

Moylan JP Jr, Bell JW, Cantrell JR, Merendino KA. The jejunal interposition operation: a follow-up on seventeen patients followed 10–17 years. Ann Surg 1970;172:205.

Orringer MB, Orringer JS. Esophagectomy without thoracotomy: a dangerous operation? J Thorac Cardiovasc Surg 1983;85:72.

Polk HC Jr. Jejunal interposition for reflux esophagitis and esophageal stricture unresponsive to valvuloplasty. World J Surg 1980;4:741.

Thomas P, Fuentes P, Giudicelli R, Reboud E. Colon interposition for esophageal replacement: current indications and long-term function. Ann Thorac Surg 1997; 64:757.

Wilkins EW Jr. Long-segment colon substitute for the esophagus. Ann Surg 1980;192:722.

6 Transabdominal Nissen Fundoplication

INDICATIONS

Gastroesophageal reflux (see Chapter 1), especially in patients in whom laparoscopic Nissen fundoplication is not applicable

PREOPERATIVE PREPARATION

Esophagogastroduodenoscopy with brushing and biopsies of any abnormal mucosa

Esophageal manometry or pH studies in selected patients

PITFALLS AND DANGER POINTS

Inadequate mobilization of gastric fundus and abdominal esophagus

Injury to spleen or to vagus nerves

Fundoplication wrap too tight or too long

Inadequate fundoplication suturing

Undiagnosed esophageal motility disorders, such as achalasia, diffuse spasm, aperistalsis, or scleroderma

Hiatal closure too tight, causing esophageal obstruction

Hiatal closure too loose, permitting postoperative paraesophageal herniation

Injury to left hepatic vein or vena cava when incising triangular ligament to liberate left lobe of liver

OPERATIVE STRATEGY

Mobilizing the Gastric Fundus

To perform a hiatus hernia repair efficiently, the lower 5–7 cm of the esophagus and the entire gastric fundus from the gastroesophageal junction down to the upper short gastric vessel must be completely mobilized from all attachments to the diaphragm and the posterior abdominal wall. Identify the gastrophrenic ligament by passing the left hand behind the stomach so the fingertips can identify this avascular ligament, which attaches the greater curvature to the diaphragm. The ligament extends from the gastroesophageal junction down to the first short gastric vessel. It is simple to divide once it has been stretched by the surgeon's left hand behind the stomach. Although in a few cases no short gastric vessels must be divided, there should be no hesitation to divide one to three proximal short gastric vessels to create a loose fundoplication.

On the lesser curvature aspect of the gastroesophageal junction, it is necessary to divide the proximal portion of the gastrohepatic ligament. This ligament often contains an accessory left hepatic artery arising from the left gastric artery and going to the left lobe of the liver and the hepatic branch of the left vagus nerve. Division of the accessory left hepatic artery has, in our experience, not proved harmful. Do not divide the left gastric artery itself. Preserving the left gastric artery and the hepatic branch of the vagus nerve helps prevent the fundoplication from slipping in a caudal direction. The lower esophagus is freed by incising the overlying peritoneum and phrenoesophageal ligaments; continue this incision in a semicircular fashion so the muscular margins of the diaphragmatic crura are exposed down to the median arcuate ligament. During all of this mobilization, look for the major branches of the anterior and posterior vagus nerves and preserve them.

Preventing Splenic Injury

Splenic trauma is a common but preventable complication of the Nissen operation. With use of the Thompson or Upper Hand retractor there is no reason for any retractor to come into contact with the spleen. The mechanism of splenic injury is usually traction on the body of the stomach toward the patient's right, which avulses that portion of the splenic capsule attached to the omentum or to the gastrosplenic ligament. Early during the operation, make it a point to look at the anterior surface of the spleen. Note where the omentum may be adherent to the splenic capsule. If necessary, divide these attachments under direct vision. Otherwise, simply apply a moist gauze pad over the spleen and avoid lateral traction on the stomach. Traction on the gastroesophageal junction in a caudal direction along the *lesser* curve of the stomach generally does not cause injury to the spleen.

If a portion of the splenic capsule has been avulsed, it can almost always be managed by applying topical hemostatic agents followed by 10 minutes of pressure. Other splenic injuries can be repaired by suturing with 2-0 chromic catgut. Extensive disruption of the spleen at its hilus may necessitate splenectomy.

Avoiding Postoperative Dysphagia

Probably secondary to local edema, transient mild dysphagia is common during the first 2–3 weeks following operation, although some patients have difficulty swallowing for many months after a hiatus hernia operation. There are several possible causes for this dysphagia. First, it is possible to make the fundoplication wrap so tight or so wide that permanent dysphagia ensues (see below). Second, the defect in the hiatus may be sutured so tightly the hiatus impinges on the lumen of the esophagus and prevents passage of food. With an 18F nasogastric tube in place, after the crural sutures have been tied to repair the defect in the hiatus it should still be possible to insert an index finger without difficulty between the esophagus and the margins of the hiatus. There is no virtue in closing the hiatus snugly around the esophagus. A final cause of dysphagia in patients who have experienced this symptom as a preoperative complaint is the presence of an esophageal motility disorder such as achalasia or aperistalsis. Patients who present to the surgeon with reflux esophagitis and who also complain of dysphagia should undergo preoperative esophageal manometry to rule out motility disorders that may require surgery in addition to the antireflux procedure or instead of it.

How Tight Should the Fundoplication Be?

The Nissen operation produces a high pressure zone in the lower esophagus by transmitted gastric pressure in the wrap, rather than by the tightness of the wrap itself. An excessively tight wrap causes dysphagia and the gas bloat syndrome. Therefore the fundoplication should be made loose, rather than tight enough to constrict the esophagus. Many surgeons use an indwelling esophageal bougie to avoid creating a wrap that is too tight. Regardless of whether the indwelling bougie is used, it is possible to judge the tightness of the wrap by applying Babcock clamps to each side of the gastric fundus and tentatively bringing them together in front of the esophagus. This mimics the effect of the sutures. The surgeon should be able to pass one or two fingers between the wrap and the esophagus without difficulty with an 18F nasogastric tube in place. Otherwise readjust the fundoplication so it is loose enough for this maneuver to be accomplished.

How Long Should the Fundoplication Be?

Another cause of postoperative dysphagia is making the fundoplication wrap too long. For the usual Nissen operation, do not wrap more than 2–3 cm of esophagus. A shorter wrap may be appropriate when esophageal dysmotility and gastroesophageal reflux coexist (e.g., when a fundoplication is added to a myotomy).

Avoiding Fundoplication Suture Line Disruption

Polk and others have noted that an important cause of failure after Nissen fundoplication has been disruption of the plication because the sutures broke. For this reason, use 2-0 sutures. Generally, the sutures that were found to have broken were silk. We have used 2-0 Tevdek because it retains its tensile strength for many years, whereas silk gradually degenerates in the tissues. It is also important not to pass the suture into the lumen of the stomach or esophagus. If this error is committed, tying the suture too tight causes strangulation and possibly leakage. Some insurance against the latter complication is to turn in the major fundoplication sutures with a layer of continuous 4-0 Prolene seromuscular Lembert sutures.

Failure to Bring the Esophagogastric Junction into the Abdomen

If it is not possible to mobilize the esophagogastric junction from the mediastinum and bring it into the abdomen while performing transabdominal repair of a hiatus hernia, it is likely that esophageal fibrosis has produced shortening. Such a situation can generally be suspected prior to operation when the lower esophagus is strictured. In our opinion, these patients require a transthoracic Collis-Nissen operation (see Chapter 9). Although it is possible to perform a Collis-Nissen procedure in the abdomen, it is difficult. If it cannot be accomplished transabdominally, it is necessary to open the chest through a separate incision or through a thoracoabdominal extension to perform the Collis-Nissen operation.

Keeping the Fundoplication from Slipping

Various methods have been advocated to keep the fundoplication from sliding in a caudal direction, where it constricts the middle of the stomach instead of the esophagus and produces an "hourglass" stomach with partial obstruction. The most important means of preventing this caudal displacement of the wrap is to include the wall of the esophagus in each of the fundoplication sutures. Also, catch the wall of the stomach just below the gastroesophageal junction within the lowermost suture. This suture anchors the lower portion of the wrap (see Fig. 6-10, below).

OPERATIVE TECHNIQUE

Incision

Elevate the head of the operating table 10°-15°. Make a midline incision beginning at the xiphoid and continue about 2-3 cm beyond the umbilicus **(Fig. 6–1)**. Explore the abdomen. Insert a Thompson or Upper Hand retractor to elevate the lower portion of the sternum. Reduce the hiatus hernia by traction along the anterior wall of the stomach. Look at the anterior surface of the spleen to determine whether there are omental adhesions to the capsule that may result in the capsule avulsing later during the operation. Place a moist gauze pad over the spleen. In most cases it is not necessary to free the left lobe of the liver; simply elevate the left lobe with a Weinberg retractor to expose the diaphragmatic hiatus.

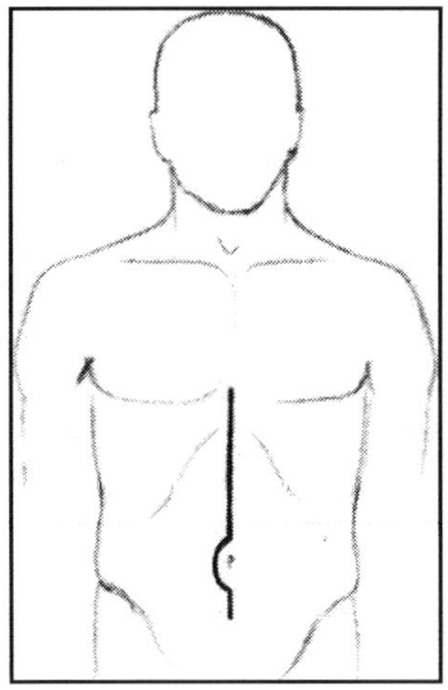

Fig. 6-1

Mobilizing the Esophagus and Gastric Fundus

Make a transverse incision in the peritoneum overlying the abdominal esophagus **(Fig. 6–2)** and continue this incision into the peritoneum overlying the right margin of the crus. Then divide the peritoneum overlying the left margin of the diaphragmatic hiatus. Separate the hiatal musculature from the esophagus using a peanut dissector until *most of the circumference of the esophagus has been exposed*. Then pass the index finger *gently* behind the esophagus and encircle it with a latex drain **(Fig. 6–3)**. Enclose both the right and left vagus nerves in the latex drain and divide all the phrenoesophageal attachments behind the esophagus. If the right (posterior) vagus trunk courses at a distance from the esophagus, it is easier to dissect the nerve away from the upper stomach and to exclude the right vagus from the fundoplication wrap. Some exclude both vagus trunks from the wrap, but we prefer to include them inside the loose wrap. Before the complete circumference of the hiatus can be visualized, it is necessary to divide not only the phrenoesophageal ligaments but also the cephalad portion of the gastrohepatic ligament, which often contains an accessory left hepatic artery that may be divided **(Fig. 6–4)**. The exposure at the conclusion of this maneuver is seen in **Figure 6–5**. Now pass the left hand behind the esophagus and behind the gastric fundus to identify the gastrophrenic ligament and divide it carefully down to the proximal short gastric vessel **(Fig. 6–6)**.

While the assistant is placing traction on the latex drain to draw the esophagus in a caudal direction, pass the right hand to deliver the gastric fundus behind the esophagus **(Fig. 6–7)**. Apply Babcock clamps to the two points on the stomach where the first fundoplication suture will be inserted and bring these two Babcock clamps together tentatively to assess whether the fundus has been mobilized sufficiently to accomplish the fundoplication without tension. **Figure 6–8**, a crosssectional view, demonstrates how the gastric fundus surrounds the lower esophagus and the vagus nerves.

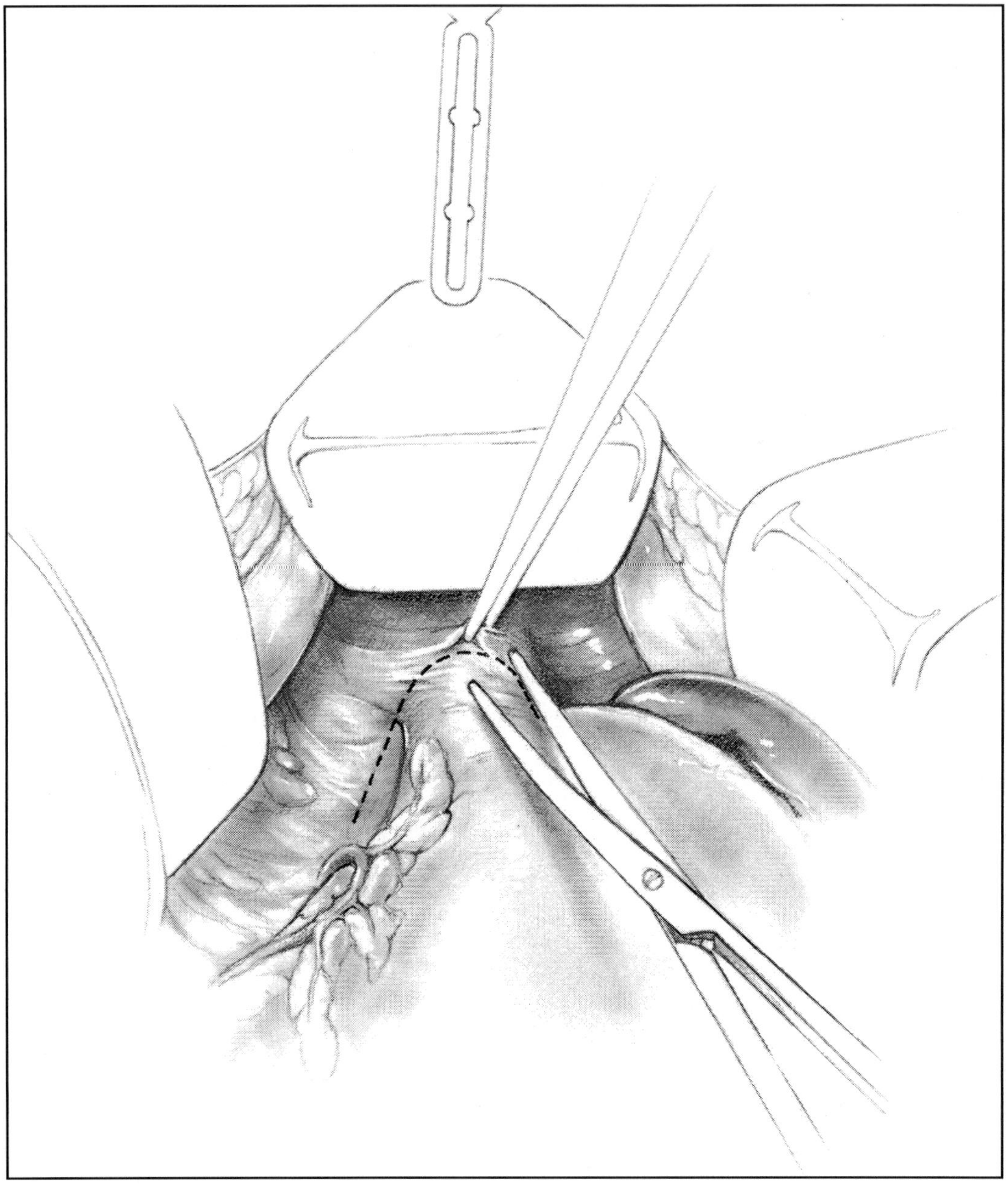

Fig. 6–2

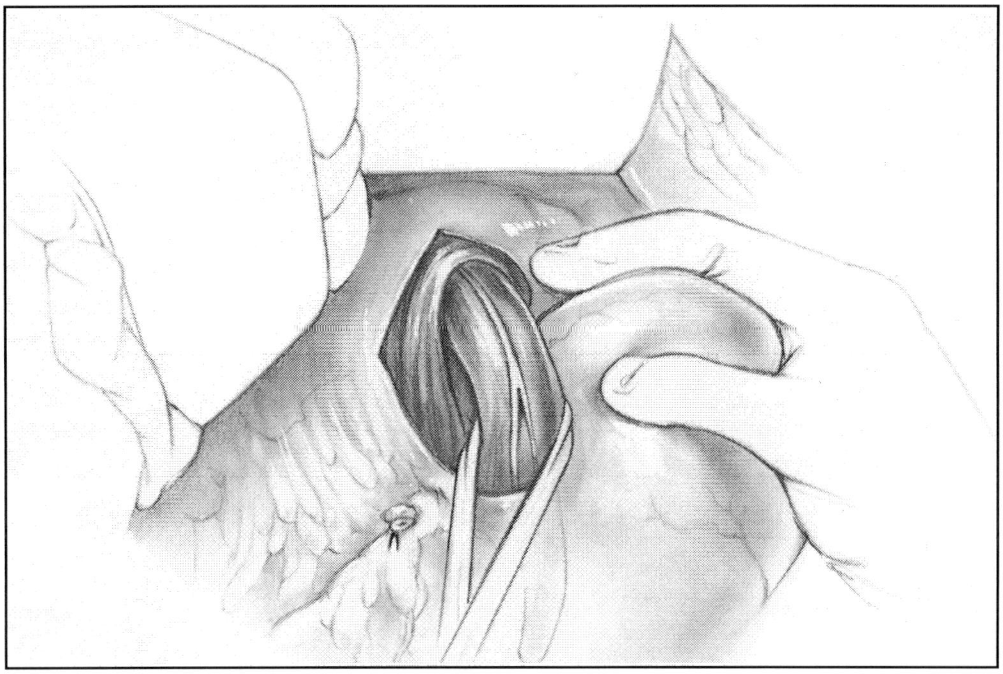

Fig. 6-3

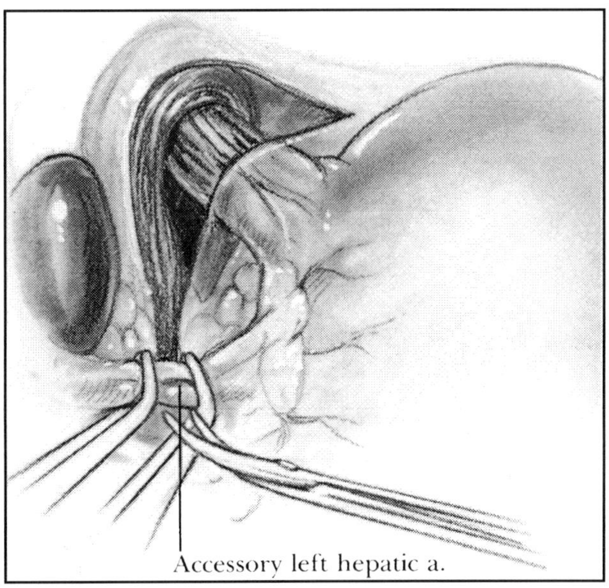

Fig. 6-4

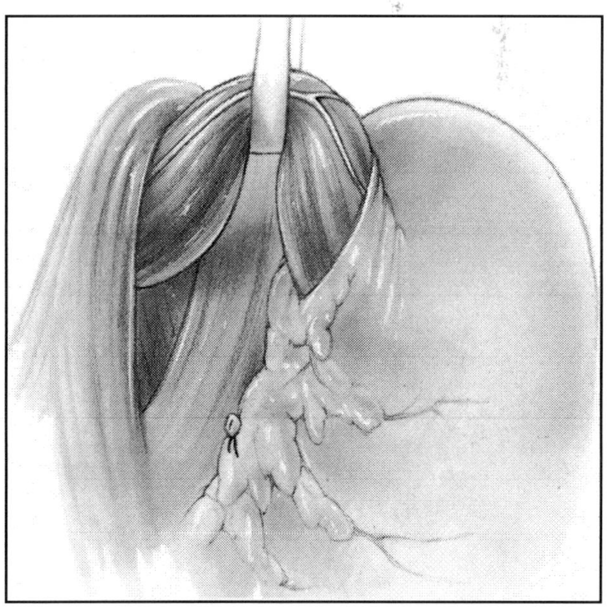

Fig. 6-5

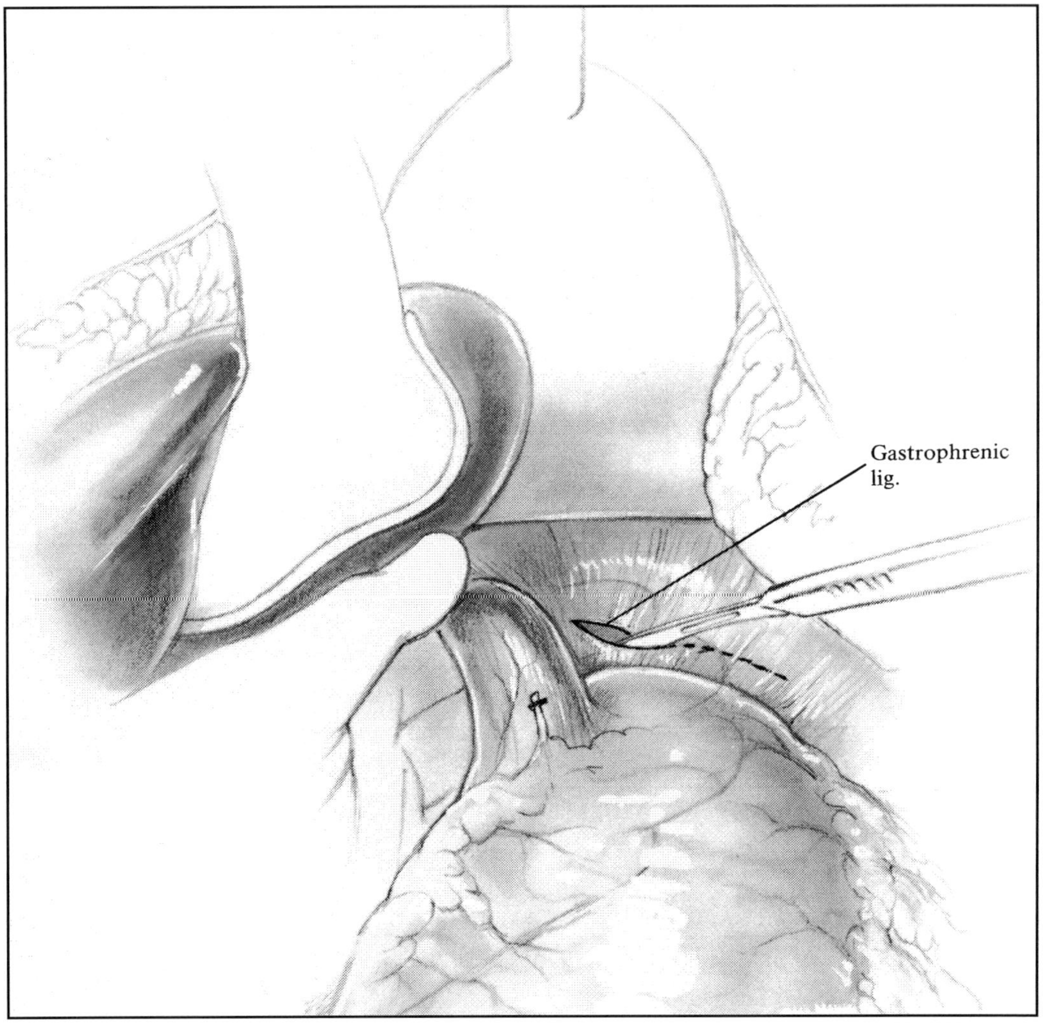

Fig. 6-6

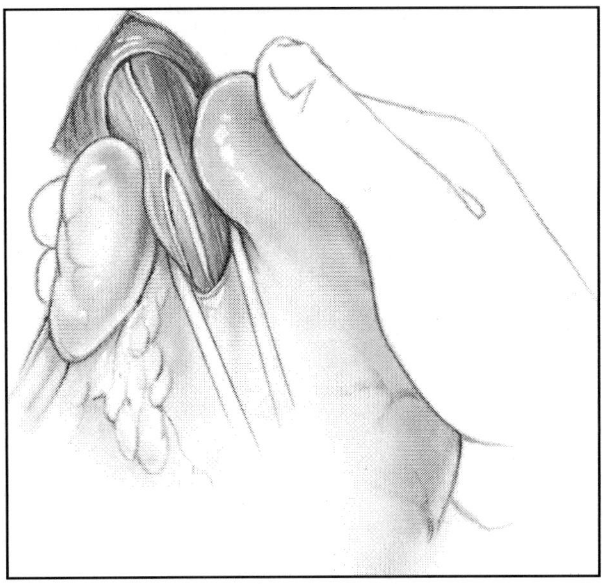

Fig. 6-7

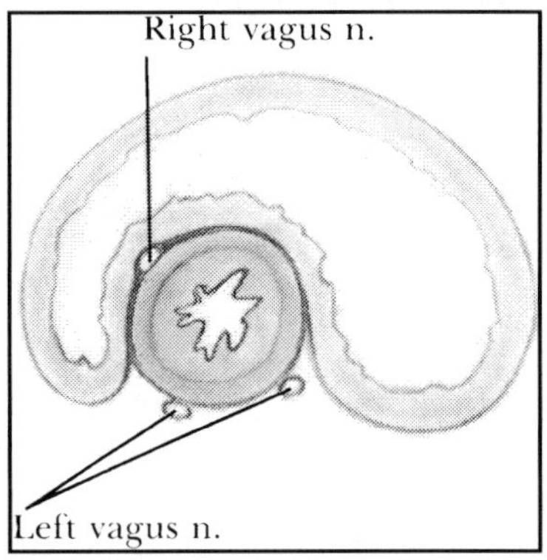

Fig. 6-8

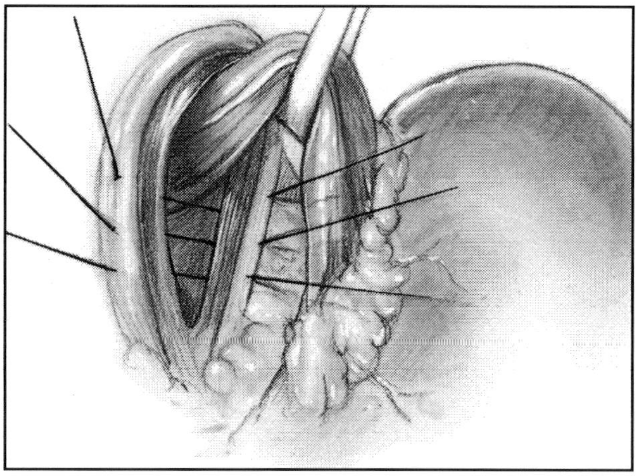

Fig. 6-9

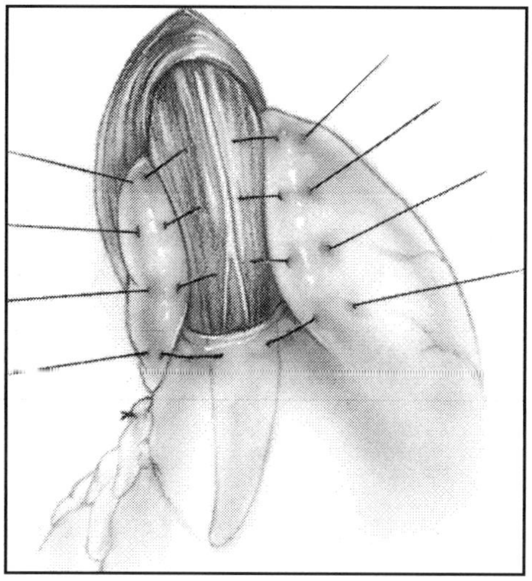

Fig. 6-10

Generally, there is inadequate mobility of the gastric fundus unless one divides the proximal one to three short gastric vessels. Ligate each with 2-0 silk.

On the greater curvature aspect of the esophagogastric junction there is usually a small fat pad. Excising the fat pad improves adhesion of the gastric wrap to the esophagus.

Repairing the Hiatal Defect

Using 0 Tevdek sutures on a large atraumatic needle, begin at the posterior margin of the hiatal defect and take a bite (1.3–2.0 cm in width) of the crus and its overlying peritoneum on each side of the hiatus. Insert the next suture about 1.0–1.2 cm cephalad and continue this process until the index finger can just be inserted *comfortably* between the esophagus and the margin of the hiatus **(Fig. 6–9)**.

Suturing the Fundoplication

Pass a 40F Maloney dilator into the stomach. Insert the first fundoplication suture by taking a bite of the fundus on the patient's left using 2-0 atraumatic Tevdek. Pass the needle through the seromuscular surface of the gastric lesser curve just distal to the esophagogastric junction; then take a final bite of the fundus on the patient's right. Attach a hemostat to tag this stitch but do not tie it. Each bite should contain 5–6 mm of tissue including submucosa, but it should not penetrate the lumen. Do not pierce any of the vagus nerves with a stitch. To perform a fundoplication without tension, it is necessary to insert the gastric sutures a sufficient distance lateral to the esophagogastric junction. Place additional sutures, as illustrated in **Figure 6–10**, at intervals of about 1 cm. Each suture should contain one bite of fundus, then esophagus, and then the opposite side of the fundus. No more than 2–3 cm of esophagus should be encircled by the fundoplication. Now tie all of these sutures **(Fig. 6–11)**. It should be possible to insert

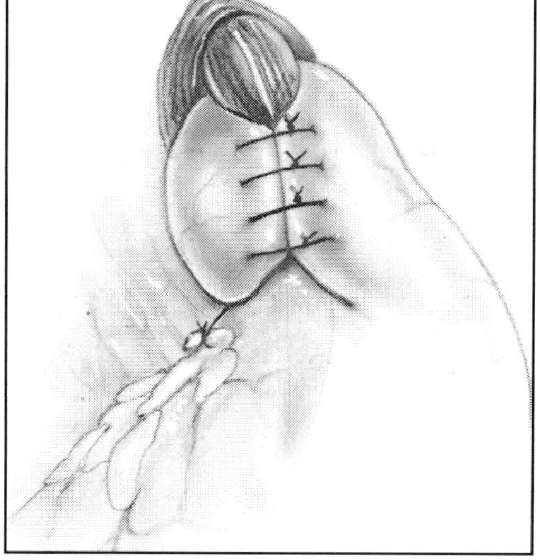

Fig. 6-11

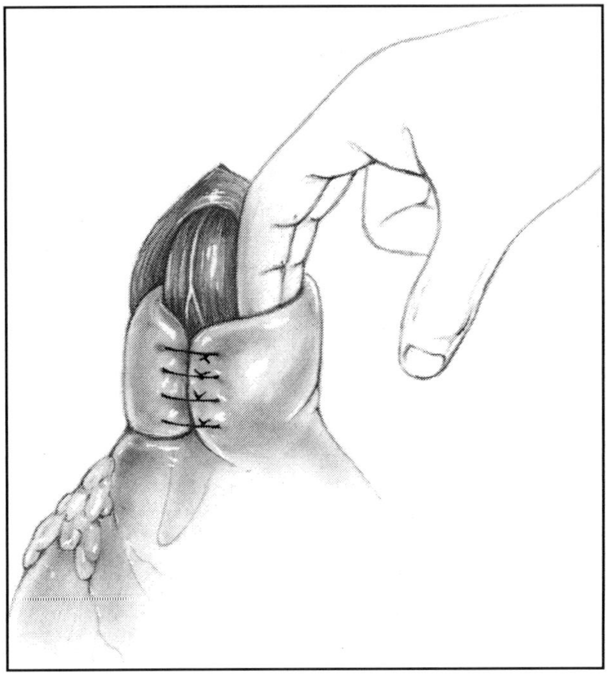

Fig. 6–12

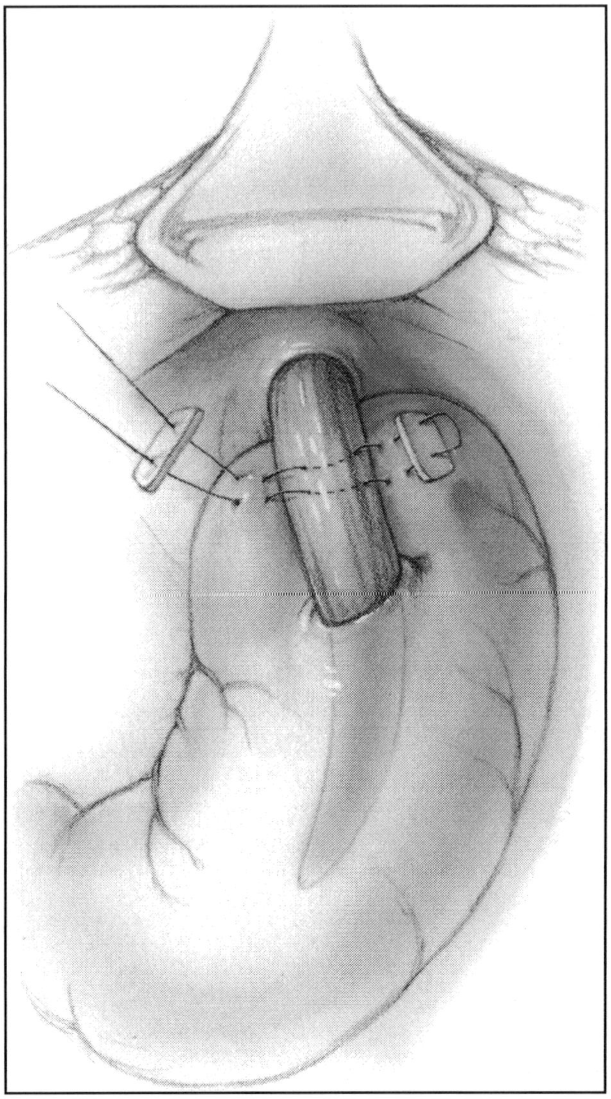

Fig. 6–13

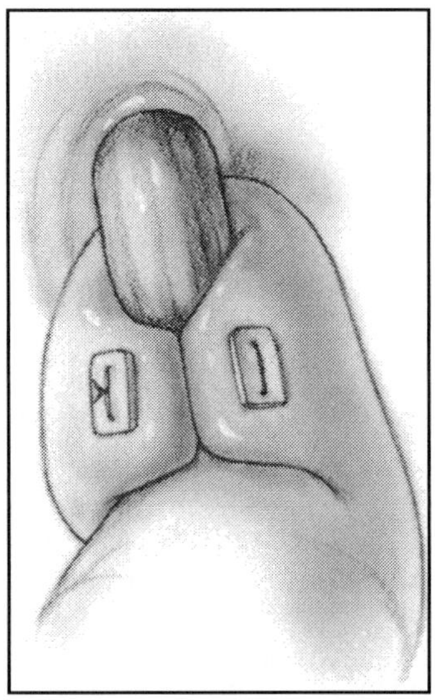

Fig. 6–14

one or two fingers between the esophagus and the Nissen wrap **(Fig. 6–12)**. If this cannot be done, the wrap is too tight.

A number of surgeons place sutures fixing the upper margin of the Nissen wrap to the esophagus to prevent the entire wrap from sliding downward and constricting the stomach in the shape of an hourglass. DeMeester and Stein, after considerable experience, advocated a Nissen wrap measuring only 1 cm in length, claiming that longer wraps produce postoperative dysphagia in a number of patients. Even with a 60F Maloney bougie in the esophagus, a 1 cm wrap has effectuated excellent control of reflux. They constructed this wrap employing one horizontal mattress suture of 2-0 Prolene buttressed with Teflon pledgets **(Figs. 6–13, 6–14)**.

Optionally, at this point one may invert the layer of fundoplication sutures by inserting a continuous seromuscular layer of 4-0 Prolene Lembert sutures (not illustrated). This layer provides protection against leakage if any of the fundoplication sutures were placed too deep.

Testing Antireflux Valve

Ask the anesthesiologist to inject 300–400 ml saline solution into the nasogastric tube and then withdraw the tube into the esophagus. Now try to expel the saline by compressing the stomach. If the saline cannot be forced into the esophagus by moderate manual compression of the stomach, the fundoplication has indeed created a competent antireflux valve.

Abdominal Closure

Close the abdomen without drainage in routine fashion.

POSTOPERATIVE CARE

Continue nasogastric suction for 1–2 days. Then initiate oral feeding. A barium esophagram is obtained before the patient is discharged. If a satisfactory repair has been accomplished, 3–4 cm of distal esophagus becomes progressively narrower, tapering to a point at the gastroesophageal junction. If this tapering effect is not noted, it suggests that the wrap may be too loose. Successful antireflux procedures, whether by the Nissen, Hill, Belsey, or Collis-Nissen technique, show similar narrowing of the distal esophagus on the postoperative esophagram. A typical postoperative barium esophagram is shown in **Figure 6–15**.

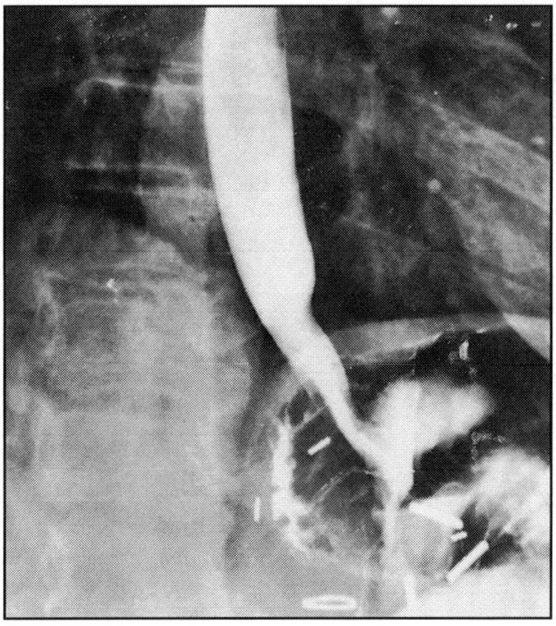

Fig. 6–15

COMPLICATIONS

Dysphagia, usually transient

"Gas bloat" (rare)

Disruption of fundoplication

Slipping downward of fundoplication with obstruction

Postoperative paraesophageal hernia if hiatal defect was not properly closed

Herniation of fundoplication into thorax

Esophageal or gastric perforation by deep necrosing sutures

Persistent gastroesophageal reflux

REFERENCES

Bais JE, Bartelsman JF, Bonjer HJ, et al. Laparoscopic or conventional Nissen fundoplication for gastrooesophageal reflux disease: randomised clinical trial; the Netherlands Antireflux Surgery Study Group. Lancet 2000; 355:170.

DeMeester TR, Stein JH. Minimizing the side effects of antireflux surgery. World J Surg 1992;16:335.

Deschamps C, Trastek VF, Allen MS, et al. Long-term results after reoperation for failed antireflux procedures. J Thorac Cardiovasc Surg 1997;113:545.

Henderson RD, Marryatt G. Total fundoplication gastroplasty; long-term follow-up in 500 patients. J Thorac Cardiovasc Surg 1983;85:81.

Herrington JR Jr. Treatment of combined sliding and paraesophageal hiatal hernia; emphasis on protection of the vagus nerves. Contemp Surg 1983;22:19.

Horgan S, Pohl D, Bogetti D, Eubanks T, Pellegrini C. Failed antireflux surgery: what have we learned from reoperations? Arch Surg 1999;134:809.

Kauer WK, Peters JH, DeMeester TR, et al. A tailored approach to antireflux surgery. J Thorac Cardiovasc Surg 1995;110:141.

Leonardi HK, Crozier RE, Ellis FH. Reoperation for complications of the Nissen fundoplication. J Thorac Cardiovasc Surg 1981;81:50.

Luostarinen ME, Isolauri JO. Randomized trial to study the effect of fundic mobilization on long-term results of Nissen fundoplication. Br J Surg 1999;86:614.

Luostarinen M, Isolauri J, Laitinen J, et al. Fate of Nissen fundoplication after 20 years: a clinical, endoscopic and functional analysis. Gut 1993;34:1015.

Peillon C, Manouvrier JL, Labreche J, et al. Should the vagus nerves be isolated from the fundoplication wrap? A prospective study. Arch Surg 1994;129:814.

Polk HC Jr. Fundoplication for reflux esophagitis: misadventures with the operation of choice. Ann Surg 1976; 183:645.

Rieger NA, Jamieson GG, Britten-Jones R, Tew S. Reoperation after failed antireflux surgery. Br J Surg 1994;81:1159.

Rogers DM, Herrington JL, Morton C. Incidental splenectomy associated with Nissen fundoplication. Ann Surg 1980;191:153.

Stirling MC, Orringer MB. Surgical treatment after the failed antireflux operation. J Thorac Cardiovasc Surg 1986; 92:667.

Urschel JD. Complications of antireflux surgery. Am J Surg 1993;166:68.

7 Laparoscopic Nissen Fundoplication

INDICATIONS

Symptomatic reflux esophagitis refractory to medical therapy

Barrett's esophagus (consider mucosal ablation)

PREOPERATIVE PREPARATION

Pass a nasogastric tube to decompress the stomach.

See Chapter 6.

PITFALLS AND DANGER POINTS

Injury to the esophagus.

Tension pneumothorax due to unrecognized entry into the mediastinal pleura. Even a relatively small tear can allow CO_2 to enter the pleural space and compromise ventilation.

Injury to spleen or stomach.

Failure to create a sufficiently floppy wrap.

OPERATIVE STRATEGY

Several laparoscopic fundoplications have been devised. We prefer the laparoscopic Nissen fundoplication because it is intended to be virtually identical to a well established open procedure when completed. The steps in the dissection are necessarily a bit different from those for the open procedure, and several additional features should be noted.

First, the hiatus is accessed by elevating the left lobe of the liver without dividing its attachments. Second, the esophagus is exposed and mobilized by dissecting the crura with minimal manipulation of the esophagus. The resulting extensive mediastinal dissection that accompanies esophageal mobilization makes approximation of the crura mandatory. Postoperative herniation of the stomach or small intestine may complicate the laparoscopic procedure when this step is omitted. Finally, several short gastric vessels *must* be divided to ensure creating a floppy wrap.

OPERATIVE TECHNIQUE

Room Setup and Trocar Placement

Position the patient with the legs slightly spread and supported on padded stirrups **(Fig. 7–1)**. Position the monitors at the head of the table. We place the primary

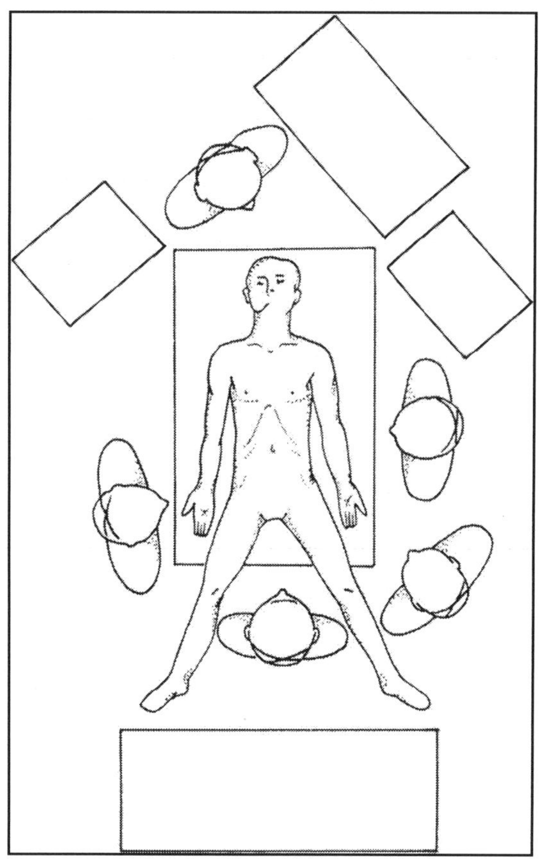

Fig. 7–1 (Reprinted with permission, from Scott-Conner CEH (ed) The SAGES Manual: Fundamentals of Laparoscopy and GI Endoscopy. New York, Springer-Verlag, 1999.)

monitor at the patient's left shoulder, with a secondary monitor at the patient's right, as shown. Some surgeons use a single monitor placed over the head of the operating table. We prefer to stand in the usual position, at the patient's side, for the initial puncture and entry into the abdomen. During dissection and suturing, the surgeon should stand between the patient's legs, directly facing the hiatus **(Fig. 7–2)**. When choosing an initial puncture site (to be used for the laparoscope) recall that the hiatus is quite high and deep. The normal umbilical port site may therefore be too low. A trocar pattern must be individualized according to the patient's body habitus. A 30° angled laparoscope is mandatory for easy visualization.

Exposure of the Hiatus

Pass a liver retractor through the right lateral port sitc. A varicty of livcr rctractors arc availablc, and which one is chosen is largely a matter of the surgeon's preference. We prefer a flexible retractor that becomes rigid and assumes the shape shown in **Figure 7–3** when a screw is turned. The particular retractor shown is composed of many short segments with an internal cable. When the tension on the cable is released, the retractor becomes limp and may be straightened out to pass it through a trocar. Once the retractor is inside the abdomen, the cable is tightened by twisting a knob on the handle. Increasing tension on the internal cable forces the articulations to bend into the shape shown. The retractor is bent into shape by tightening the cable in the commodious right subphrenic space and is then passed underneath the liver.

The liver retractor is properly placed when stable exposure is obtained and the diaphragmatic surface is seen behind the left lobe of the liver. It may not be possible to distinguish the actual hiatus at this point. This exposure generally requires that the retractor be "toed in" so the part of the retractor closest to the hiatus has maximal lift applied. The laparoscope and instruments are then insinuated underneath the left lobe of the liver in the working space thus created.

Generally, the stomach and some omentum partially or completely obscure the hiatus even with the liver retracted. Therefore the second part of obtaining exposure entails placing an endoscopic Babcock clamp on the stomach and pulling toward the left lower quadrant **(Fig. 7–4)**.

Dissecting the Hiatus

The esophagus is dissected by clearing the peritoneum off the hiatus and carefully exposing the

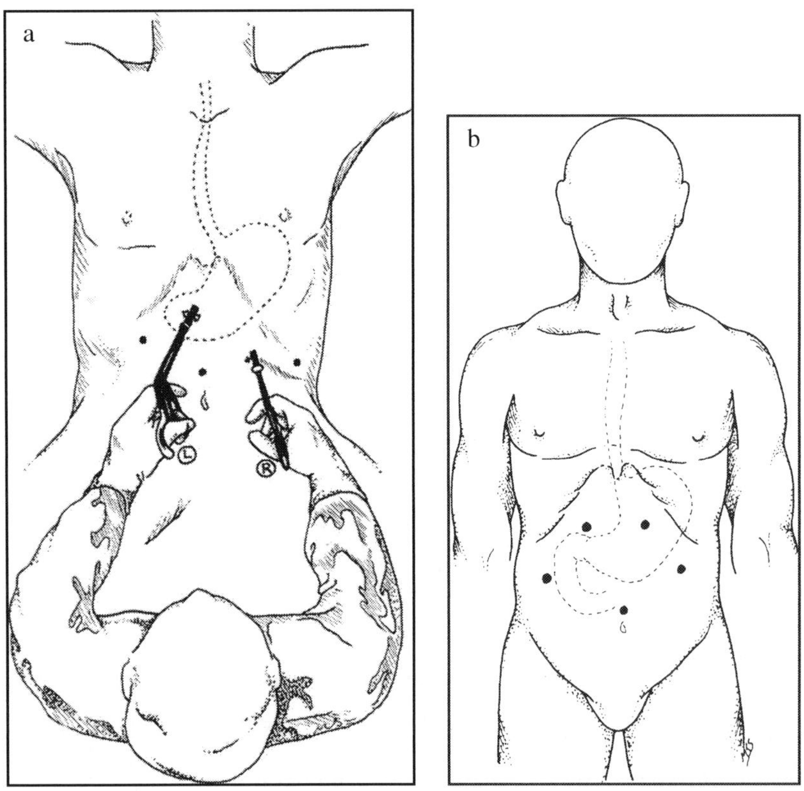

Fig. 7-2 (Reprinted with permission, from Scott-Conner CEH (ed) The SAGES Manual: Fundamentals of Laparoscopy and GI Endoscopy. New York, Springer-Verlag, 1999.)

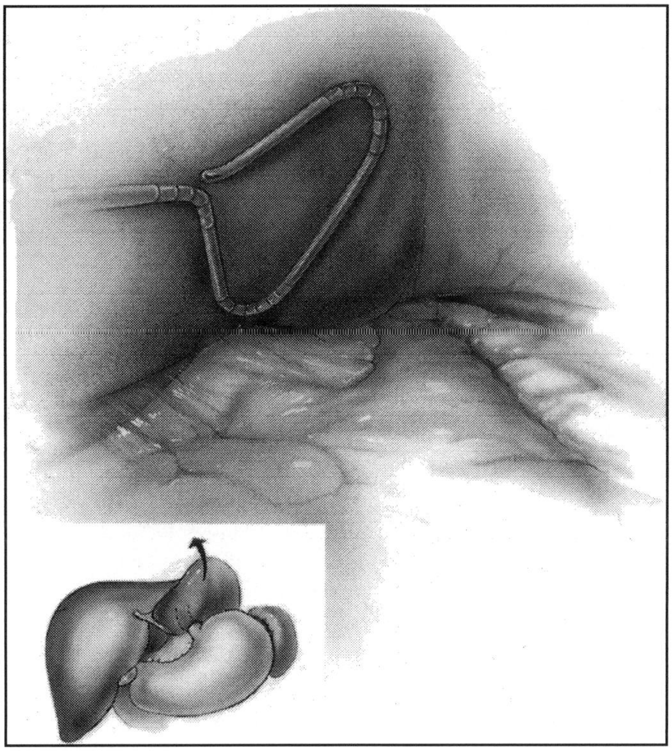

Fig. 7-3

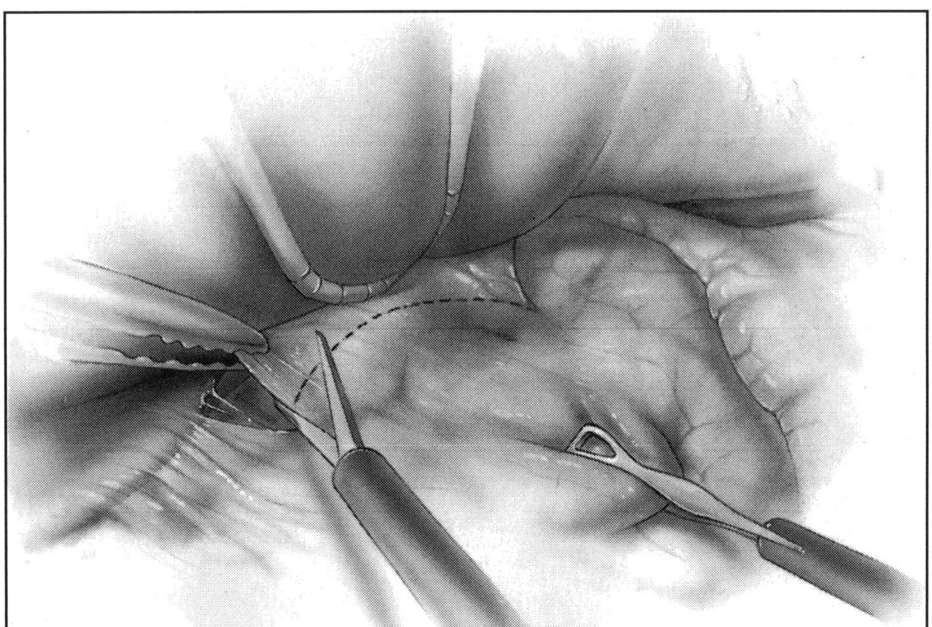

Fig. 7-4

muscular crura. Properly performed, this maneuver automatically exposes the esophagus and creates a posterior window.

Begin the dissection by exposing the right crus. Start by opening the peritoneum just to the right of the probable hiatus. The first step involves dividing the lesser omentum. A grasper is used to elevate the flimsy lesser omentum close to the hiatus, and ultrasonic dissecting scissors are used to divide the omentum (Fig. 7-4).

It is tempting to begin this dissection by opening the transparent part of the omentum farther to the right. If you begin your omental window high, however, near the hiatus, you are less likely to encounter a hepatic artery. This has the additional advantage of keeping the window in the lesser omentum relatively small, which helps anchor the wrap and prevents slipping.

Do not try to identify and dissect the esophagus at this stage. To do so risks perforation. A far safer approach is to dissect and clearly define the muscular hiatus and both crura. First identify the right crus after dividing the peritoneum. Next carry the dissection up over the arch of the crura, concentrating on exposing the muscle fibers of the diaphragm. During this dissection the esophagus becomes obvious by its orientation, longitudinal muscle, and overlying vagus nerve; it may also be gently displaced downward **(Fig. 7–5)** and to the left. The esophagus has a light pink to reddish pink color and characteristic longitudinal striations. If there is uncertainty as to the location of the esophagus, the nasogastric tube may be palpable to light touch with a grasper, or an esophagogastroduodenoscopy (EGD) scope may be passed and used to elevate and transilluminate the esophagus. These maneuvers are rarely needed.

A closed grasper is used to push the esophagus down. This grasper is introduced parallel to the esophagus through one of the left-sided trocars and is used to probe into the mediastinum by gently pushing the esophagus down.

When the upper part of the hiatus has been cleaned thoroughly, elevate the esophagus gently with a closed grasper and clean the lower part of the *left* crus from the *right* side by working underneath the esophagus **(Fig. 7–6)**. This maneuver produces a window behind the esophagus while minimizing the risk of perforating the esophagus. The esophagus is *never actually grasped*; rather, it is gently displaced to one side or the other using a closed grasper. Frequently the anterior vagus nerve is seen on the right side of the esophagus.

It is fairly common to encounter a sizable vessel next to the esophagus on the right side **(Fig. 7–7)**.

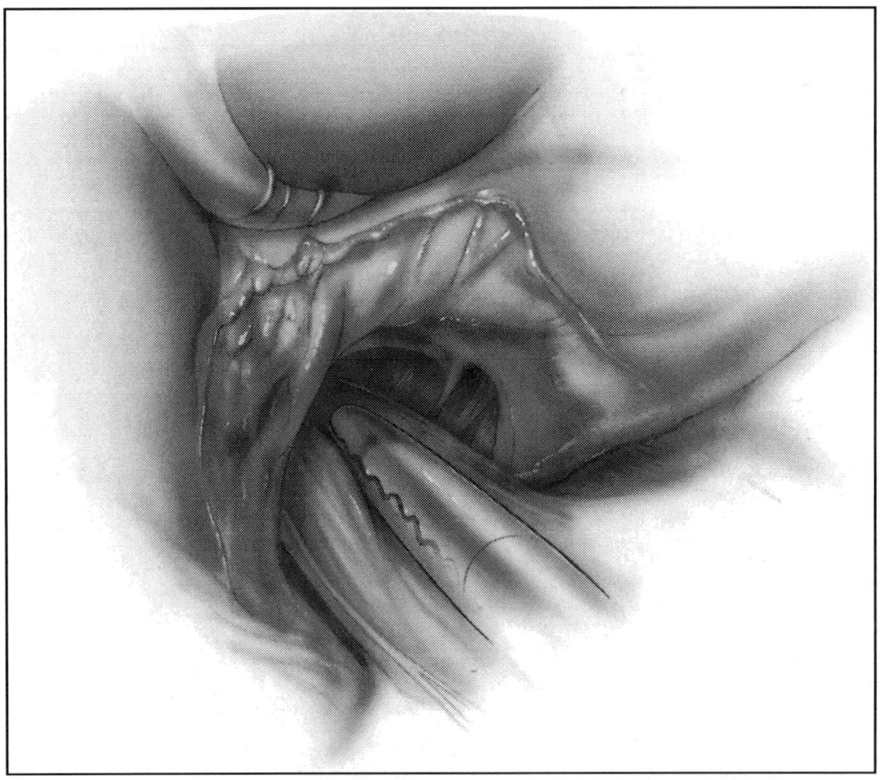

Fig. 7-5

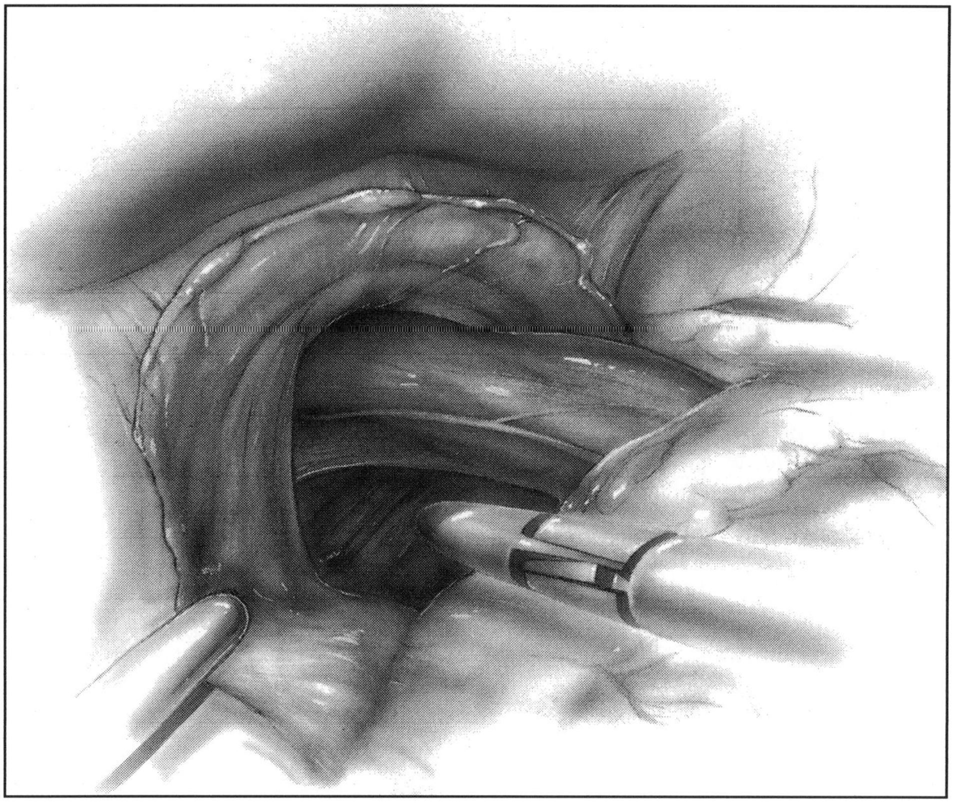

Fig. 7-6

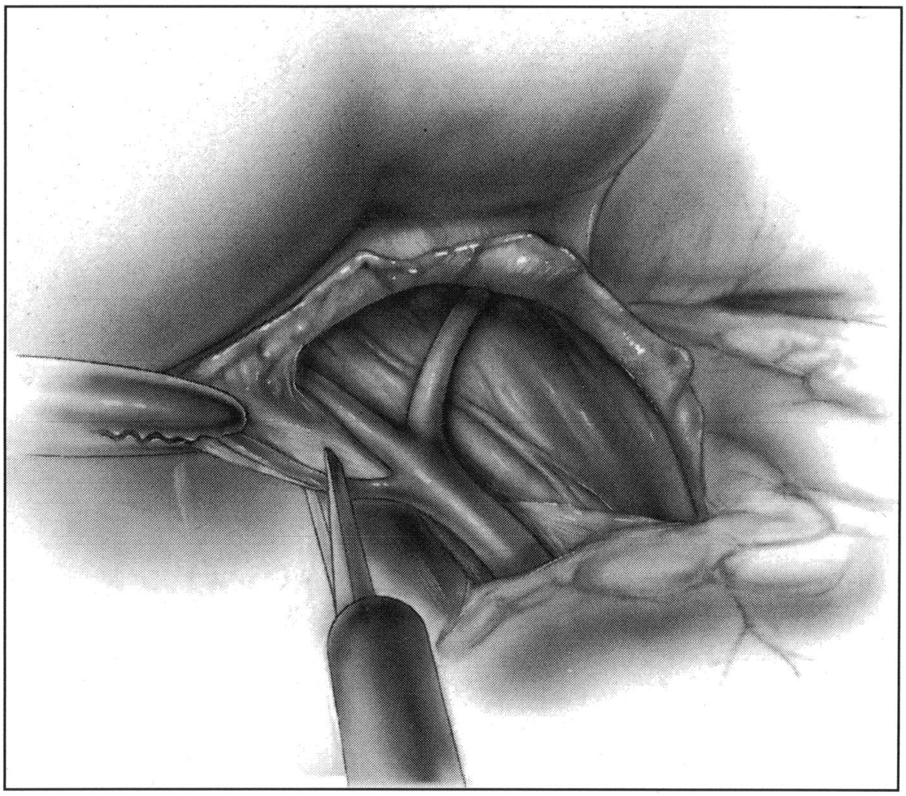

Fig. 7-7

The vessel is smaller than it appears; it looks large because it is closer to the scope than the esophagus. This vessel is usually a branch of the inferior phrenic artery. It must be carefully secured with ultrasonic shears **(Fig. 7–8)**. A replaced hepatic artery, sometimes encountered in this region, is usually larger and is seen to curve away toward the liver rather than pass cephalad toward the diaphragm. If a replaced hepatic artery is encountered, gently displace it to the right (out of the field of surgery) and protect it.

Mobilizing the Esophagus

If the crura have been carefully dissected to create an adequate posterior window, there should be a clear space behind the esophagus and retractors should pass easily. The retractors we prefer are curved and paired. They are designed to be inserted from the left and right sides.

Pass the first retractor from the left side. The design of the retractor shown is similar to that of the liver retractor. It is passed into the abdomen limp, and the cable is tightened to make it assume its working configuration. Once the curve is set, the retractor is rigid and ready for use.

Follow the arc of the circle while passing the retractor. Gently swing it from behind. Do not attempt to create a window with the retractor—the window should already be there. Do not attempt to "hook up" under the esophagus; to do so risks posterior perforation. When the tip of the retractor is seen to emerge from the right side of the space behind the esophagus, lift the esophagus with the retractor **(Fig. 7–9)**.

Pass the second esophageal retractor from the right. Follow the first retractor around, concentrating on the feel of metal on metal as the second retractor "rides" along parallel to the first. Maintain traction on the stomach to help generate a sufficient length of esophagus **(Fig. 7–10)**.

Move the two retractors apart in a spreading movement, parallel to the long axis of the esophagus **(Fig. 7–11)** to enlarge the window behind the esoph-

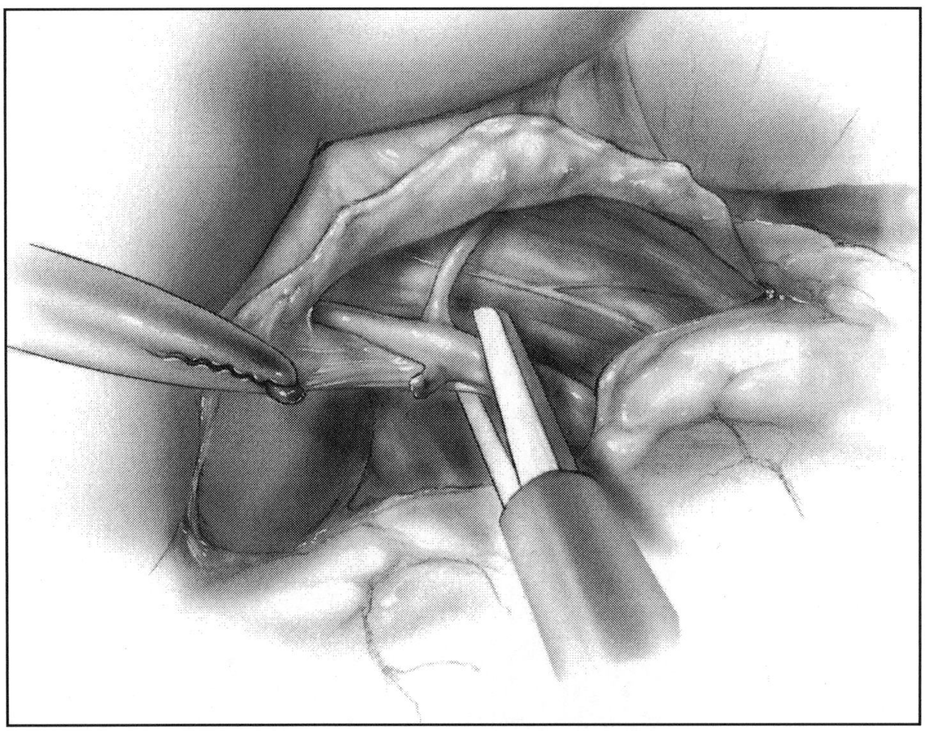

Fig. 7-8

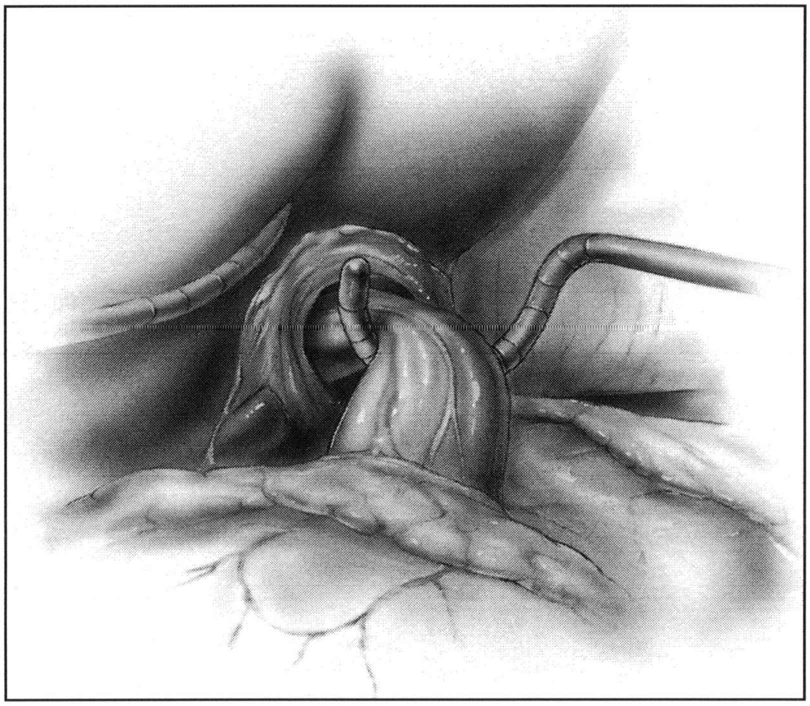

Fig. 7-9

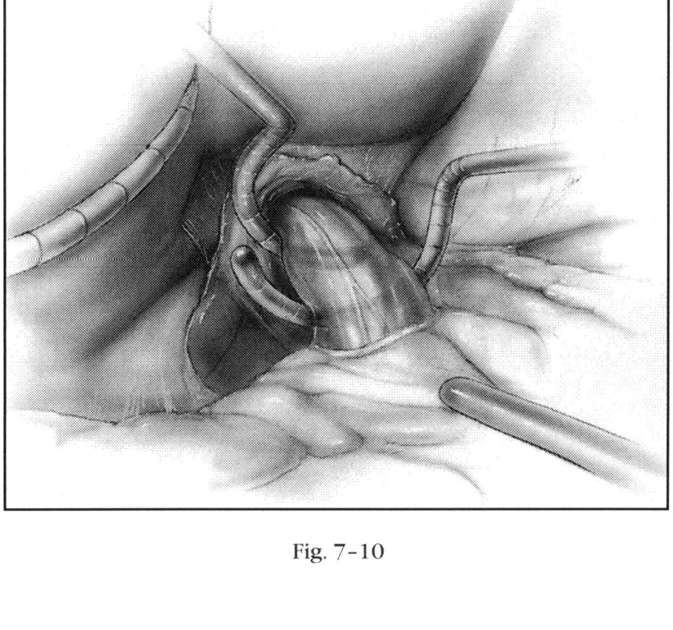

Fig. 7-10

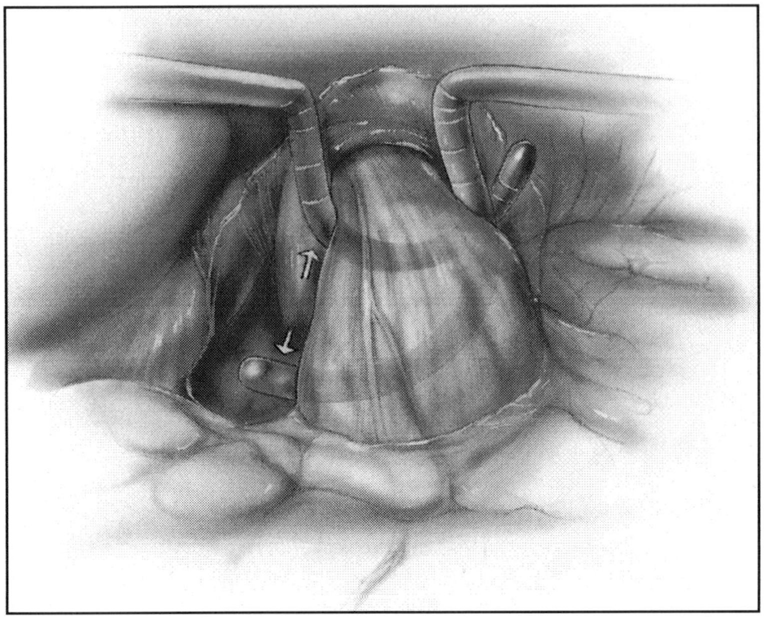

Fig. 7-11

agus if needed. Generally only one of the retractors is needed for the remainder of the procedure.

Closing the Hiatus

The hiatus must be closed to avoid herniation of the stomach or small intestine. Place one or two simple sutures of 0 or 2-0 silk and tie them **(Fig. 7–12)**. Leave a gap to avoid overtightening the hiatus, which may cause postoperative dysphagia.

Dividing the Short Gastric Vessels

The short gastric vessels tether the fundus of the stomach to the spleen **(Fig. 7–13a)**. Begin dividing these vessels at a convenient point high on the fundus and work cephalad **(Fig. 7–13b)**. We prefer ultrasonic shears for this division. Test the mobility of the fundus by passing it back and forth anterior to the esophagus **(Figs. 7–14a, 7–14b)**.

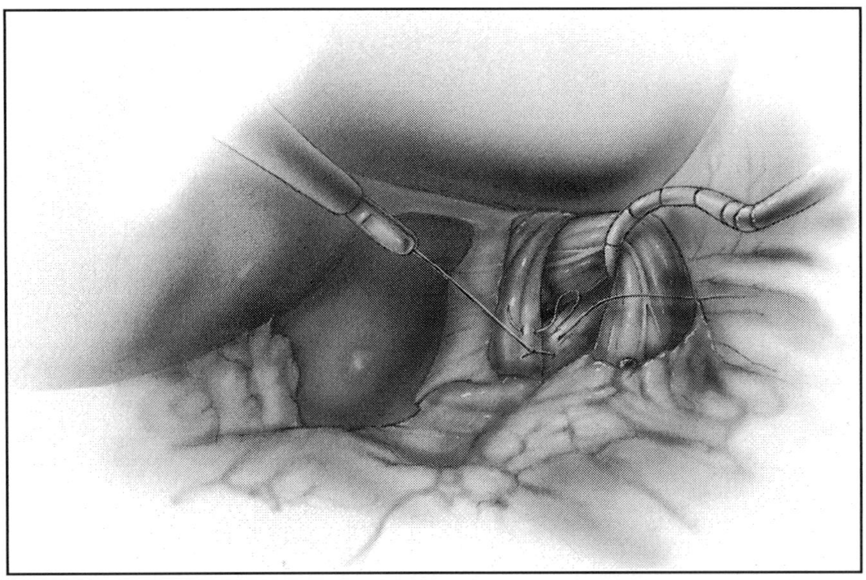

Fig. 7-12

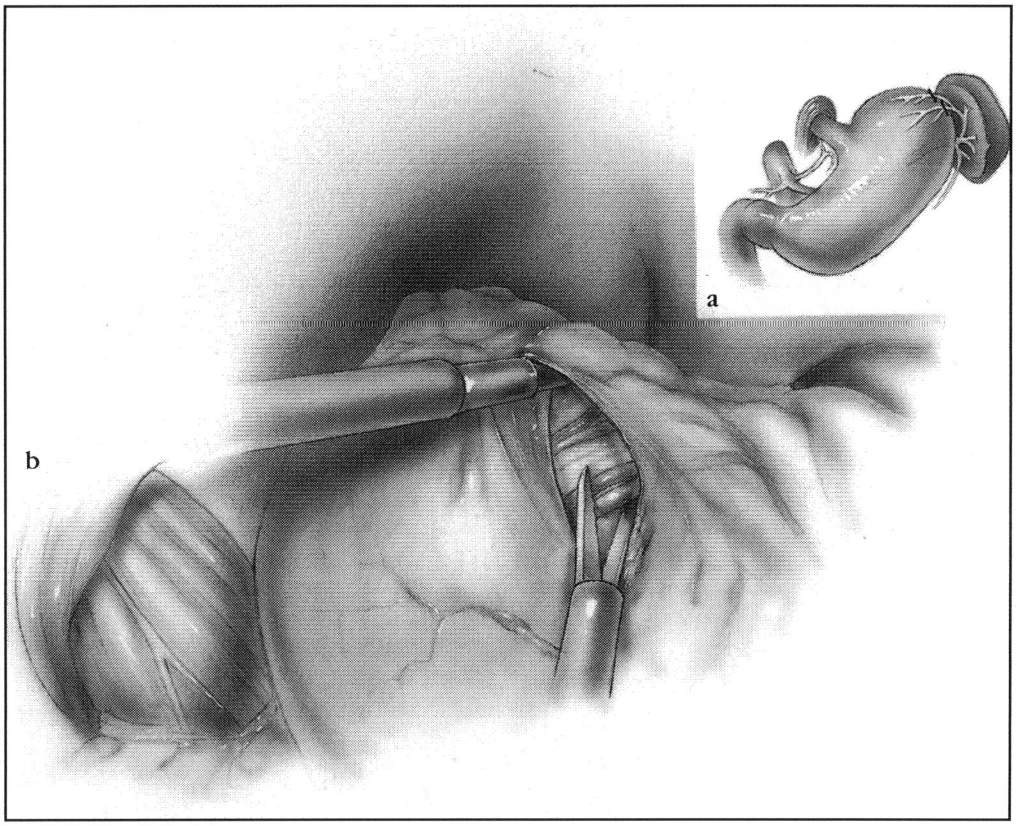

Fig. 7-13a,b

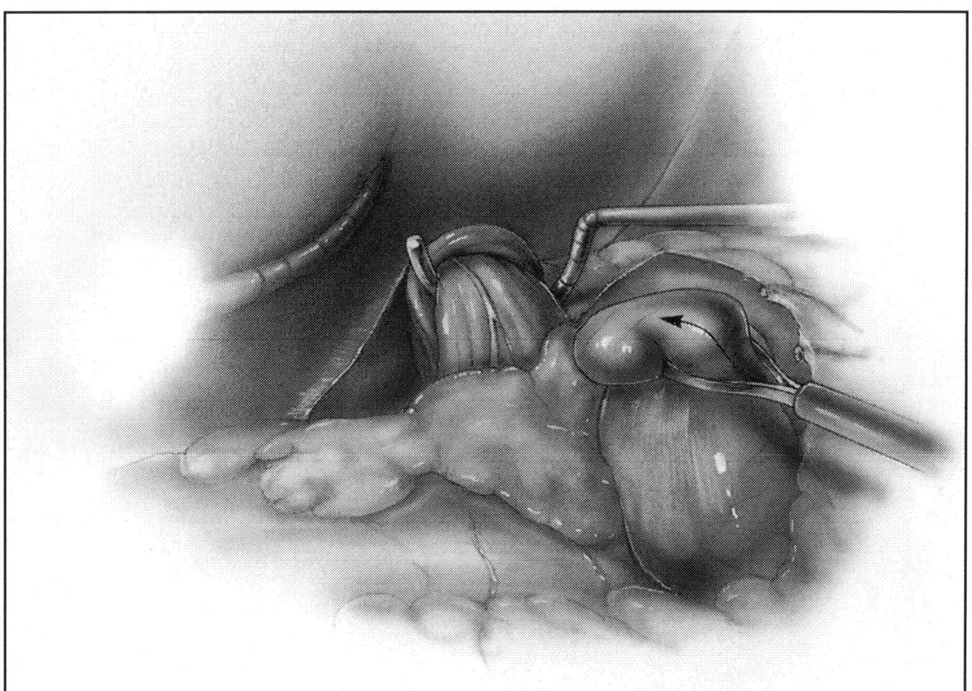

Fig. 7-14a

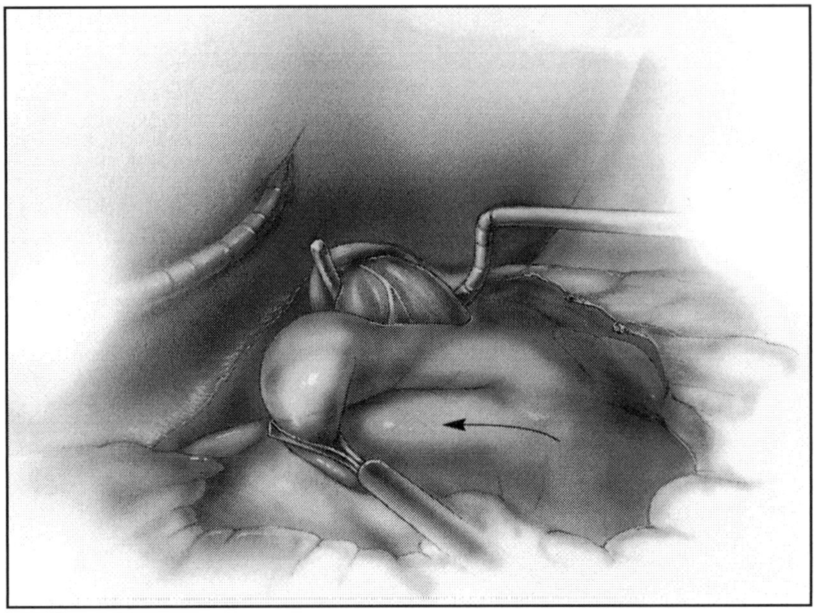

Fig. 7-14b

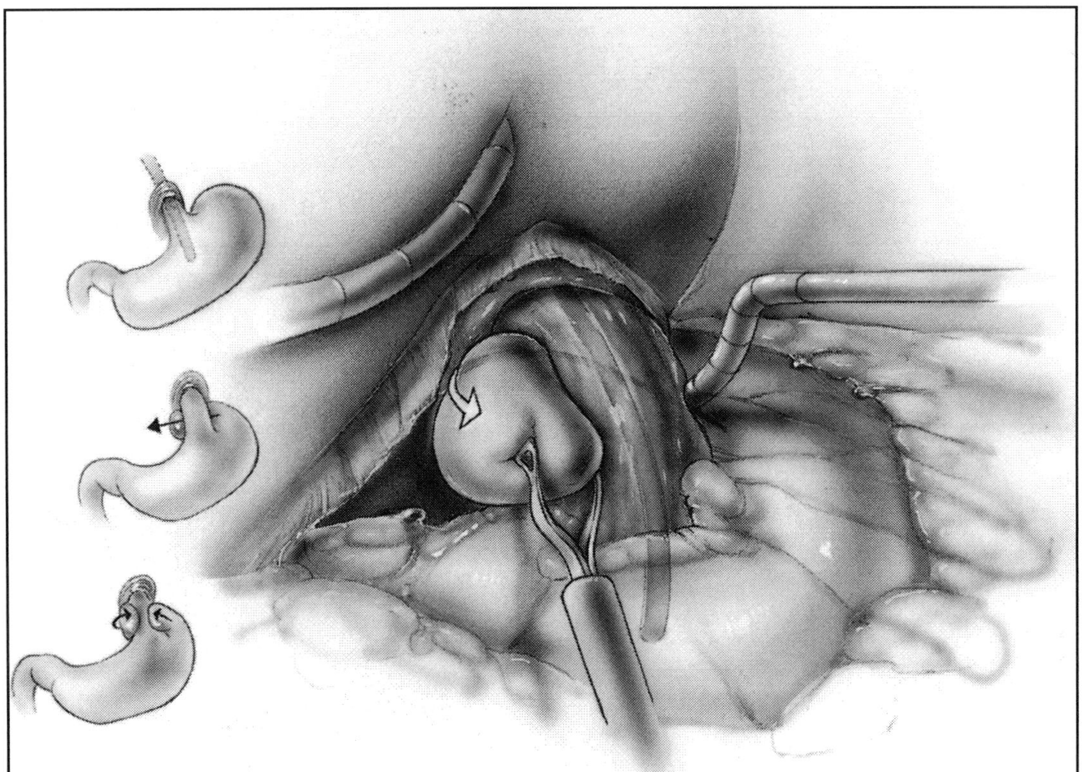

Fig. 7-15a,b,c,d

If at any time there has been concern about injury to the esophagus or stomach, have the anesthesiologist instill methylene blue into the nasogastric tube and look for staining. Repair any areas of concern at this time. Use the wrap to buttress any esophageal repair.

Creating the Wrap

Remove the esophageal retractors and allow the esophagus to return to its normal anatomic position. Pass Maloney dilators from above. For most adults, sequentially pass dilators until a 56-60F dilator is in place **(Fig. 7–15a)**.

Replace the left esophageal retractor and elevate the esophagus. Use an angled grasper to reach behind the esophagus from right to left. Grasp the fundus and pull it behind the esophagus. It should pass easily **(Fig. 7–15b, 7–15c, 7–15d)**.

Bring additional fundus over from the left side to meet the portion that has been passed behind **(Fig. 7–16)**. The wrap should meet easily and feel "floppy." Avoid the error of creating a twist by pulling the posterior part of the wrap too far to the right. Such a twist may contribute to postoperative dysphagia.

Place three sutures to complete the wrap. Catch a bit of the esophagus with the first suture or two to anchor the wrap well above the stomach **(Fig. 7–17)**. Take care not to take an excessively deep bite and create a perforation. Some surgeons place clips on the knots to mark the location of the wrap. It facilitates postoperative evaluation with barium swallow. The completed wrap should lie easily below the diaphragm **(Fig. 7–18)**.

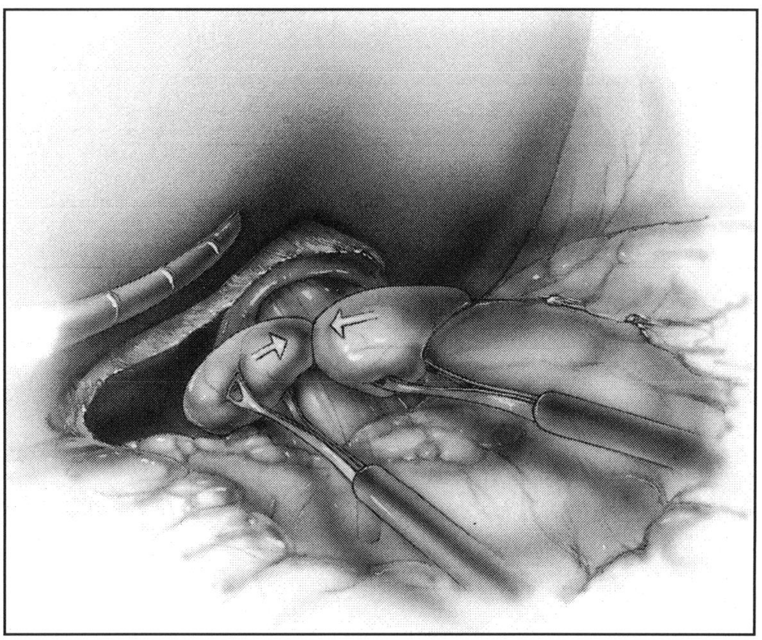

Fig. 7-16

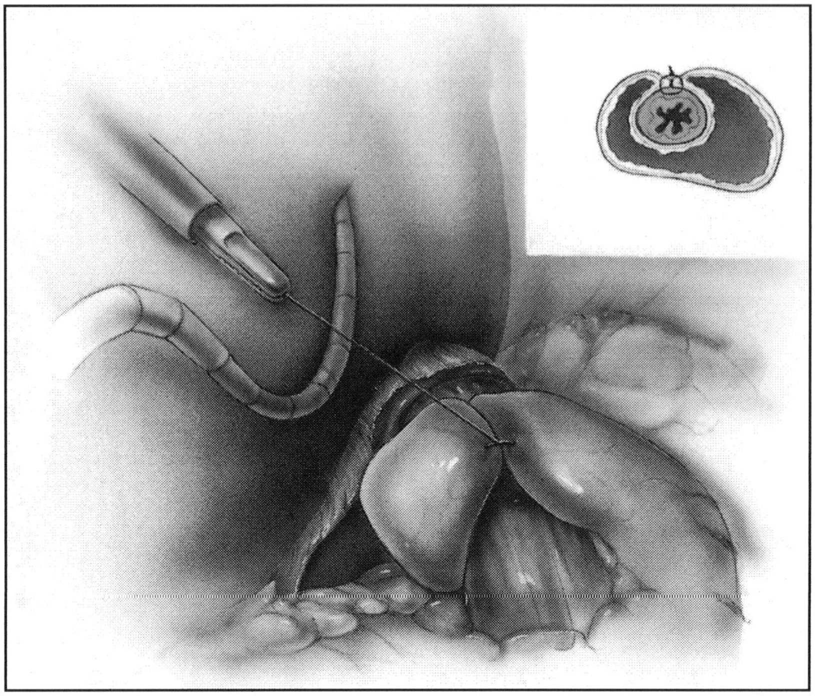

Fig. 7-17

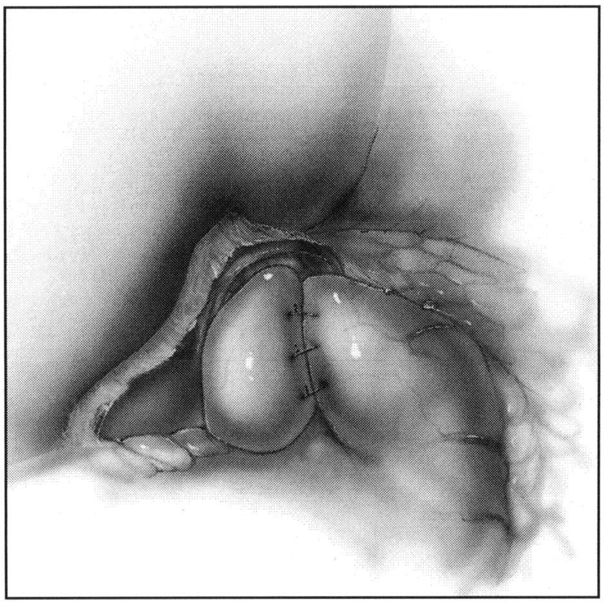

Fig. 7-18

POSTOPERATIVE CARE

We keep the nasogastric tube in place for the first 24 hours to avoid gastric dilatation. A Hypaque swallow the first postoperative day should demonstrate free passage of Hypaque without extravasation. This is particularly important if there is any question of the integrity of the wrap or esophagus.

COMPLICATIONS

Esophageal perforation

Herniation of viscera through the hiatal opening

Slipped wrap

Dysphagia

REFERENCES

Hunter JG, Trus TL, Branum GD, Waring JP, Wood WC. A physiologic approach to laparoscopic fundoplication for gastroesophageal reflux disease. Ann Surg 1996; 223:673.

Peters JH. Laparoscopic treatment of gastroesophageal reflux and hiatal hernia. In: Scott-Conner CEH (ed) The SAGES Manual: Fundamentals of Laparoscopy and GI Endoscopy. New York, Springer-Verlag, 1999, pp 196–212.

Schauer PR, Meyers WC, Eubanks S, et al. Mechanisms of gastric and esophageal perforations during laparoscopic fundoplication. Ann Surg 1996;223:43.

8 Posterior Gastropexy (Hill Repair)

Surgical Legacy Technique

INDICATIONS

See Chapter 6.

Gastroesophageal reflux.

Successful execution of this operation requires that the esophagus be long enough to suture the esophagogastric junction to the level of the median arcuate ligament without tension (5–7 cm of intraabdominal esophagus).

PREOPERATIVE PREPARATION

See Chapter 6.

PITFALLS AND DANGER POINTS

Hemorrhage from laceration of celiac or inferior phrenic artery

Injury to spleen

Improper calibration of lumen of lower esophageal sphincter

Excessive narrowing of diaphragmatic hiatus

Failure to identify the median arcuate ligament

Injury to left hepatic vein or vena cava when incising triangular ligament to liberate left lobe of liver

OPERATIVE STRATEGY

Dissecting the Median Arcuate Ligament

The median arcuate ligament constitutes the anterior portion of the aortic hiatus, the aperture in the diaphragm through which the aorta passes. The ligament, a condensation of preaortic fascia, arches over the anterior surface of the aorta just cephalad to the origin of the celiac artery and joins the right crus of the diaphragm at its insertion onto the vertebral column. This band of fibrous tissue covers about 3 cm of the aorta above the celiac axis and is in turn covered by crural muscle fibers. It can be identified by exposing the celiac artery and pushing it posteriorly with the finger at the inferior rim of the median arcuate ligament. For Hill's operation, the surgeon dissects the celiac artery and celiac ganglion away from the overlying median arcuate ligament in the midline, avoiding the two inferior phrenic arteries that arise from the aorta just to the right and just to the left of the midline. Nerve fibers from the celiac ganglion must be cut to liberate the median arcuate ligament.

An alternative method for identifying the median arcuate ligament is to visualize the anterior surface of the aorta above the aortic hiatus. A few fibers of preaortic fascia may have to be incised. Then with the left index fingernail pushing the anterior wall of the aorta posteriorly, pass the fingertip in a caudal direction. The fingertip passes behind a strong layer of preaortic fascia and median arcuate ligament. At a point about 2–3 cm caudal to the upper margin of the preaortic fascia, blocking further passage of the fingertip, is the attachment of the inferior border of the median arcuate ligament to the aorta at the origin of the celiac artery. The pulsation of the celiac artery is easily palpated by the fingertip, which is lodged between the aorta and the overlying ligament. Vansant and colleagues believed that the foregoing maneuver constitutes sufficient mobilization of the median arcuate ligament and that the ligament need not be dissected free from the celiac artery and ganglion to perform a posterior gastropexy. We believe that a surgeon who has not had considerable experience liberating the median arcuate ligament from the celiac artery may find Vansant's modification to be safer than Hill's approach. If one succeeds in catching a good bite of the preaortic fascia and median arcuate ligament by Vansant's technique, the end result should be satisfactory.

If the celiac artery or the aorta is lacerated during the course of the Hill operation, do not hesitate to divide the median arcuate ligament and preaortic fascia in the midline. This step may be necessary to expose the full length of the laceration.

Calibrating the Esophagocardiac Orifice

In addition to fixing the esophagocardiac junction to the median arcuate ligament, the Hill operation serves to narrow the entrance of the lower esophagus into the stomach by partially turning in the lesser curvature aspect of the esophagogastric junction. Calibration of this turn-in is important if reflux is to be prevented without at the same time causing chronic obstruction. Hill (1977) used intraoperative manometry to measure the pressure at the esophagocardiac junction before and after completing the gastropexy. He believed that a pressure of 50–55 mm Hg ensures that the calibration is proper. Orringer et al. reported that intraoperative pressures did not correlate at all with pressures obtained at postoperative manometry, perhaps because of the variable influence of preoperative medication and anesthetic agents.

If intraoperative manometry is not used, the adequacy of the repair should be tested by invaginating the anterior wall of the stomach along the indwelling nasogastric tube upward into the esophagogastric junction. Prior to the repair, the index finger can pass freely into the esophagus because of the incompetent lower esophageal sphincter. After the sutures have been placed and drawn together but not tied, the tip of the index finger should be able to palpate the esophageal orifice but should not quite be able to enter the esophagus alongside the 18F nasogastric tube. This method of calibration has been successful in our hands.

Liberating Left Lobe of Liver

As discussed in Chapter 6, liberating the left lobe of the liver is rarely needed.

OPERATIVE TECHNIQUE

Incision and Exposure

With the patient in the supine position, elevate the head of the table about 10°–15° from the horizontal. Make a midline incision from the xiphoid to a point about 4 cm below the umbilicus **(Fig. 8–1)**. Insert a Thompson or Upper Hand retractor to elevate the lower portion of the sternum and draw it forcefully in a cephalad direction. Explore the abdomen for incidental pathology, such as a duodenal ulcer, cholelithiasis, chronic pancreatitis, or colon disease.

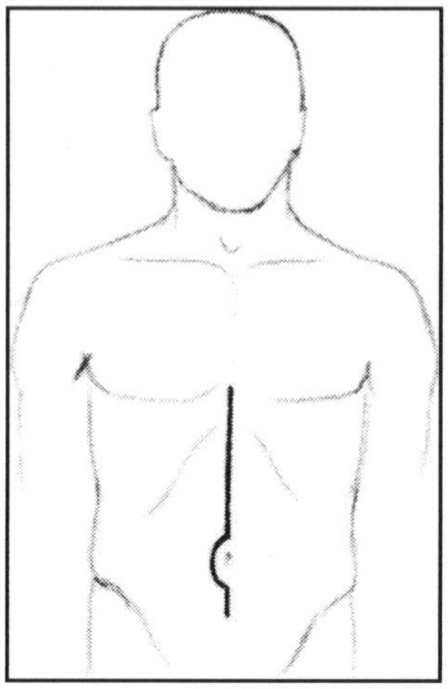

Fig. 8–1

Mobilizing the Esophagogastric Junction

Identify the peritoneum overlying the abdominal esophagus by palpating the indwelling nasogastric tube. Divide this peritoneum with Metzenbaum scissors and continue the incision over the right and left branches of the crus **(Fig. 8–2)**. After exposing the crus, elevate this muscle by inserting a peanut sponge dissector between the crus and the esophagus, first on the right and then on the left. Then insert the left index finger to encircle the esophagus by *gentle* dissection. If the esophagus is inflamed owing to inadequately treated esophagitis, it is easy to perforate it by rough finger dissection. Identify and protect both the right and left vagus nerves. Then encircle the esophagus with a latex drain and free it from posterior attachments by dividing the phrenoesophageal ligaments **(Fig. 8–3)**.

Make an incision in the avascular portion of the gastrohepatic ligament. Continue this incision in a cephalad direction toward the right side of the hiatus. When dividing the gastrohepatic ligament it is often necessary to divide an accessory left hepatic branch of the left gastric artery **(Fig. 8–4)**. At the conclusion of this step, the muscular portion of the crura surrounding the hiatus should be clearly visible throughout the circumference of the hiatus.

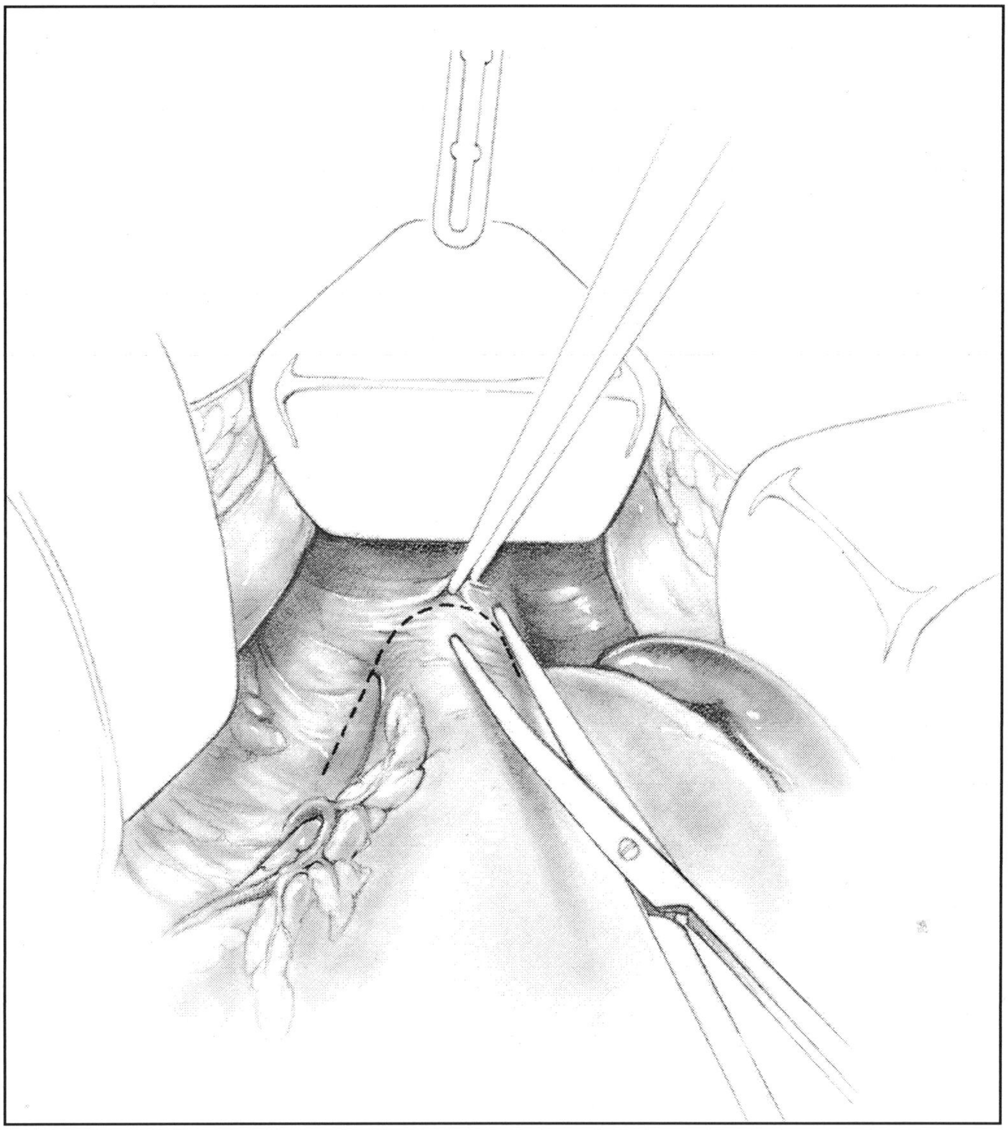

Fig. 8–2

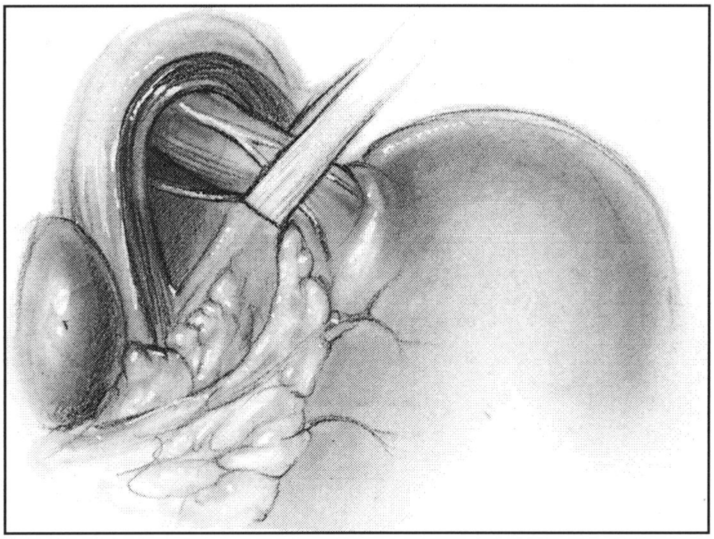

Fig. 8–3

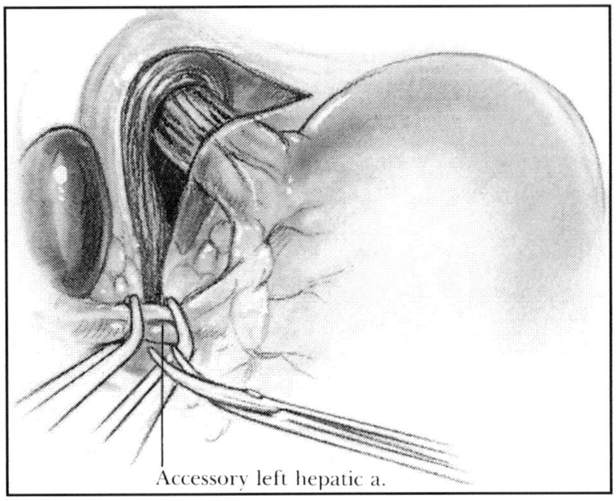

Fig. 8–4

The only structure binding the gastric fundus to the posterior abdominal wall now is the gastrophrenic ligament. The best way to divide this ligament is to insert the left hand behind the esophagogastric junction and then bring the left index finger between the esophagogastric junction and the diaphragm. This places the ligament on stretch. Divide this avascular ligament **(Fig. 8–5)** from the esophagogastric junction along the greater curvature down to the first short gastric artery. It is often necessary to divide the first two short gastric vessels to achieve proper mobilization. This may be done by applying a Hemoclip to the splenic side and a 2-0 silk ligature to the gastric side of the short gastric vessel.

Avoid injuring the spleen by carefully inspecting the anterior surface of this organ prior to dissection in this region. Divide any attachments between the

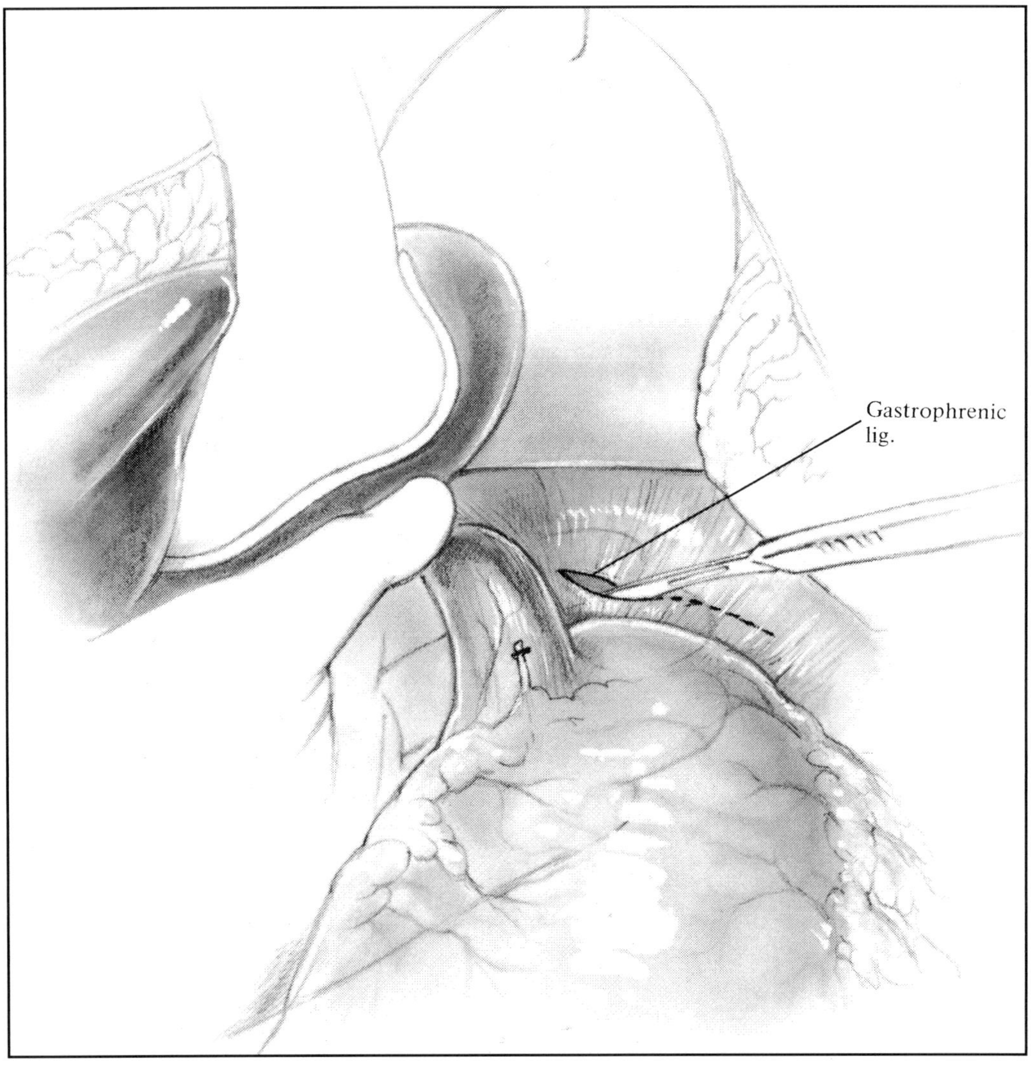

Fig. 8–5

omentum and the splenic capsule, as traction on the omentum would otherwise cause avulsion of the capsule and bleeding.

Inserting the Crural Sutures

Ask the first assistant to retract the esophagus toward the patient's left; then narrow the aperture of the hiatus by approximating the crural bundles behind the esophagus. Use 0 Tevdek atraumatic sutures on a substantial needle. Take a bite of 1.5–2.0 cm of crus on the left and a similar bite on the right. Include the overlying peritoneum together with the crural muscle **(Fig. 8–6)**. Do not tie these sutures at this time but tag each with a small hemostat. It is sometimes helpful to grasp the left side of the crus with a long Babcock or Allis clamp. Do not apply excessive traction with these clamps or sutures, as the crural musculature tends to split along the line of its fibers. Insert three or four sutures of this type as necessary. Then tentatively draw the sutures together and insert the index finger into the remaining hiatal aperture. It should be possible to insert a fingertip into the remaining aperture alongside the esophagus with its indwelling nasogastric tube. Narrowing the hiatal aperture more than this may cause permanent dysphagia and does not help reduce reflux. Do not tie the crural sutures at this point.

Identifying the Median Arcuate Ligament

Hill's Method

After the lower esophagus and proximal stomach have been completely freed, identify the celiac artery and use the left index finger to press it posteriorly into the aorta. If the index finger slides in a cephalad direction, its tip meets the lower border of the median arcuate ligament. Between the aorta and median arcuate ligament are branches of the celiac ganglion as well as the right and left inferior phrenic arteries, which arise from the aorta in this vicinity. It is necessary to divide some of the nerve fibers; but once the inferior margin of the ligament is freed from the aorta in the midline, it is possible to pass an instrument in a cephalad direction without encountering any further resistance. Hill passed a Goodell cervical dilator between the median arcuate ligament and the aorta to protect the aorta while sutures were being inserted into the lower border of the ligament. He stated that if a small diaphragmatic branch of the aorta is disrupted the bleeding often subsides with pressure. However, it is possible for the inexperienced surgeon to induce major hemorrhage by traumatizing the arteries in this vicinity. Caution is indicated.

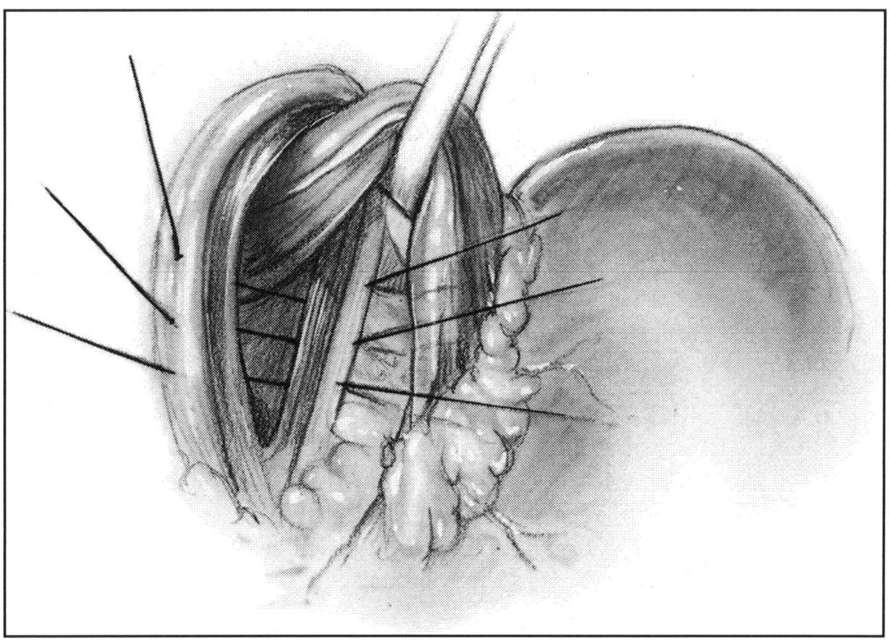

Fig. 8-6

Vansant's Method

Vansant and colleagues described another technique for identifying and liberating the median arcuate ligament by approaching it from its superior margin: Identify the anterior surface of the aorta in the hiatal aperture between the right and left branches of the crus. Occasionally, it is necessary to dissect away some areolar tissue. With the left index fingernail pressing posteriorly against the aorta about 4 cm cephalad to the diaphragm, slide the index finger in a caudal direction. Deep behind the confluence of the diaphragmatic crura, the tip of the index finger passes behind a dense band of preaortic fascia that crosses over the aorta as the aorta passes through the aortic hiatus in the posterior diaphragm. The width of this band is variable but averages perhaps 3 cm. At the lower margin of this band the fingertip encounters pulsation of the celiac artery, which arises from the anterior wall of the aorta at the inferior margin of the median arcuate ligament. The median arcuate ligament lies between the fingertip and a thin layer of muscle fibers representing the caudal confluence of the diaphragmatic crura. With the index finger in place, Vansant and associates inserted three interrupted atraumatic sutures of no. 1 braided silk into the median arcuate ligament. Each suture is tagged with a hemostat, leaving each needle attached for later use when suturing the posterior gastropexy.

Suturing Posterior Gastropexy

Rotate the esophagogastric junction so the lesser curvature aspect of the stomach faces anteriorly. Then place a large Babcock clamp on the anterior and another clamp on the posterior phrenoesophageal bundle. Between these two bundles the longitudinal muscle fibers of the esophagus can be seen as they join the lesser curvature of the stomach. Where to place the proximal suture is an important consideration. Placing it too high causes excessive narrowing of the esophageal lumen; placing it too low does not increase the intraluminal pressure adequately in the lower esophageal sphincter area. We use 2-0 atraumatic Tevdek and include a few millimeters of adjacent gastric wall together with the phrenoesophageal bundle to ensure that the submucosa has been included in the suture. After placing the upper suture, cross the two ends or insert the first throw of a tie. Then estimate the lumen of the esophagastric junction by invaginating the stomach with the index finger along the indwelling nasogastric tube. If this maneuver is attempted before tying down the suture, the finger passes easily into the lumen of the esophagus in patients who have an incompetent lower esophageal sphincter. After the first suture is tentatively closed, only the tip of the index finger should be able to enter the esophagus. In the absence of intraoperative esophageal manometry, this is the best method for calibrating proper placement of the gastropexy sutures.

If the first suture has been judged to be properly placed, tag it with a hemostat and insert three additional sutures of atraumatic 2-0 Tevdek into the phrenoesophageal bundles, at intervals of about 1 cm, caudal to the first suture. Place a hemostat on each suture as a tag. After all the sutures have been placed, tighten each and again use the index finger to calibrate the lumen of the esophagogastric junction. If it is satisfactory, expose the anterior wall of the aorta in the hiatal aperture behind the esophagus. With the index fingernail closely applied to the anterior wall of the aorta, pass the fingertip in a caudal direction underneath the preaortic fascia and median arcuate ligament down to the point where the fingertip palpates the pulsation of the celiac artery. Then remove the index finger and replace it with a narrow right-angled retractor such as the Army-Navy retractor **(Fig. 8–7)**. Be certain that the retractor is indeed deep to the median arcuate ligament. This retractor serves to protect the aorta while the gastropexy sutures are being inserted through the preaortic fascia.

Identify the proximal suture that has already been placed in the phrenoesophageal bundles and pass the suture through the preaortic fascia. Be sure to take a substantial bite of the tissue anterior to the Army-Navy retractor. Pass the needle deep enough so it makes contact with the metal retractor; otherwise, only some overlying crural muscle fibers may be included in the stitch, which is then not strong enough to ensure a long-term successful result. After the first stitch has been passed through the preaortic fascia, tag it with a hemostat; pass each of the remaining phrenoesophageal sutures through the preaortic fascia by the same technique and tag each with a hemostat (Fig. 8–7).

Another good method to expedite suturing of the median arcuate ligament is to use a large right-angle bronchus clamp. Insert the tip of the clamp behind the median arcuate ligament instead of behind the Army-Navy retractor. Use the clamp to draw the median arcuate ligament vigorously anteriorly. Pass the needle with the suture through the median arcuate ligament just deep to the clamp, which ensures that a large bite of ligament is included in each stitch. Be certain not to injure the underlying aorta with the needle.

At this point check the entire area for hemostasis. Then tie the previously placed crural sutures (Fig.

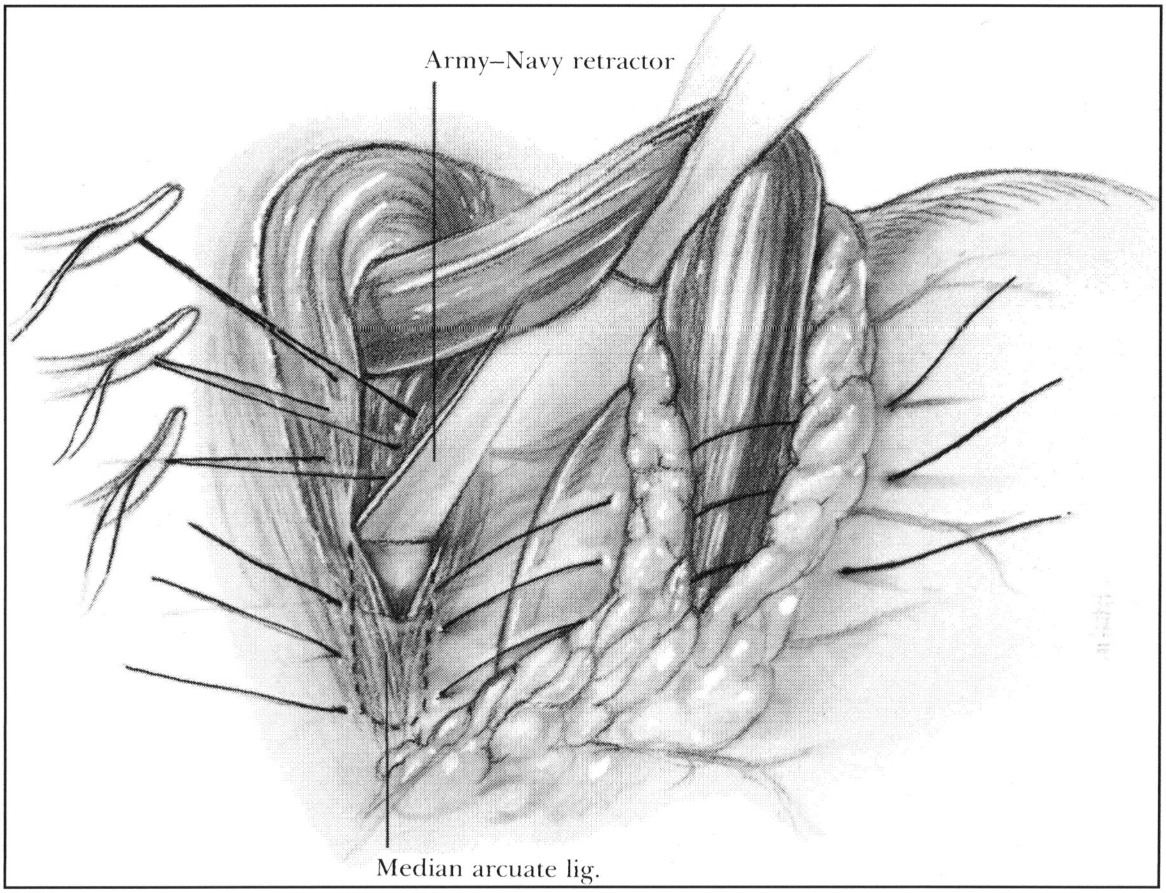

Fig. 8-7

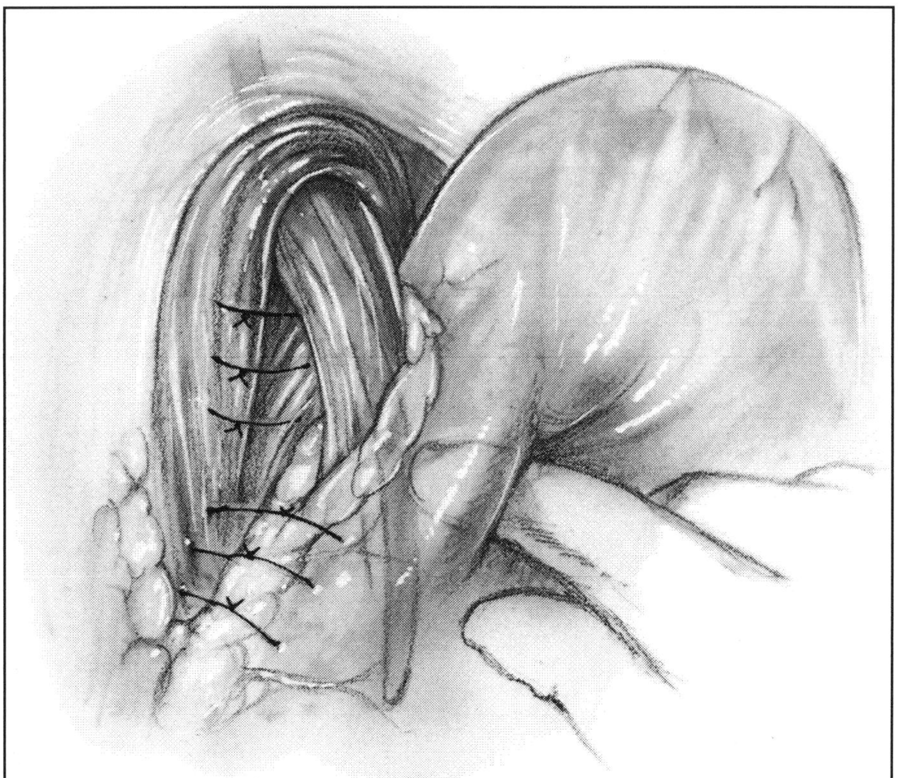

Fig. 8-8

8-6), narrowing the aperture of the hiatus. After these sutures have been tied, the index finger should pass freely into the hiatal aperture with an indwelling 18F nasogastric tube in the esophagus. If this is not the case, replace the proximal crural suture as necessary. Now tie each of the previously placed *gastropexy* sutures and cut all the ends **(Fig. 8–8)**.

Testing the Antireflux Valve

A simple method for testing the efficacy of the antireflux valve is to have the anesthesiologist inject about 500 ml of saline into the nasogastric tube and then withdraw the tube to a point above the esophagogastric junction. In the presence of a competent antireflux valve, compressing the saline-filled stomach fails to force the saline into the esophagus.

Abdominal Closure

Close the abdomen without drainage in routine fashion.

POSTOPERATIVE CARE

Continue nasogastric suction for 1-2 days.

Obtain a radiograph of the esophagogastric junction after a barium swallow before the patient is discharged from the hospital.

COMPLICATIONS

Dysphagia (usually transient).

Persistence or recurrence of gastroesophageal reflux. This and other complications following the Hill operation, are uncommon.

REFERENCES

Aye RW, Hill LD, Kraemer SJ, Snopkowski P. Early results with the laparoscopic Hill repair. Am J Surg 1994;167:542.

Aye RW, Mazza DE, Hill LD. Laparoscopic Hill repair in patients with abnormal motility. Am J Surg 1997;173:379.

Hill LD. An effective operation for hiatal hernia; an eight year appraisal. Ann Surg 1967;166:681.

Hill LD. Progress in the surgical management of hiatal hernia. World J Surg 1977;1:425.

Orringer MB, Schneider R, Williams GW, Sloan H. Intraoperative esophageal mamometry: is it valid? Ann Thorac Surg 1980;30:13.

Vansant JH, Baker JW, Ross DG. Modification of the Hill technique for repair of hiatal hernia. Surg Gynecol Obstet 1976;143:637.

9 Transthoracic Gastroplasty (Collis) and Nissen Fundoplication

INDICATIONS

Short esophagus due to reflux esophagitis

Recurrent gastroesophageal reflux with stricture after an antireflux procedure

Previous subtotal gastrectomy generally contraindicates a Collis-Nissen procedure

PREOPERATIVE PREPARATION

Dilate the esophageal stricture up to 40F. It can generally be done with Maloney dilators.

Insert a nasogastric tube down to the stricture.

Assessment for colon interposition is prudent in difficult cases (see Chapter 5). Bowel preparation allows colon to be used as a conduit if needed.

When esophagoscopy reveals severe acute ulcerative esophagitis with inflammation and bleeding, a 2- to 3-week period of preoperative intensive medical treatment with cimetidine, omeprazole, or both reduces inflammation and lessens the risk of intraoperative perforation of the esophagus.

PITFALLS AND DANGER POINTS

Esophageal perforation

Hemorrhage resulting from traumatizing or avulsing the accessory left hepatic artery, inferior phrenic artery, ascending branch of the left gastric artery, short gastric vessel, or inferior pulmonary vein

Laceration of spleen

Inadvertent vagotomy

Inadequate suturing, permitting the fundoplication to slip postoperatively

OPERATIVE STRATEGY

Performing an Adequate Gastroplasty

The object of performing a gastroplasty is to lengthen a shortened esophagus for an extent sufficient to prevent tension from being exerted on the antireflux operation and hernia repair. This newly constructed esophagus ("neoesophagus") consists of a tube made from the lesser curvature of the stomach. A 56F Maloney dilator is passed into the stomach, and the tube is constructed by applying an 80 mm linear cutting stapler precisely at the esophagogastric junction parallel to and snugly alongside the Maloney dilator. When the stapler is fired, the esophageal tube is lengthened by as much as 7 cm. If the stapler has been placed snugly against the esophagogastric junction, there are no irregularities or outpouchings at this point.

Mobilizing the Esophagus and Stomach

Not only is it important to mobilize the distal esophagus completely, at least as far up as the inferior pulmonary vein, but the proximal stomach must be entirely free of attachments, just as when a Nissen fundoplication is being performed through an abdominal approach. This operation can be accomplished without tension only with full mobilization. It requires dividing the phrenoesophageal and gastrophrenic ligaments, freeing the hiatus throughout its complete circumference from any attachments to the stomach or lower esophagus, and dividing an accessory left hepatic artery, which courses from the left gastric artery across the proximal gastrohepatic ligament to help supply the left lobe of the liver. After mobilization has been accomplished, the remaining maneuvers in the Collis-Nissen operation are not difficult.

If the esophagus is inadvertently perforated during the dissection, exercise careful judgment when deciding whether it is safe to suture the esophageal laceration or a resection and colon or jejunum interposition is necessary. If it is elected to suture the laceration, try to cover the suture line with a flap of parietal pleura (see Figs. 14-1 to 14-3).

Avoiding Hemorrhage

Avoiding unnecessary bleeding during any operation requires a careful dissection and a knowledge of vascular anatomy. This is especially important when mobilizing the stomach through a thoracic approach because losing control of the accessory left hepatic, short gastric, or inferior phrenic artery causes the proximal bleeding arterial stump to retract deep into the abdomen. Controlling these retracted vessels is difficult and may require laparotomy or at least a peripheral incision in the diaphragm. Preventing this complication is not difficult if the dissection is orderly and the surgeon is aware of the anatomic location of these vessels. Similarly, careful dissection and avoidance of traction along the greater curvature of the stomach helps prevent damaging the spleen.

Avoiding Esophageal Perforation

When the distal esophagus is baked into a fibrotic mediastinum, sharp scalpel dissection is safer than blunt dissection if injury to the esophagus and the vagus nerves is to be avoided. Sometimes the fibrosis terminates 8–9 cm above the diaphragm. If so, the esophagus and the vagus nerves can easily be encircled at this point, which provides a plane for subsequent dissection of the distal esophagus.

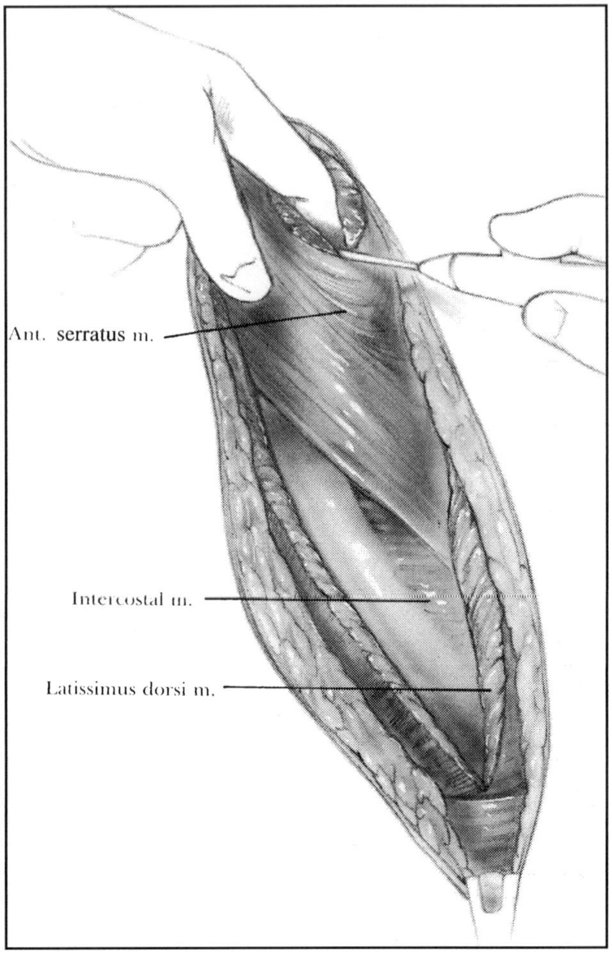

Fig. 9-2

OPERATIVE TECHNIQUE

Incision

With the patient under one-lung anesthesia in the lateral position, left side up, make a skin incision in the sixth intercostal space from the costal margin to the tip of the scapula **(Fig. 9–1)**. Then identify the latissimus dorsi muscle and insert the index finger underneath it. Transect this muscle with electrocautery; then divide the underlying anterior serratus muscle in similar fashion **(Fig. 9–2)**. In both cases it is preferable to divide these muscles somewhat caudal to the skin incision, as it helps preserve muscle function. Then use electrocautery to divide the intercostal muscles along the upper border of the seventh rib **(Fig. 9–3)** and open the pleura. Complete this opening from the costal margin to the region of the lateral spinal muscles. Separate the periosteum and surrounding tissues from a 1 cm segment of the posterior portion of the seventh rib lateral to the spinal muscles. Excise a 1 cm segment of this rib **(Fig. 9–4)**. Then divide the intercostal neurovascular bundle that runs along the inferior border of this rib **(Fig. 9–5)**.

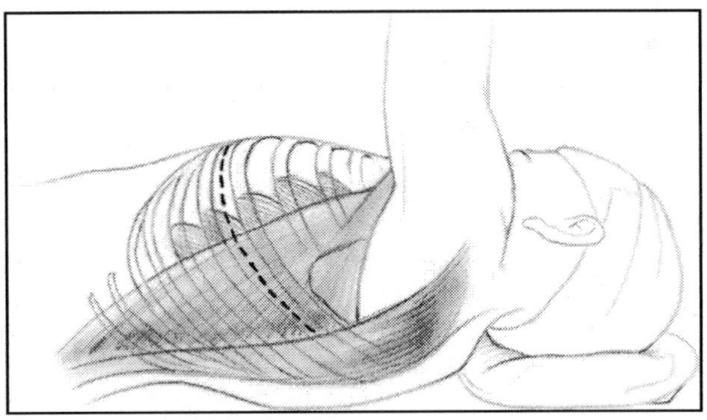

Fig. 9-1

Insert a Finochietto retractor into the incision and gradually increase the distance between the blades of the retractor over a 10-minute period to avoid causing rib fractures. In patients who have undergone previous surgery of the distal esophagus or proximal stomach, do not hesitate to continue this incision across the costal margin, converting it into a thoracoabdominal incision to facilitate dissection

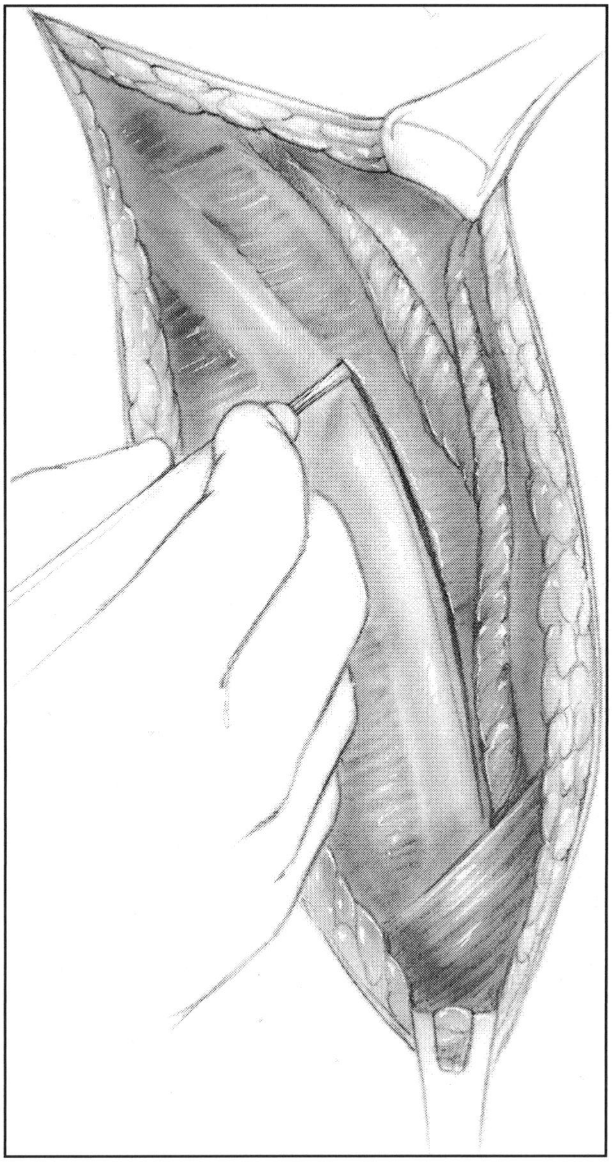

Fig. 9-3

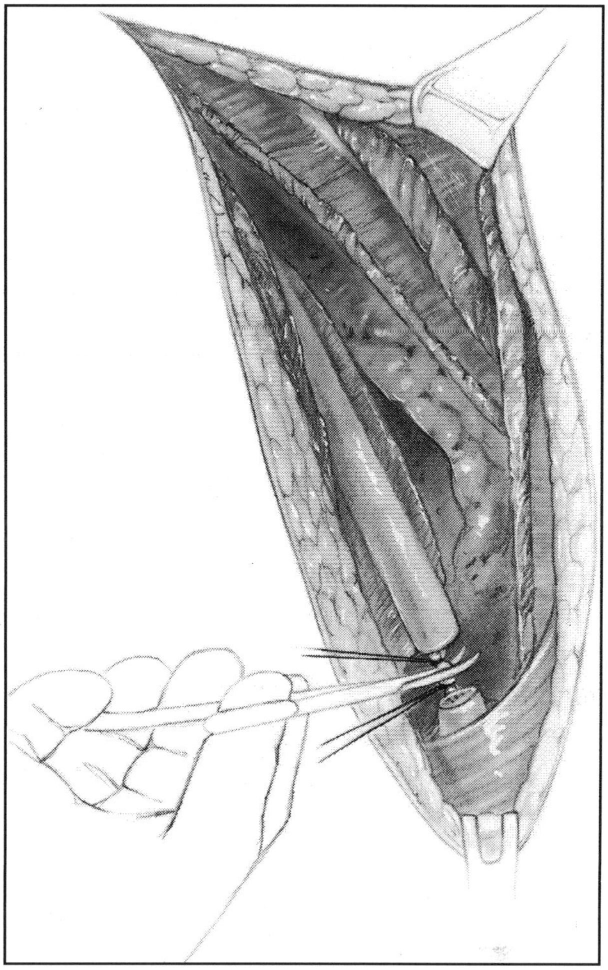

Fig. 9-5

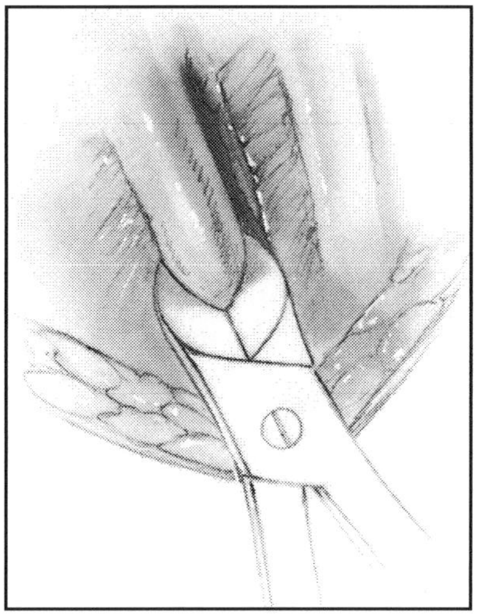

Fig. 9-4

on the abdominal aspect of the diaphragmatic hiatus (see Figs. 3-6, 3-7).

Liberating the Esophagus

Incise the inferior pulmonary ligament with electrocautery and then compress the lung and retract it in anterior and cephalad directions using moist gauze pads and Harrington retractors. Incise the mediastinal pleura just medial to the aorta **(Figs. 9–6, 9–7)**. Encircle the esophagus with the index finger using the indwelling nasogastric tube as a guide. If this cannot be done easily, it may be necessary to initiate sharp dissection at a somewhat higher level, where the fibrosis may be less advanced. Encircle the esophagus and the vagus nerves with a latex drain. Continue the dissection of the esophagus from the inferior pulmonary vein down to the diaphragmatic hiatus. After the mediastinal pleura has been incised down to the hiatus, continue the incision anteriorly and divide the pleura of the pericardiophrenic sulcus (Fig. 9-6); otherwise, the medial aspect of the hiatal ring is not visible. If the right pleural cavity has been inadvertently entered, simply place a moist gauze pad over the rent in the pleura to prevent excessive seepage of blood into the right chest and continue the dissection.

Excising the Hernial Sac

Identify the point at which the left branch of the crus of the diaphragm meets the hernial sac. Any attenuated fibers of the phrenoesophageal ligament and preperitoneal fat are made apparent by applying traction to the diaphragm. Incise these tissues and the underlying peritoneum **(Fig. 9–8)**. Continue the incision in the peritoneum in a circumferential fashion, opening the lateral and anterior aspects of the hernial sac; expose the greater curvature of the stomach. Insert the left index finger into the sac and continue the incision along the medial (deep) margin of the hiatus using the finger as a guide **(Fig. 9–9)**. A branch of the inferior phrenic artery may be noted posterolaterally near the left vagus nerve; it is divided and ligated with 2-0 silk. While attempting to circumnavigate the proximal stomach, the index finger in the hernial sac encounters an obstruction on the lesser curvature side of the esophagogastric junction. It represents the proximal margin of the gastrohepatic ligament, which often contains a 2- to 4-mm accessory left hepatic artery coming off the ascending left gastric artery. By hugging the lesser curvature side of the cardia with the index finger, this finger can be passed between the stomach and the

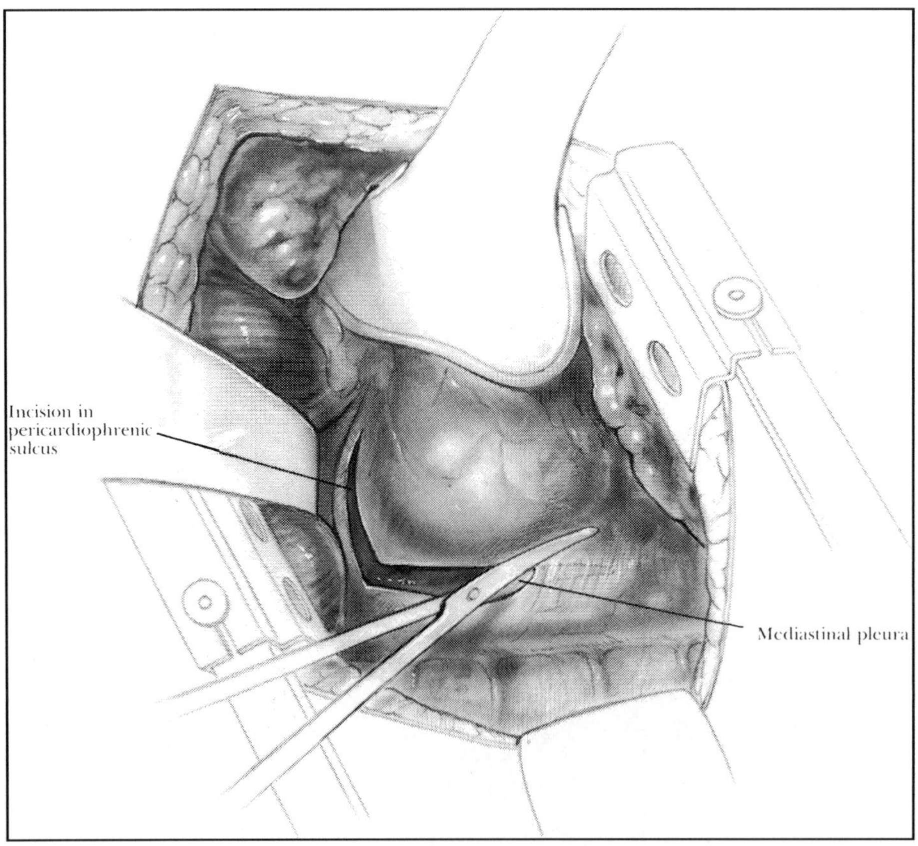

Fig. 9-6

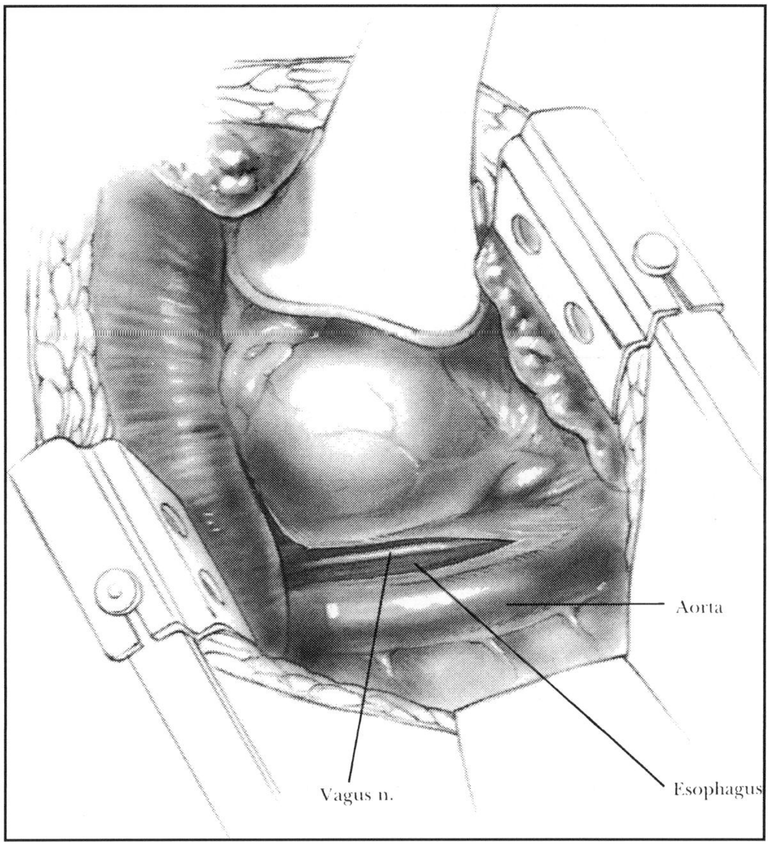

Fig. 9-7

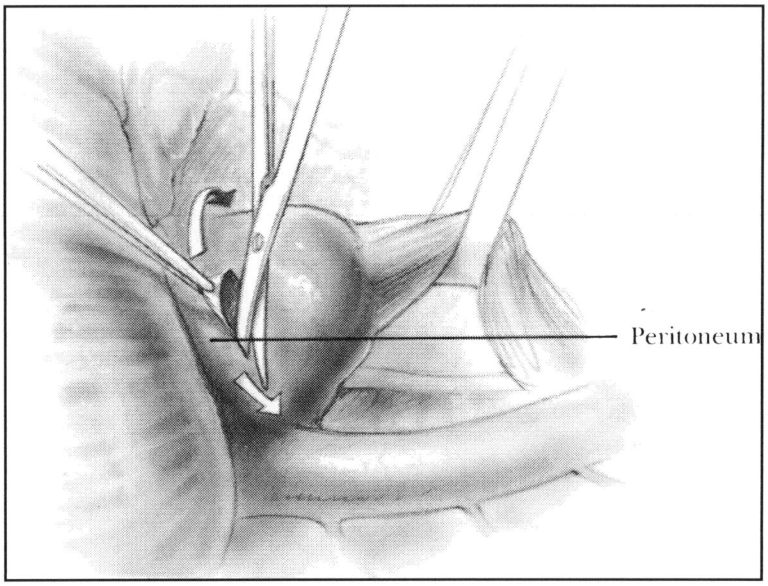

Fig. 9-8

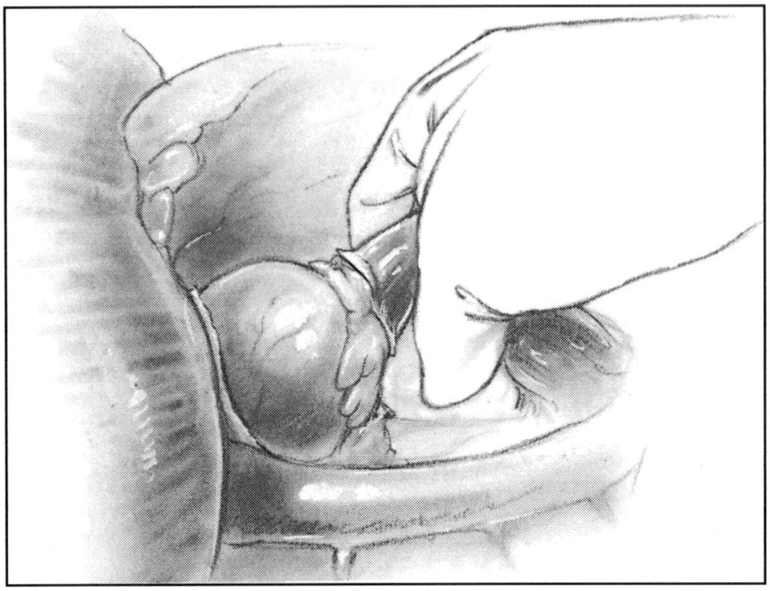

Fig. 9–9

gastrohepatic ligament, delivering the ligament into the chest, deep to the stomach. Identify the artery and ligate it proximally and distally with 2-0 silk. Divide it between the two ligatures **(Fig. 9–10)**. After this step, it should be possible to pass the index finger around the entire circumference of the proximal stomach and encounter no attachments between the stomach and the hiatus. Throughout these maneuvers, repeatedly check on the location of the vagus nerves and preserve them. Excise the peritoneum that constituted the hernial sac.

Dilating an Esophageal Stricture

Ascertain that the esophagus is lying in a straight line in the mediastinum. Ask the anesthesiologist or a surgical assistant to pass Maloney dilators into the esophagus through the mouth after removing the indwelling nasogastric tube. As the dilator is passed down the esophagus, guide it manually into the lumen of the stricture. Successively larger bougies are passed, up to size 50–60F, which can be successfully accomplished in probably 95% of cases. Occasionally, forceful dilata-

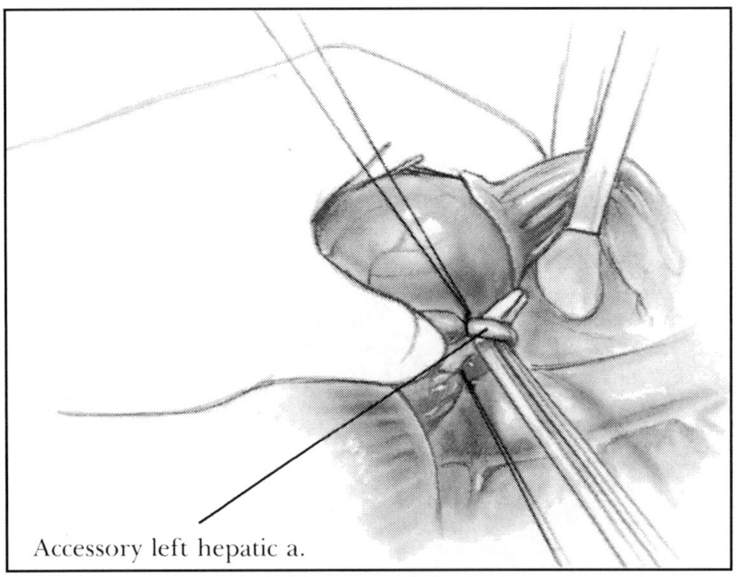

Fig. 9–10

tion of this type causes the lower esophagus to burst in the presence of unyielding transmural fibrosis. In this case, resect the damaged esophagus and perform a colonic or jejunal interposition between the healthy esophagus and the stomach (see Chapter 5).

Dividing the Short Gastric Vessels

Continue the dissection along the greater curvature of the stomach in an inferior direction until the first short gastric vessel is encountered. Use a long right-angled Mixter clamp to encircle this vessel with two 2-0 silk ligatures. Tie each ligature, leaving at least 1 cm between them. Divide between ligatures. Continue this process until about five proximal short gastric vessels have been divided and about 12–15 cm of greater curvature has been mobilized.

Gastroplasty

Verify that the esophagogastric junction has indeed been completely mobilized. Identify the point at which the greater curvature of the stomach meets the esophagus. Overlying this area is a thin fat pad perhaps 3 cm in diameter. Carefully dissect this fat pad away from the serosa of the stomach and the longitudinal muscle of the esophagus **(Fig. 9–11)**. Avoid damaging the anterior vagus nerve.

Pass a 56–60F Maloney dilator into the stomach and position it along the lesser curvature. Then apply

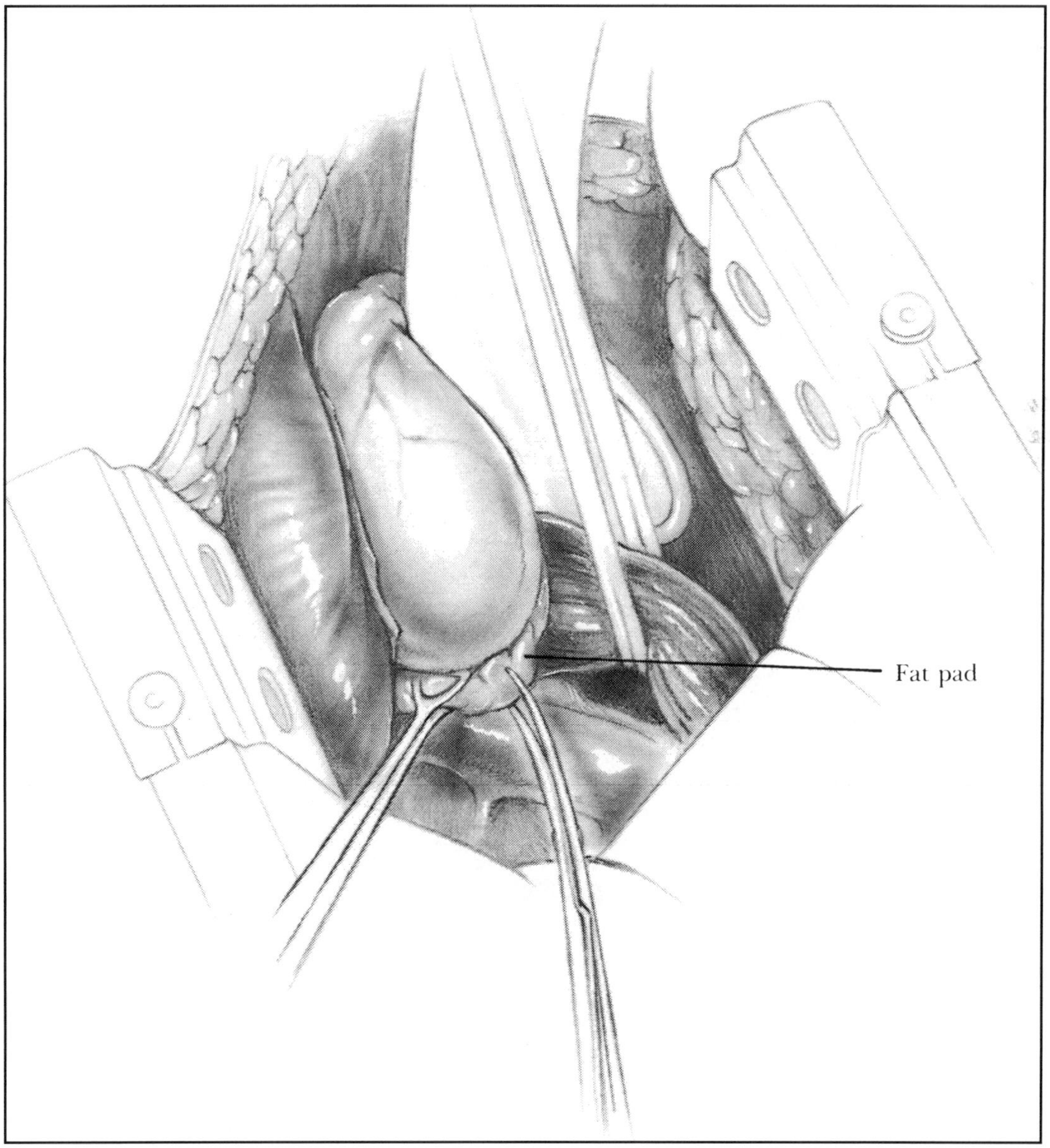

Fig. 9–11

an 80 mm linear cutting stapler parallel and closely adjacent to the Maloney dilator; a Babcock clamp retracts the greater curvature of the stomach in a lateral direction **(Fig. 9–12)**. Fire the stapler and remove it. Verify that the staples have been shaped into an adequate B and that there are no leaks. Lightly electrocoagulate the everted mucosa. This maneuver will have lengthened the esophagus by approximately 6–7 cm **(Fig. 9–13)**. In most cases no additional length of neoesophagus is necessary because of the greater lengths now available in these stapling devices. Although this step is not shown here, it is wise as a precautionary measure to oversew the staple lines with two continuous Lembert sutures of 4-0 Prolene or PDS: one continuous suture to invert the staple line along the neoesophagus and a second continuous suture to invert the staple line along the gastric fundus. A continuous suture of the Lembert type is suitable, taking care not to turn in an excessive amount of tissue, as it would narrow the neoesophagus unnecessarily.

Performing a Modified Nissen Fundoplication

Because the neoesophagus has utilized a portion of the gastric fundus, there may not be sufficient remaining stomach to perform the Nissen fundoplication in the classic manner. Instead, as seen in **Figure 9–14**, the apex of the gastric fundus is wrapped around the neoesophagus in a counter-clockwise fashion.

Before inserting any sutures, remove the indwelling large Maloney dilator and replace it with one of 50F. Place a large hemostatic clip at the site of the new esophagogastric junction (i.e., the junction of the neoesophagus with the stomach) as a radiographic marker. The fundoplication should encircle the neoesophagus in a loose wrap for a distance of 3 cm **(Fig. 9–15)**.

Figure 9–15 illustrates insertion of the first Nissen fundoplication stitch including a 5- to 6-mm bite of gastric wall, then a bite of the neoesophagus, and finally a bite of the opposite wall of the gastric fundus.

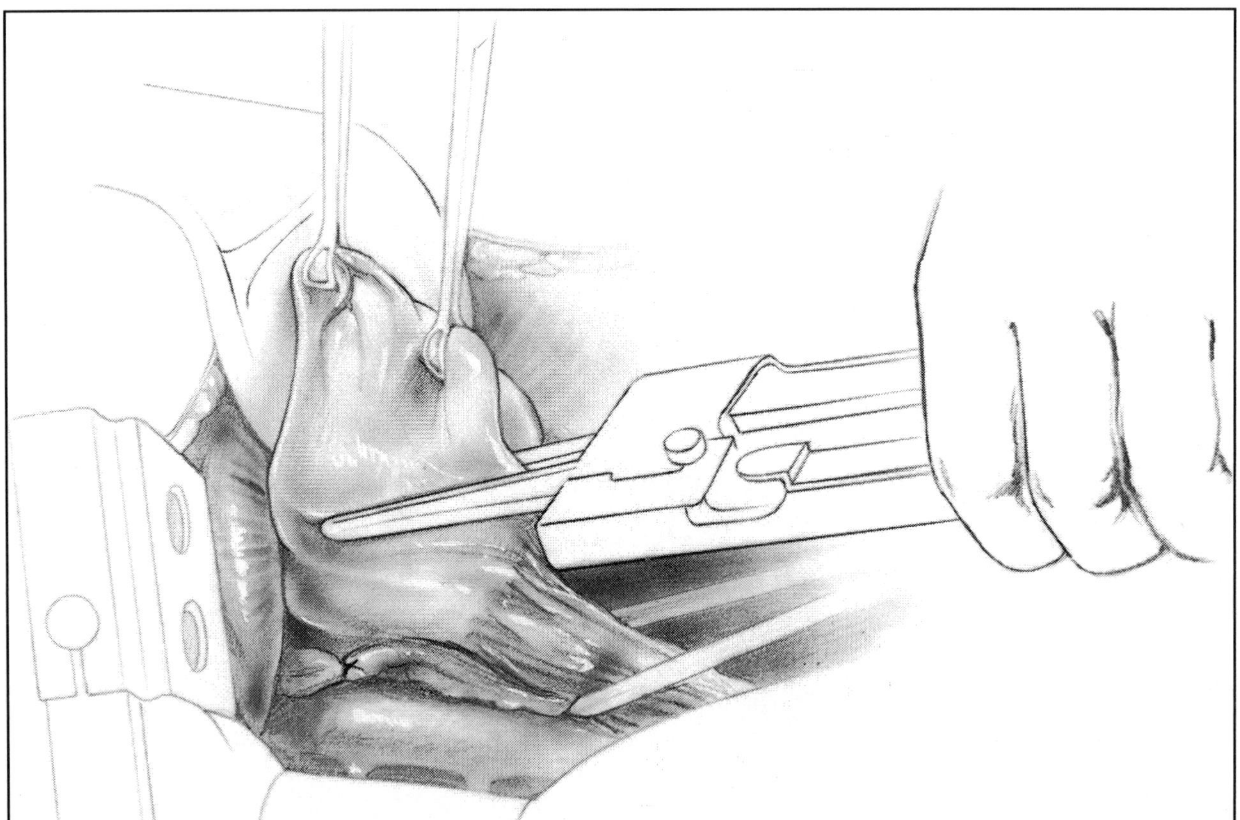

Fig. 9–12

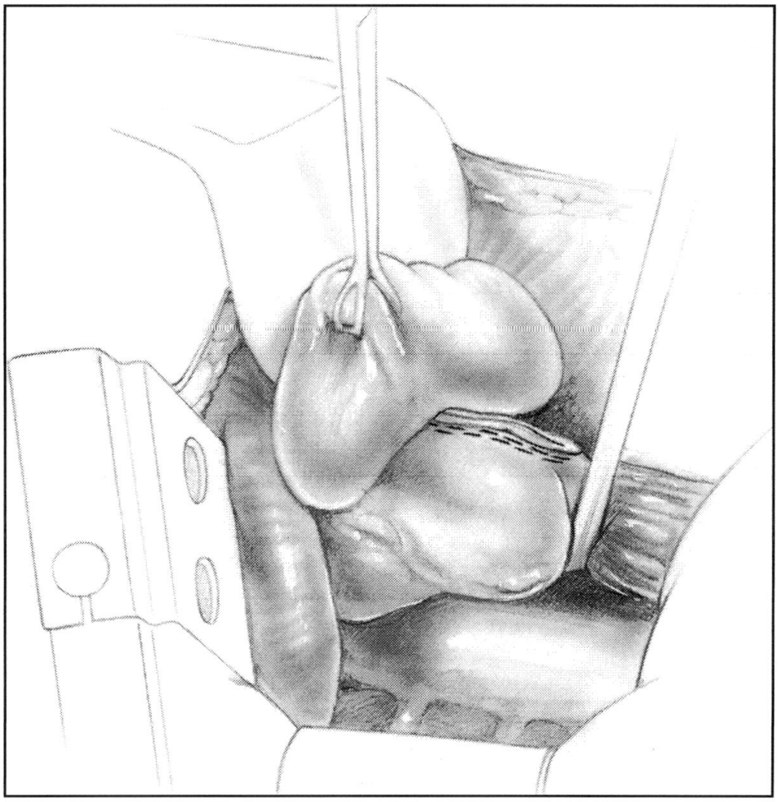

Fig. 9–13

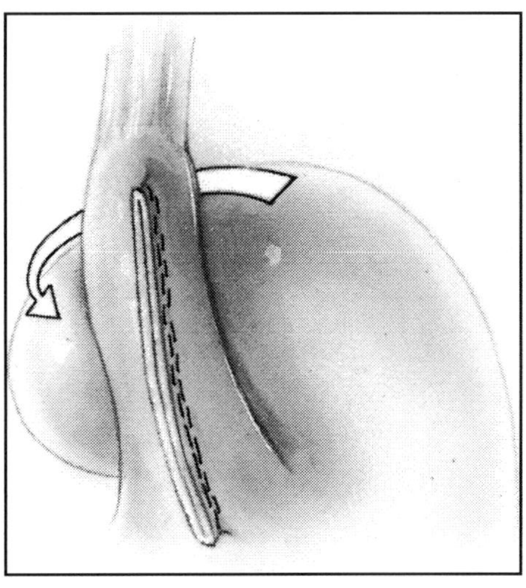

Fig. 9–14

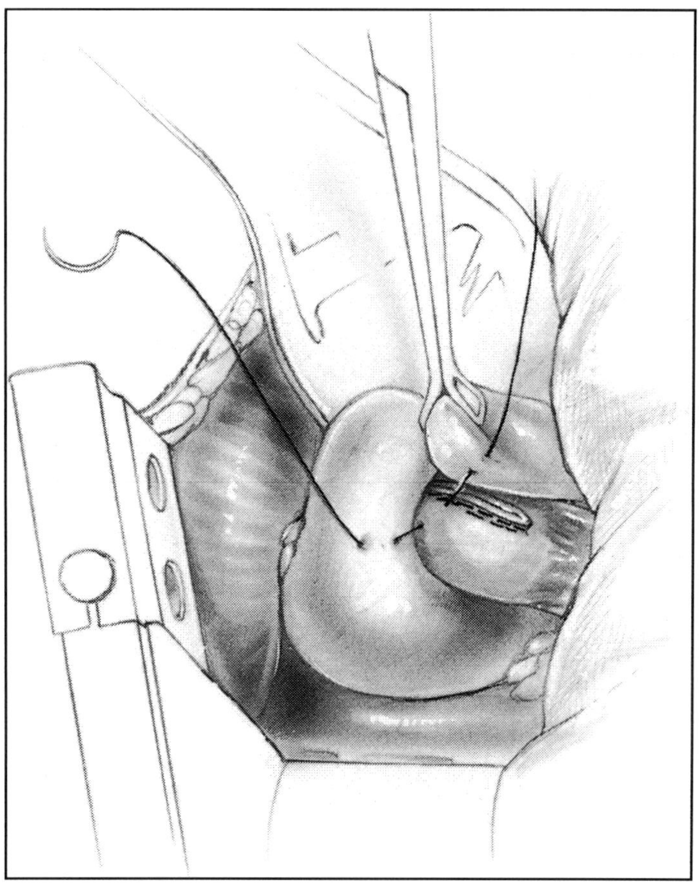

Fig. 9–15

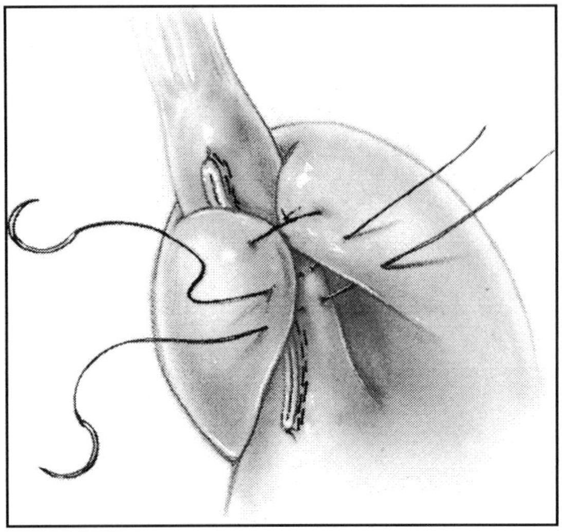

Fig. 9-16

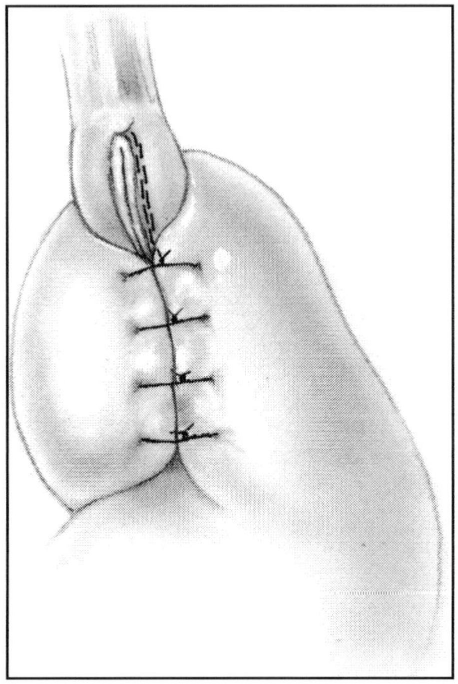

Fig. 9-17

These bites should be deep to the submucosa but not into the lumen of the stomach. We prefer 2-0 Tevdek for these sutures. A total of three or four fundoplication sutures are used at 1 cm intervals **(Figs. 9–16, 9–17)**. Now remove the Maloney dilator from the esophagus and replace it with a nasogastric tube. **Figure 9–18** illustrates that the fundoplication wrap around the neoesophagus is loose enough to admit the fingertip. Optionally, invert the layer of fundoplication sutures by oversewing it with a continuous Lembert seromuscular suture of 4-0 Prolene (not illustrated).

Closing the Hiatal Defect

Close the defect in the posterior portion of the hiatus by inserting 0 Tevdek interrupted sutures through the right and left margins of the hiatus. Take a bite 1.5–2.0 cm in width and include overlying parietal pleura. After checking for hemostasis, reduce the fundoplication into the abdomen. It should slide down with ease. Then tie each of the sutures, leaving space for the surgeon's fingertip alongside the esophagus or neoesophagus with a nasogastric tube in place **(Figs. 9–19, 9–20)**. Place a hemostatic clip at the edge of the hiatus as a marker. It is not necessary to resuture the incision in the mediastinal pleura.

Irrigate the mediastinum and thoracic cavity with warm saline and check for complete hemostasis. Insert a 36F chest tube through a puncture wound below the level of the incision and bring the tube up the posterior gutter above the hilus of the lung. Insert three to five interrupted no. 2 PDS pericostal sutures and tie them to approximate the ribs. Close the overlying serratus and latissimus muscles in two layers with 2-0 PG continuous sutures. Close the skin with continuous or interrupted fine nylon sutures.

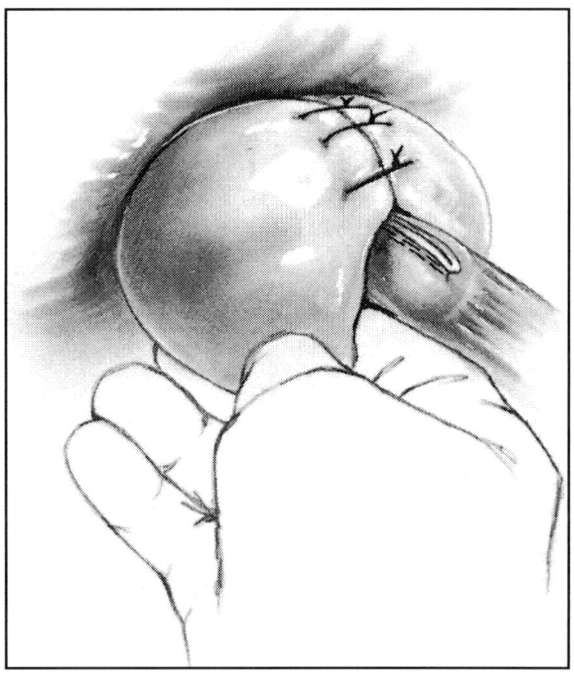

Fig. 9-18

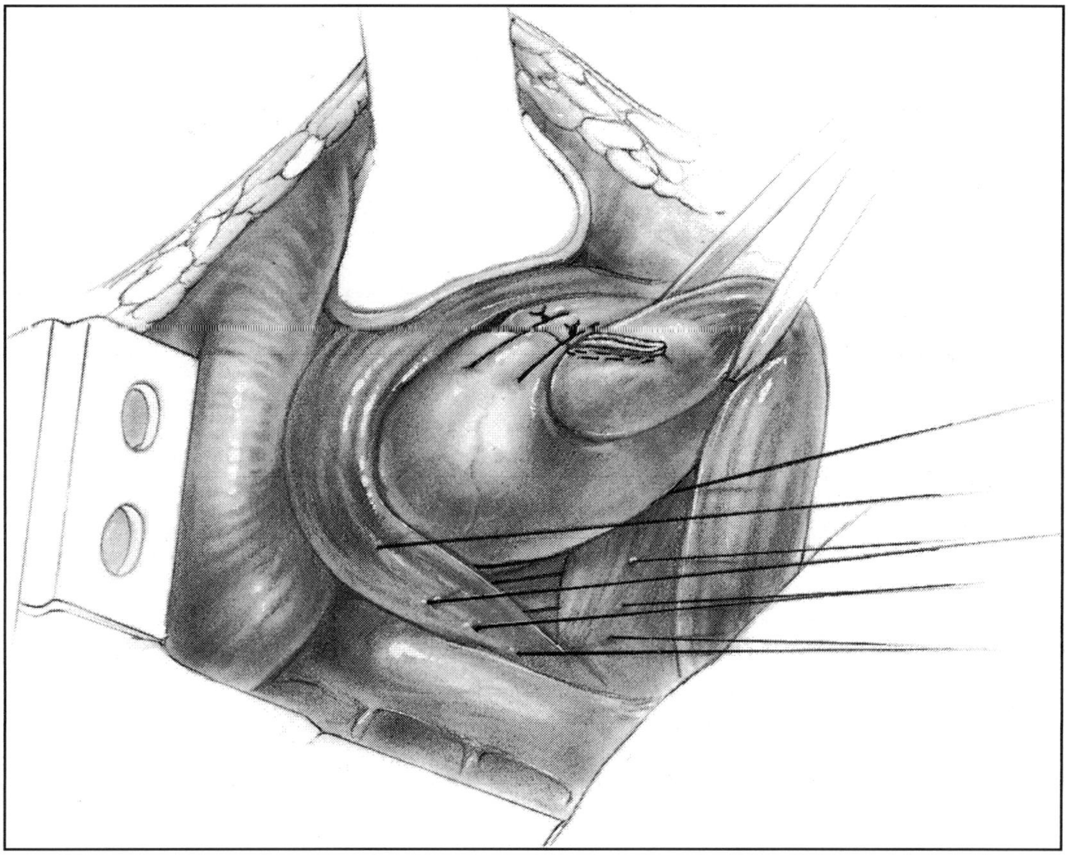

Fig. 9–19

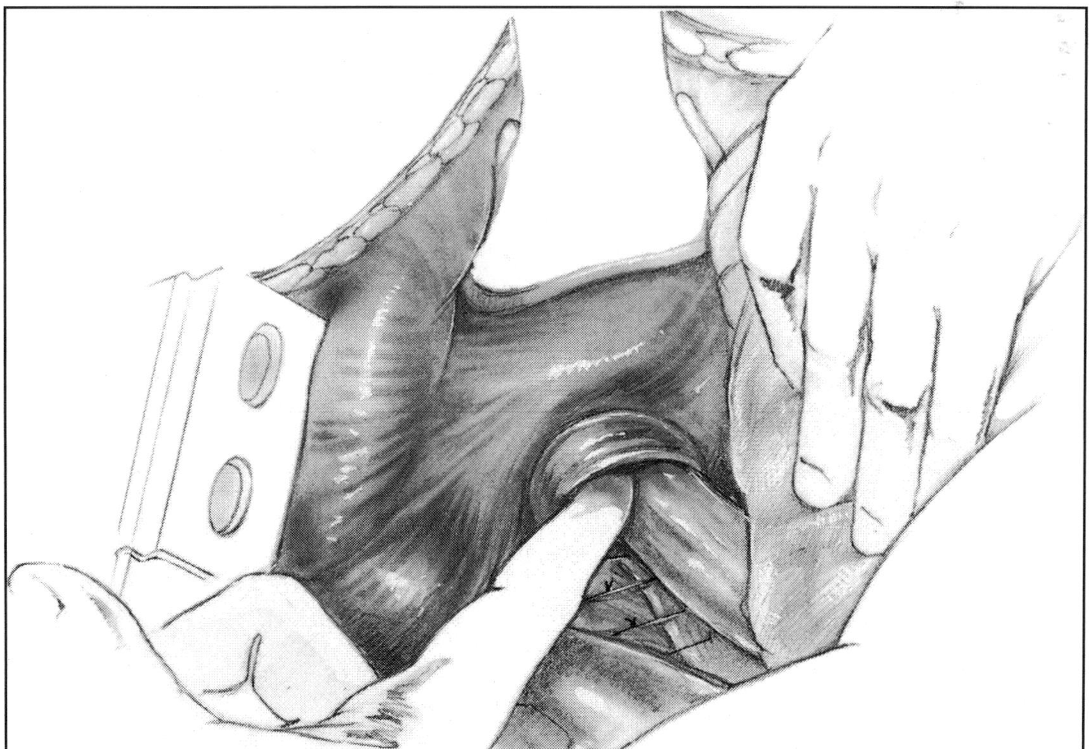

Fig. 9–20

POSTOPERATIVE CARE

Continue nasogastric suction for 1-3 days.

Continue perioperative antibiotics for 24 hours.

Obtain an esophagram (first water-soluble then thin barium) on postoperative day 7.

Remove the chest drainage tube on day 3 unless drainage is excessive.

COMPLICATIONS

Obstruction. Occasionally there is a partial obstruction at the area of the fundoplication due to edema during the first 2 weeks following surgery. If the wrap is too tight, this obstruction may persist.

Recurrent gastroesophageal reflux. This is uncommon after the Collis-Nissen procedure unless the fundoplication suture line disrupts.

Leakage from the gastroplasty or fundoplication sutures. This complication is rare. If the fundoplication sutures are inserted into the lumen of the stomach and the suture is tied with strangulating force, a leak is possible. The risk of this occurring may be reduced by oversewing the fundoplication suture line with a continuous Lembert seromuscular suture.

Necrosis of the gastroplasty tube. This complication was reported by Orringer and Orringer during an operation for recurrent hiatus hernia. They warned that traumatizing the lesser curve of the stomach may doom a gastroplasty tube.

REFERENCES

Gastal OL, Hagan JA, Peters JH, et al. Short esophagus: analysis of predictors and clinical implications. Arch Surg 1999;134:633.

Jobe BA, Horvath KD, Swanstrom LL. Postoperative function following laparoscopic Collis gastroplasty for shortened esophagus. Arch Surg 1998;133:867.

Orringer MB, Orringer JS. The combined Collis-Nissen operation: early assessment of reflux control. Ann Thorac Surg 1982;33:534.

Stirling MC, Orringer MB. Continued assessment of the combined Collis-Nissen operation. Ann Thorac Surg 1989;47:224.

Urschel HC, Razzuk MA, Wood RE, et al. An improved surgical technique for the complicated hiatal hernia with gastroesophageal reflux. Ann Thorac Surg 1973;15:443.

10 Bile Diverting Operations for Management of Esophageal Disease

INDICATIONS

Disabling bile reflux symptoms after esophageal surgery

PREOPERATIVE PREPARATION

Confirm bile reflux by visual inspection at endoscopy, radionuclide scan, or 24-hour pH monitoring.

Insert a nasogastric tube.

PITFALLS AND DANGER POINTS

Injury to liver, pancreas, or stomach

Damaging blood supply to residual gastric pouch

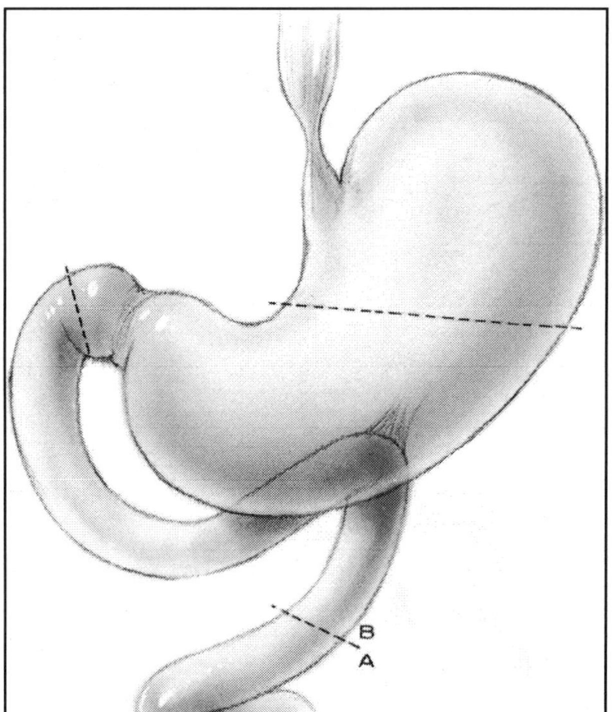

Fig. 10-1

OPERATIVE STRATEGY

Bile Diversion after Failed Antireflux Procedures

Bile diversion is considered only after multiple failed antireflux procedures. Generally vagotomy and antrectomy with bile diversion via a Roux-en-Y reconstruction **(Figs. 10–1, 10–2)** is the procedure of choice. If transabdominal vagotomy does not appear feasible because of excessive scar tissue around the abdominal esophagus, transthoracic or thoracoscopic vagotomy is an alternative.

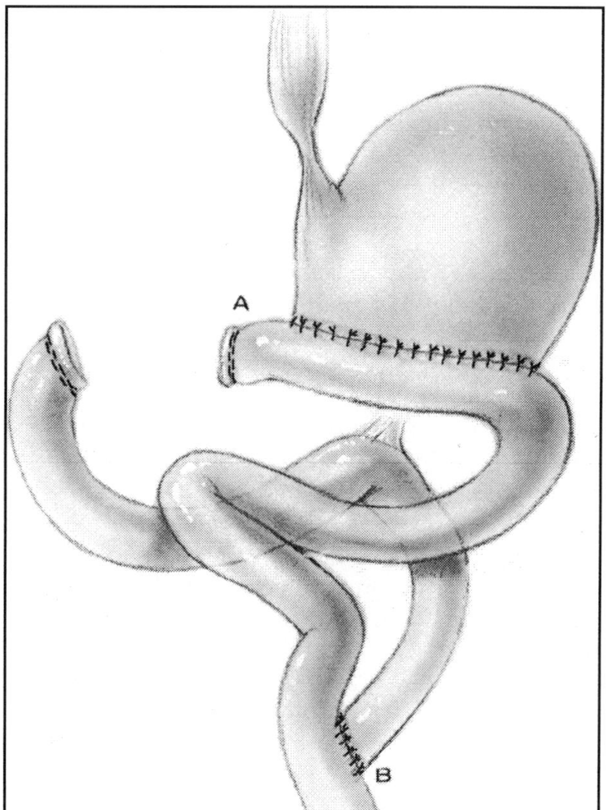

Fig. 10-2

Bile Diversion after Esophagogastrectomy

Bile diversion after esophagogastrectomy is used when bile reflux complicates otherwise successful esophageal resection with esophagogastrectomy. Perform the dissection with extreme care to avoid traumatizing the blood supply to the residual stomach. Generally, the gastric remnant is supplied only by the right gastric and right gastroepiploic vessels. A variation of this procedure, the duodenal switch procedure, is also illustrated.

OPERATIVE TECHNIQUE

Vagotomy and Antrectomy with Bile Diversion

Incision and Exposure

Ordinarily a long midline incision from the xiphoid to a point about 5 cm below the umbilicus is adequate for this operation. Divide the many adhesions and expose the stomach. Evaluate the difficulty of performing a hemigastrectomy, rather than other available operations. Insert an Upper Hand or Thompson retractor and determine if a transabdominal vagotomy is feasible.

Vagotomy

If dissecting the area of the esophagogastric junction appears too formidable a task, thoracoscopic or transthoracic vagotomy is an option.

Hemigastrectomy

Close the duodenal stump by stapling or suturing.

Roux-en-Y Gastrojejunostomy

Create a Roux-en-Y limb of jejunum and then perform an end-to-side gastrojejunostomy using sutures or staples. Position this anastomosis so it sits about 1 cm proximal to the stapled closed end of the jejunum. Complete construction of the Roux-en-Y segment by anastomosing the proximal cut end of the jejunum near the ligament of Treitz to the side of the descending segment of jejunum at a point 60 cm distal to the gastrojejunostomy. Close the defect in the jejunal mesentery with interrupted sutures.

Closure

Close the abdominal wall without drainage in the usual fashion.

Bile Diversion Following Esophagogastrectomy

Incision and Exposure

Make a midline incision from the xiphoid to a point somewhat below the umbilicus. Divide the various adhesions subsequent to prior surgery and expose the pyloroduodenal region. Because of the previous surgery (esophagogastrectomy) **(Fig. 10–3)** this area is now located 5–8 cm from the diaphragmatic hiatus.

Dividing the Duodenum, Duodenojejunostomy, Roux-en-Y Reconstruction

Divide the duodenum at a point 2–3 cm beyond the pylorus. Be careful not to injure the right gastric or right gastroepiploic vessels, as they constitute the entire blood supply of the residual gastric pouch. To divide the duodenum, first free the posterior wall of the duodenum from the pancreas for a short distance. If possible, pass one jaw of a 55/3.5 mm linear stapler behind the duodenum, close the device, and fire the stapler. Then divide the duodenum flush with the stapling device. Lightly cauterize the everted mucosa

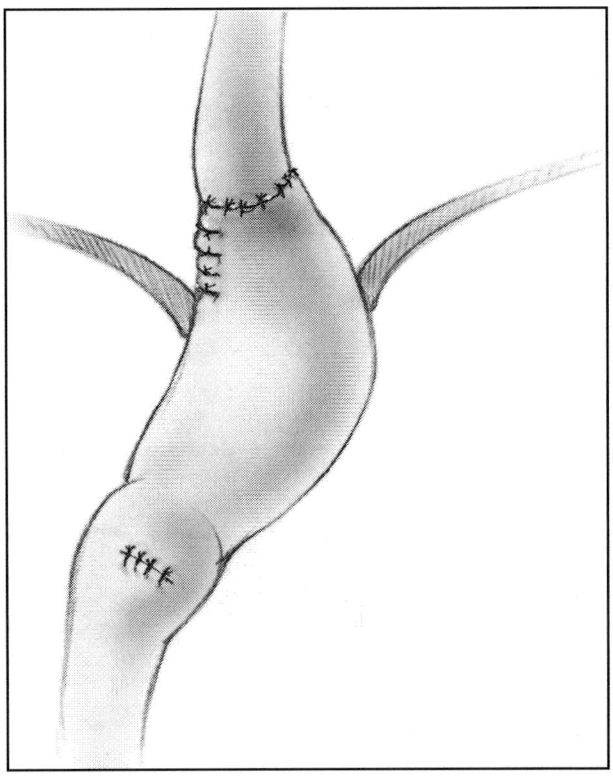

Fig. 10-3

and remove the stapler, which leaves the proximal duodenum open. Leave 1 cm of the posterior wall of the duodenum free (**Fig. 10–4**, point A) to construct an anastomosis with the jejunum.

Develop a Roux-en-Y limb of jejunum then bring the open distal end of the divided jejunum (Fig. 10–4, point D) to the level of the duodenum. Generally it most comfortably assumes an antecolic position, but occasionally it is feasible to bring it through an incision in the mesocolon (retrocolic).

Establish an end-to-end duodenojejunostomy (**Fig. 10–5**, point A to point D) utilizing one layer of interrupted 4-0 silk for the seromuscular layer and continuous or interrupted sutures of atraumatic 5-0 PG for the mucosal layers.

Complete the construction of the Roux-en-Y segment by creating an end-to-side jejunojejunostomy at a point 60 cm distal to the duodenojejunostomy. Close the defect in the jejunal mesentery with interrupted sutures.

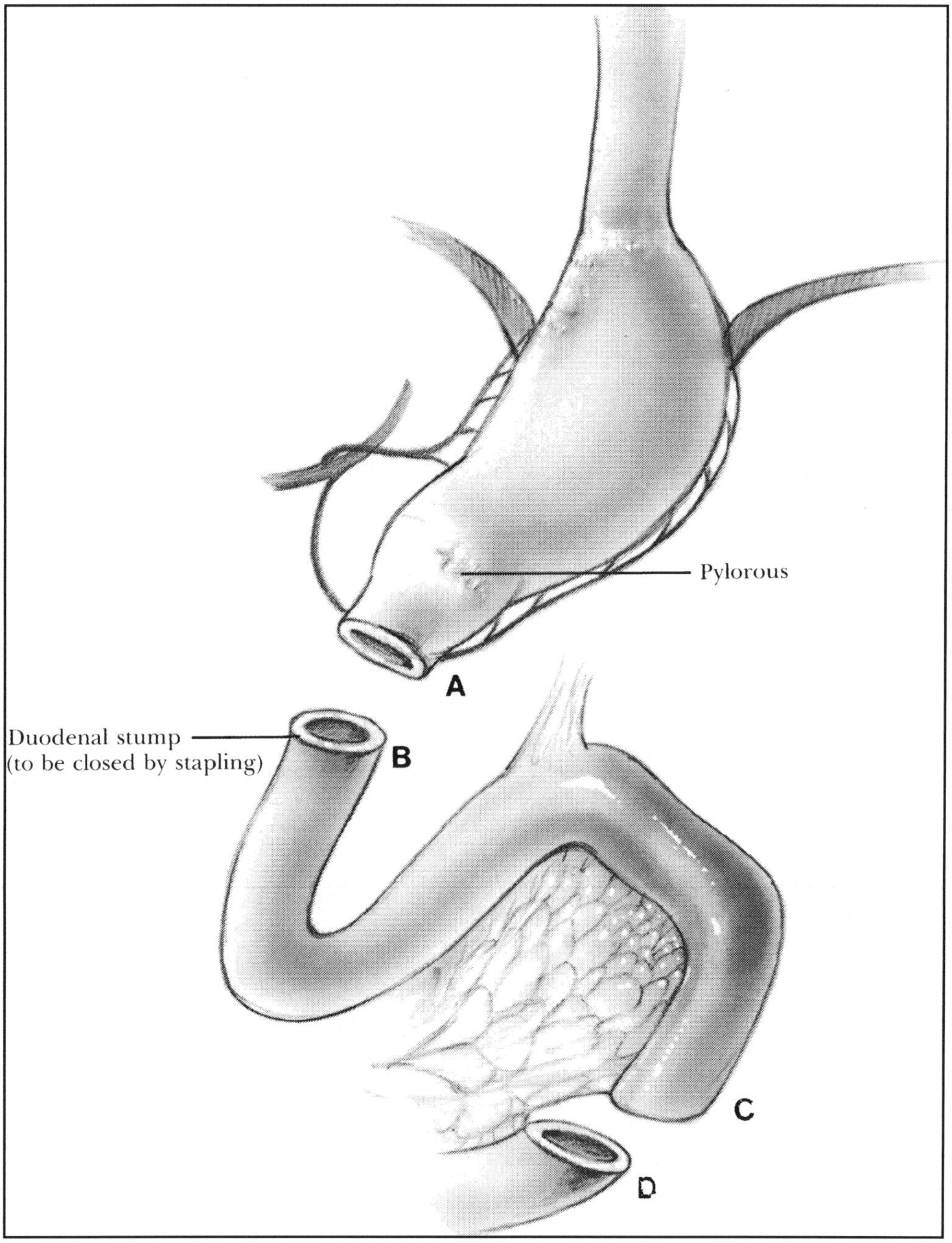

Fig. 10–4

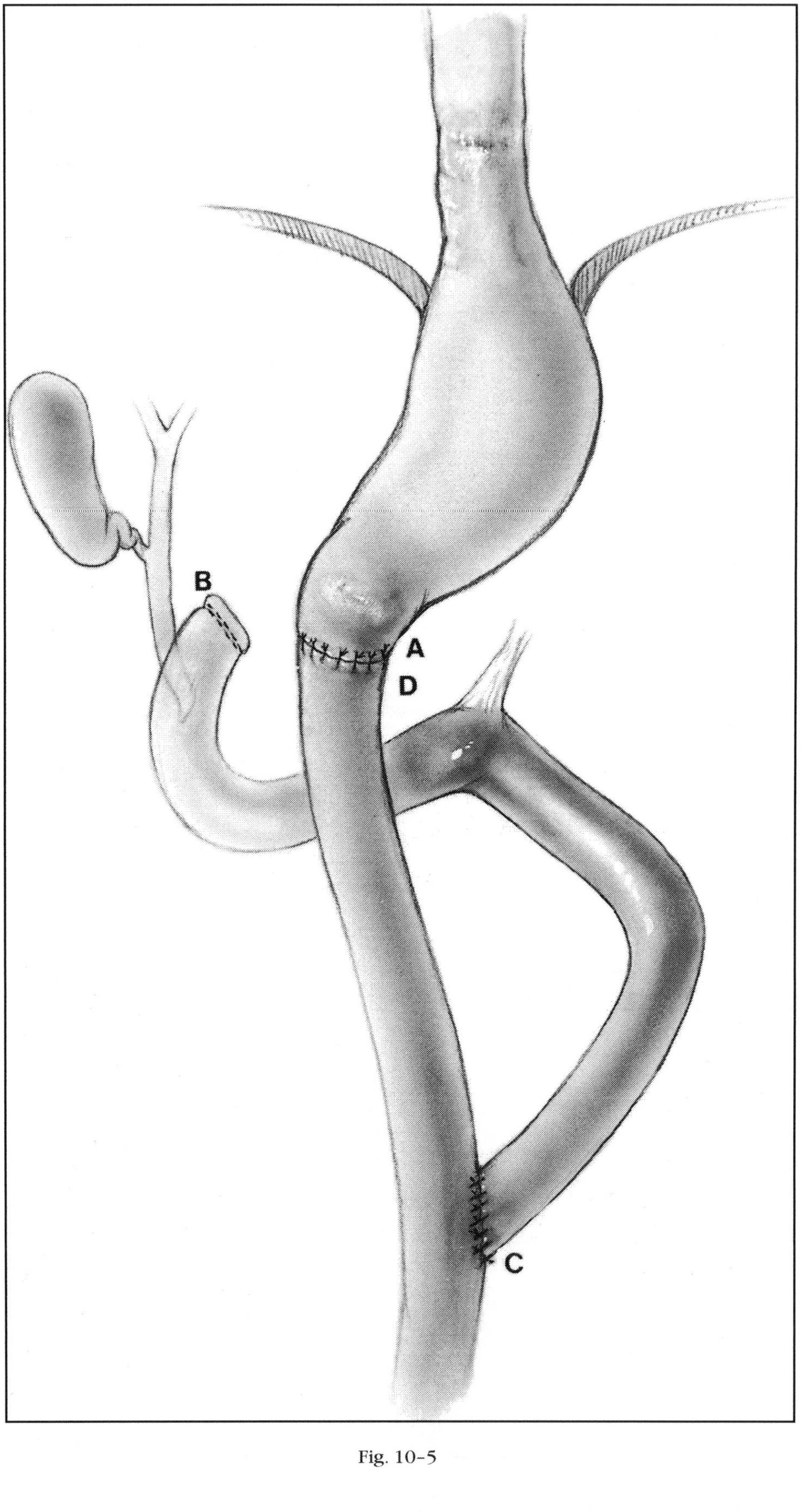

Fig. 10-5

Bile Diversion by Duodenojejunostomy Roux-en-Y Switch Operation

Incision and Exposure

Make a midline incision from the xiphoid to a point about 3–4 cm below the umbilicus.

Duodenojejunostomy

Perform a thorough Kocher maneuver, freeing the head of the pancreas and duodenum anteriorly and posteriorly. Place a marking suture on the anterior wall of the duodenum precisely 3 cm distal to the pylorus. This represents the probable point at which the duodenum will be transected. Now approach the point at which the duodenum and pancreas meet. Divide and carefully ligate the numerous small vessels emerging from the area of the pancreas and entering the duodenum on both anterior and posterior surfaces until a 2 cm area of the posterior wall of duodenum has been cleared. Do not dissect the proximal 2–3 cm of duodenum from its attachment to the pancreas. Dissecting the next 2 cm of duodenum free of the pancreas provides enough length to allow stapled closure of the duodenal stump and a duodenojejunal end-to-end anastomosis. Be careful not to injure the pancreatic segment of the distal common bile duct or the duct of Santorini, which enters the duodenum at a point about 2 cm proximal to the papilla of Vater.

After this step has been completed, make a 2 cm transverse incision across the anterior wall of the duodenum near the marking suture **(Fig. 10–6)**.

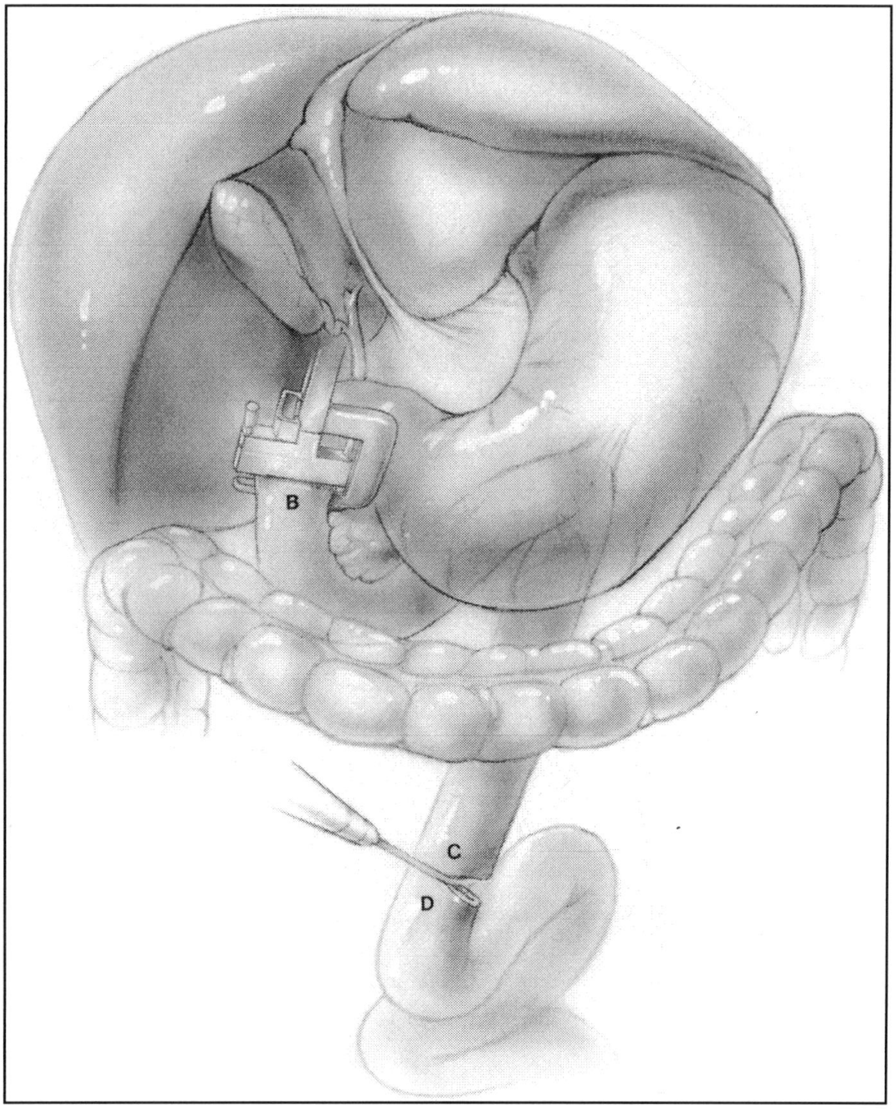

Fig. 10–6

Insert an index finger and palpate the ampulla. Confirm its location by compressing the gallbladder and liver, observing the influx of bile into the distal duodenum. Now use a 55/3.5 mm linear stapler to occlude the duodenal stump just distal to the marking suture. Complete the transection of the duodenum after the stapler has been fired by cutting along the stapling device with a scalpel, cauterize the mucosa and check the staple line in the usual fashion.

At a point 20 cm distal to the ligament of Treitz, transect the jejunum and incise its mesentery down to, but not across, the arcade vessel (**Fig. 10–7**, C and D). Limiting the incision in the mesentery to 3 cm helps preserve the innervation of the intestinal pacemaker in the upper jejunal mesentery. Bring the distal transected end of the jejunum through a small incision in the mesocolon and make an end-to-end anastomosis between the proximal transected duodenum to the jejunum using 4-0 interrupted silk sutures for the seromuscular layer and 5-0 Vicryl sutures for the mucosa (**Fig. 10–8**, A and C). Then perform an end-to-side jejunojejunostomy to the descending limb of jejunum (Fig. 10–8) at a point 60 cm distal to the duodenojejunostomy. Eliminate any defect in the mesocolon or the jejunal mesentery by suturing. Irrigate the abdominal cavity and abdominal wound and close the abdomen in the usual fashion without drainage.

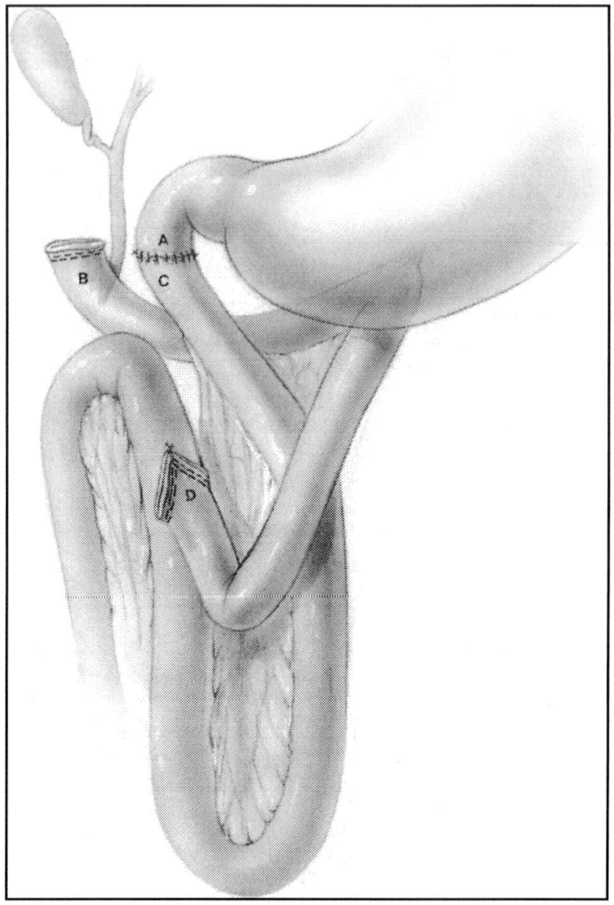

Fig. 10–8

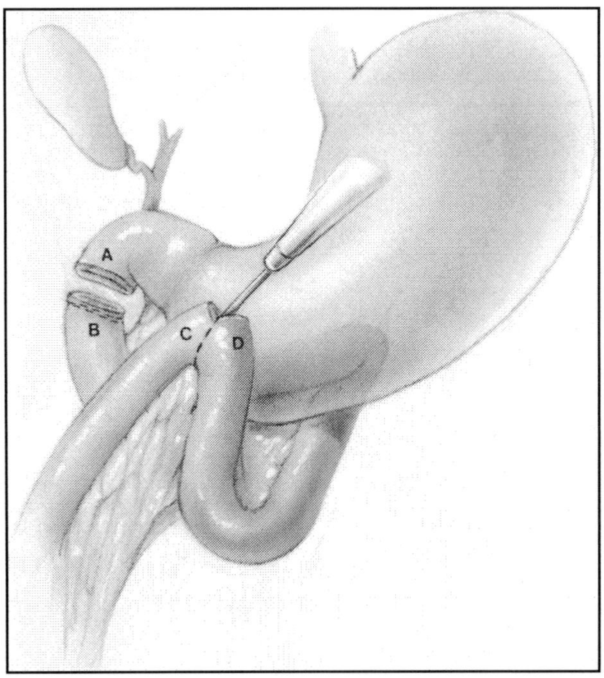

Fig. 10–7

COMPLICATIONS

Intestinal obstruction

Anastomotic leak

REFERENCES

Appleton BN, Beynon J, Harikrishnan AB, Manson JM. Investigation of oesophageal reflux symptoms after gastric surgery with combined pH and bilirubin monitoring. Br J Surg 1999;86:1099.

Critchlow JF, Shapiro ME, Silen W. Duodenojejunostomy for the pancreaticobiliary complications of duodenal diverticulum. Ann Surg 1985;202:56.

DeLangen ZL, Slooff MJ, Jansen W. The surgical treatment of postgastrectomy reflux gastritis. Surg Gynecol Obstet 1984;158:322.

DeMeester TR, Fuchs KH, Ball CS, et al. Experimental and clinical results with proximal end-to-end duodenojejunostomy for pathological duodenogastric reflux. Ann Surg 1987;206:414.

Mason RJ, DeMeester TR. Importance of duodenogastric reflux in the surgical outpatient practice. Hepatogastroenterology 1999;46:48.

Oberg S, Peters JH, DeMeester TR, et al. Determinants of intestinal metaplasia within the columnar-lined esophagus. Arch Surg 2000;135:651.

Oberg S, Ritter MP, Crookes PF, et al. Gastroesophageal reflux disease and mucosal injury with emphasis on short-segment Barrett's esophagus and duodenogastroesophageal reflux. J Gastrointest Surg 1998;2:547.

Smith J, Payne WS. Surgical technique for management of reflux esophagitis after esophagogastrectomy for malignancy: further application of Roux-en-Y principle. Mayo Clin Proc 1975;50:588.

Stein HJ, Barlow AP, DeMeester TR, et al. Complications of gastroesophageal reflux disease: role of the lower esophageal sphincter, esophageal acid and acid/alkaline exposure, and duodenogastric reflux. Ann Surg 1992; 216:35.

11 Cricopharyngeal Myotomy and Operation for Pharyngoesophageal (Zenker's) Diverticulum

INDICATIONS

Symptomatic Zenker's diverticulum

PREOPERATIVE PREPARATION

Perioperative antibiotics

OPERATIVE STRATEGY

Adequate Myotomy

Performing a cricopharyngeal myotomy is similar to performing a cardiomyotomy. The physiologic upper esophageal sphincter is considerably wider than the anatomic cricopharyngeus muscle. The transverse muscle fibers are only about 2.0–2.5 cm wide, whereas the high pressure zone corresponding to the cricopharyngeus area can be 4 cm wide. Consequently, a proper cricopharyngeal myotomy should not only transect all of the transverse fibers of the cricopharyngeus muscle but also 1–2 cm of the proximal esophagus so the myotomy is at least 4 cm long. The incision in the muscle is carried down to the mucosa of the esophagus, which should bulge out through the myotomy after all the muscle fibers have been divided. Additionally, the mucosa is freed from the overlying muscle over the posterior half of the esophagus.

Is Diverticulectomy Necessary?

If the pharyngoesophageal diverticulum is a small diffuse bulge measuring no more than 2–3 cm in diameter, we perform only a myotomy and make no attempt to excise any part of the diverticulum because after the myotomy there is only a gentle bulge of mucosa and no true diverticulum. On the other hand, longer, finger-like projections of mucosa should be amputated because there have been a few case reports of recurrent symptoms due to the persistence of diverticula left behind in patients in whom an otherwise adequate myotomy had been done. Belsey advocated suturing the most dependent point of the diverticulum to the prevertebral fascia in the upper cervical region. This procedure effectively upends the diverticulum so it can drain freely into the esophageal lumen by gravity. We prefer to amputate diverticula larger than 3 cm rather than perform a diverticulopexy. With application of a stapling device, amputation of the diverticulum takes only about 1 minute of additional operating time, and the results have been excellent.

OPERATIVE TECHNIQUE

Incision and Exposure

With the patient's head turned somewhat toward his or her right, make an incision along the anterior border of the left sternomastoid muscle beginning at a point 2–3 cm above the clavicle **(Fig. 11–1)**. Divide the platysma muscle. Electrocoagulate the bleeding points. Free the anterior border of the sternomastoid muscle and retract it laterally, exposing the omohyoid

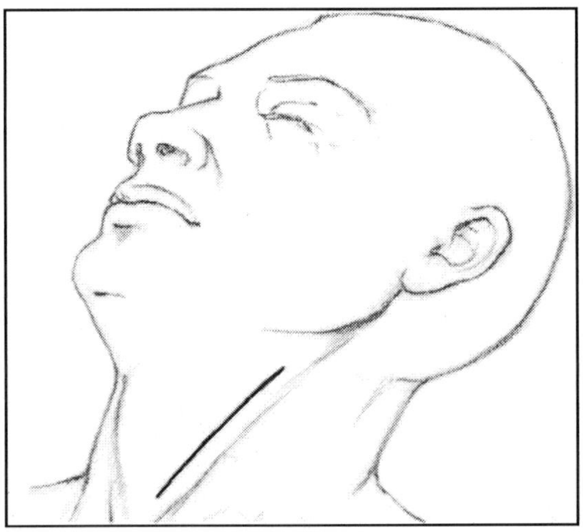

Fig. 11-1

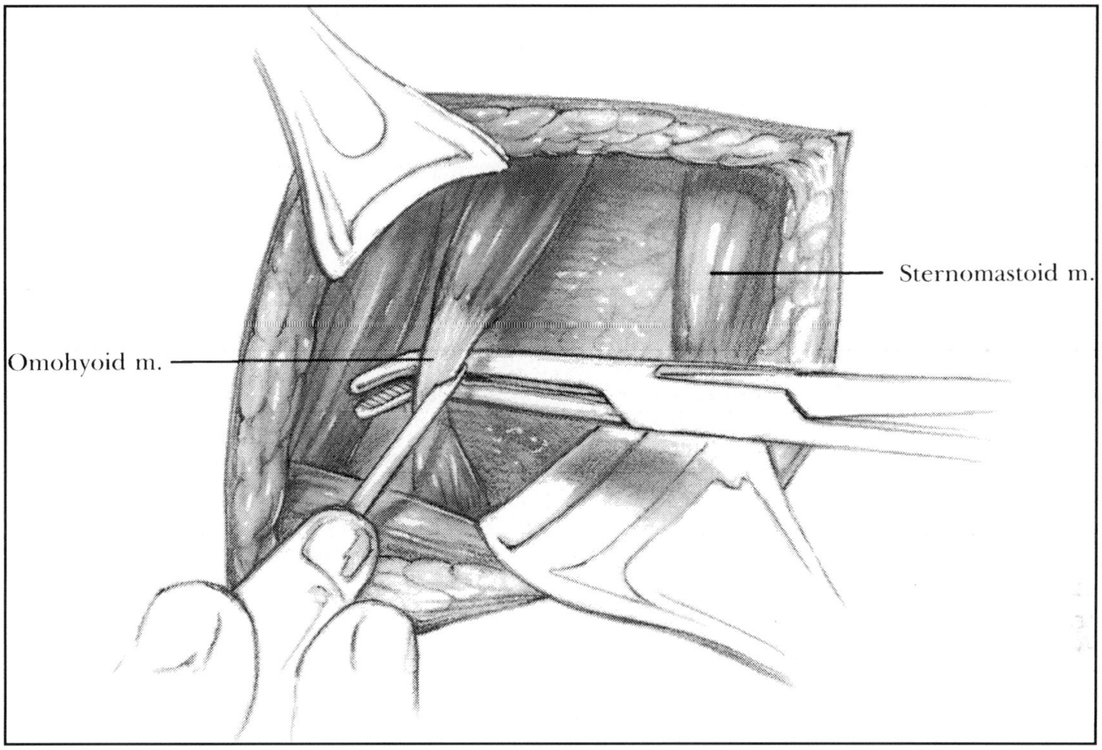

Fig. 11–2

muscle crossing the field from medial to lateral. Transect this muscle **(Fig. 11–2)**. The diverticulum is located deep to the omohyoid muscle. Identify the carotid sheath and the descending hypoglossal nerve and retract these structures laterally. The thyroid gland is seen in the medial portion of the operative field underneath the strap muscles. Retract the thyroid gland and the larynx in a medial direction, revealing in most cases a prominent middle thyroid vein **(Fig. 11–3)**. Ligate and divide this vein.

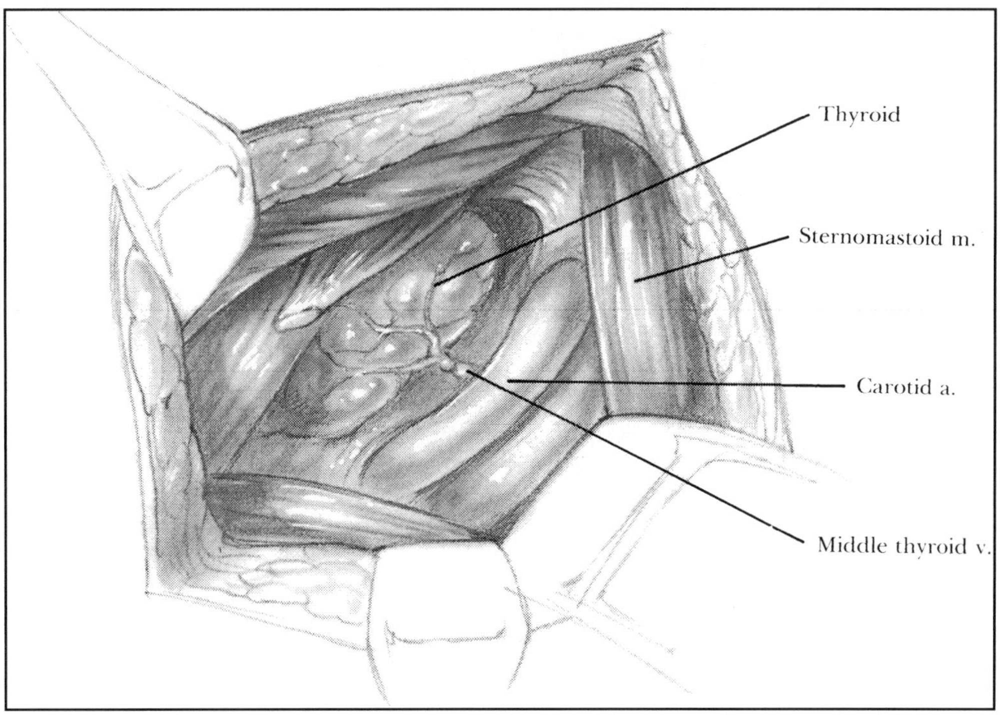

Fig. 11–3

Divide the areolar tissue anterior to the carotid artery and identify the inferior thyroid artery and the recurrent laryngeal nerve. In some patients there appears to be no true left inferior thyroid artery arising from the thyrocervical trunk, in which case the lower thyroid is supplied by branches of the superior thyroid artery. In most patients with the inferior thyroid artery emerging from underneath the carotid artery and crossing the esophagus to supply the lower thyroid, divide and ligate this vessel after identifying the recurrent laryngeal nerve. After this step has been completed, retracting the larynx in an anteromedial direction and the carotid artery laterally exposes the lateral and posterior aspects of the cervical esophagus and the pharyngoesophageal junction. Often it is not necessary to divide the inferior thyroid artery or its branches to develop adequate exposure for diverticulectomy.

Dissecting the Pharyngoesophageal Diverticulum

The pharyngoesophageal diverticulum emerges posteriorly between the pharyngeal constrictor and the cricopharyngeus muscles. Its neck is at the level of the cricoid cartilage, and the dependent portion of the diverticulum descends between the posterior wall of the esophagus and the prevertebral fascia overlying the bodies of the cervical vertebrae. Blunt dissection with the index finger or a peanut sponge generally identifies the most dependent portion of the diverticulum. Grasp it with a Babcock clamp and elevate the diverticulum in a cephalad direction. Mobilize the diverticulum by sharp and blunt dissection down to its neck. If there is any confusion about the anatomy, especially in patients who have undergone previous operations in this area, ask the

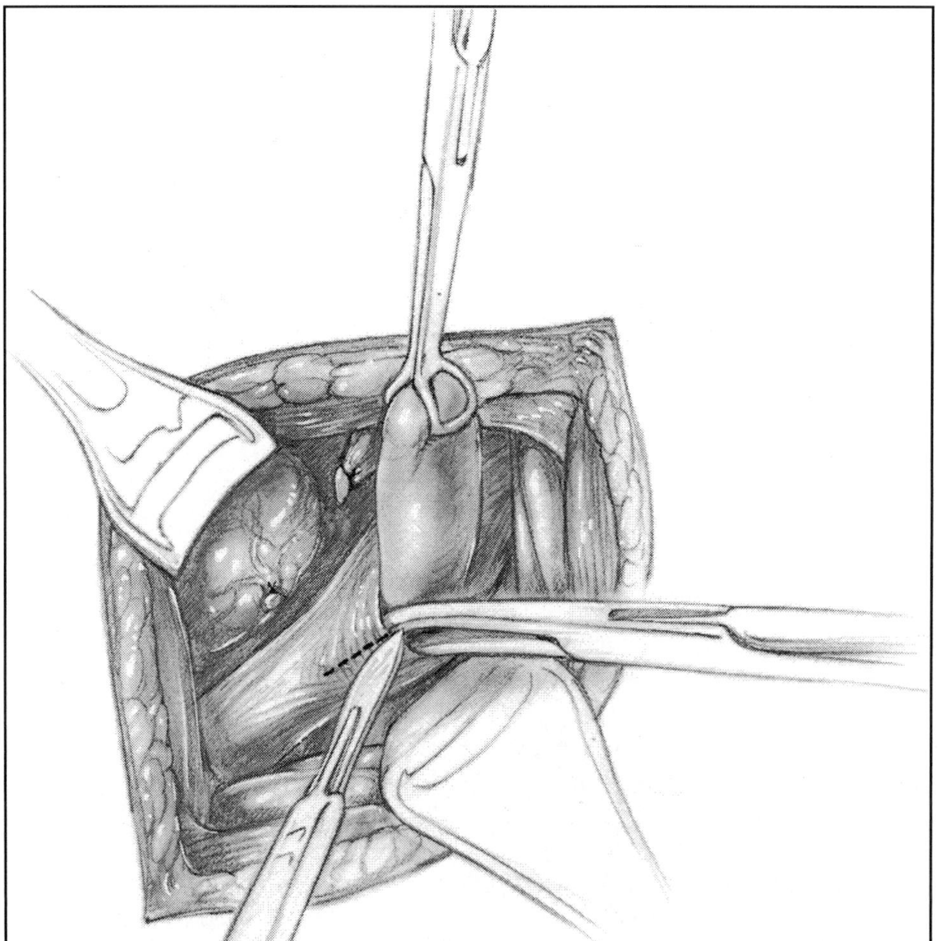

Fig. 11-4

anesthesiologist to pass a 40F Maloney bougie through the mouth into the cervical esophagus. Guide the tip of the bougie past the neck of the diverticulum so it enters the esophagus. The exact location of the junction between the esophagus and the diverticulum can then be identified. There is generally some fibrous tissue overlying the mucosa of the diverticulum. Lightly incise it with a scalpel near the neck of the sac down to the submucosa. At this point the transverse fibers of the cricopharyngeus muscle are easily identified.

Cricopharyngeal and Esophageal Myotomy

Insert a blunt-tipped right-angled hemostat between the mucosa and the transverse fibers of the cricopharyngeus muscle just distal to the neck of the diverticulum **(Fig. 11–4)**. Elevate the hemostat in the posterior midline and incise the fibers of the cricopharyngeus muscle with a scalpel. Continue this dissection down the posterior wall of the esophagus for a total distance of about 5–6 cm. Now elevate the incised muscles of the cricopharyngeus and the upper esophagus from the underlying mucosal layer over the posterior half of the esophageal circumference by blunt dissection.

After the mucosa has been permitted to bulge out through the myotomy, determine whether the diverticulum is large enough to warrant resection. If so, apply a 30- or 55-mm linear stapler with 3.5 mm staples across the neck of the diverticulum **(Fig. 11–5)**. Close the stapler. Fire the staples and amputate the diverticulum flush with the stapling device. The 40F Maloney dilator in the lumen of the esophagus protects against excising too much mucosa and narrowing the lumen. After removing the stapling device, carefully inspect the staple line and the staples for proper closure. Check for complete hemostasis **(Fig. 11–6)**.

An alternative method for performing the myotomy is illustrated in **Figure 11–7**, where the incision is initiated 1.0–1.5 cm cephalad to the cricopharyngeus muscle, in the pharyngeal constrictor muscle. It is

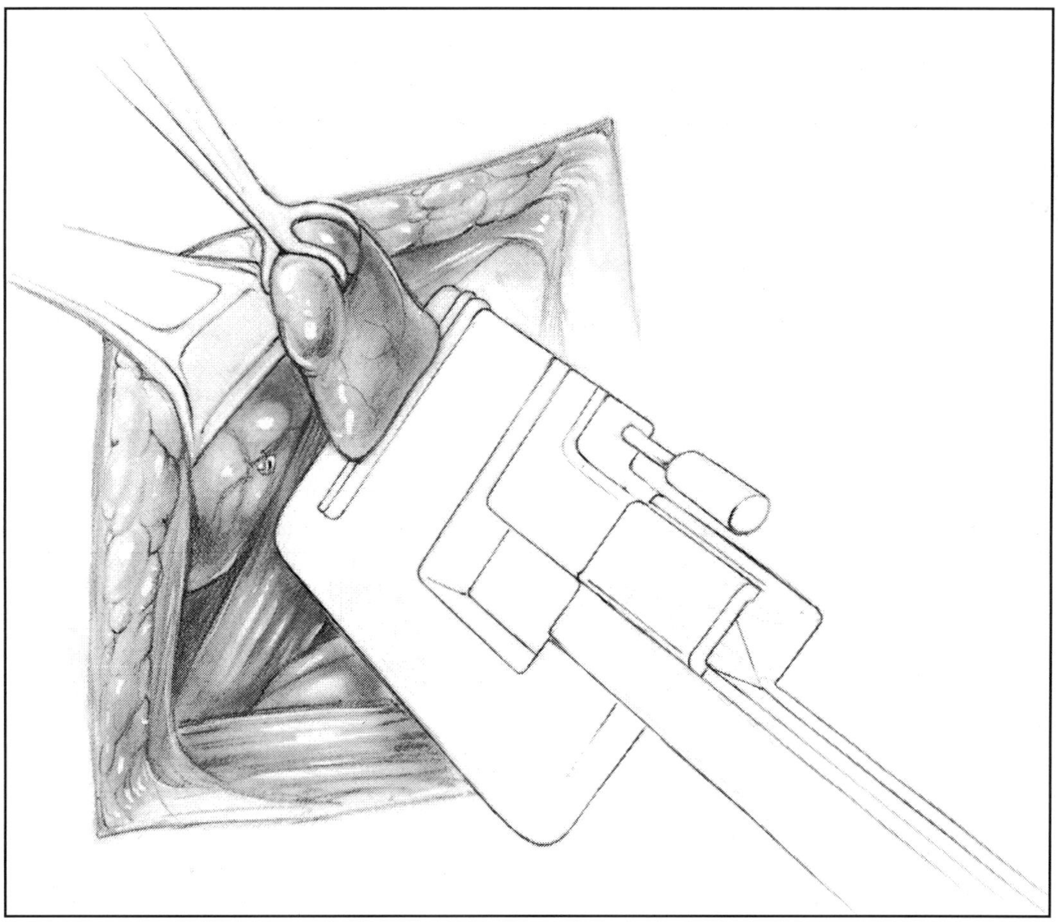

Fig. 11-5

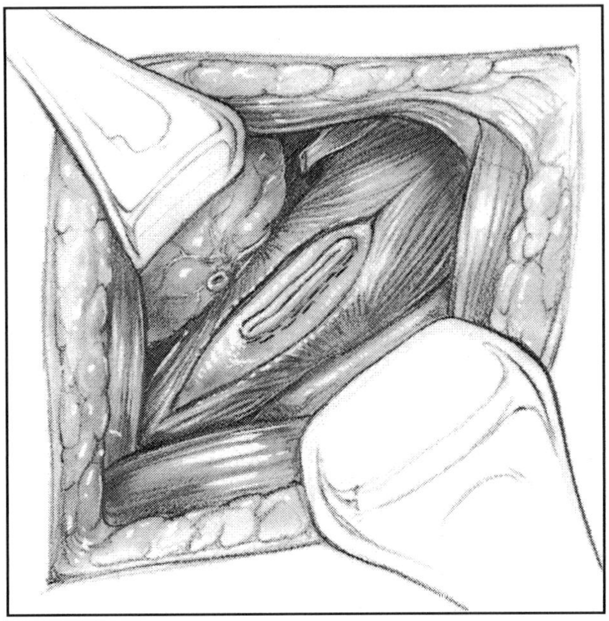

Fig. 11-6

then continued downward for 4–5 cm. Remove the diverticulum in the usual fashion.

Drainage and Closure

After carefully inspecting the area and ensuring complete hemostasis, insert a medium-size latex drain into the prevertebral space just below the area of the diverticulectomy. Bring the drain out through the lower pole of the incision.

Close the incision in layers with interrupted 4-0 PG sutures to the muscle fascia and platysma. Close the skin with continuous subcuticular sutures of 4-0 PG, interrupted nylon sutures, or skin staples.

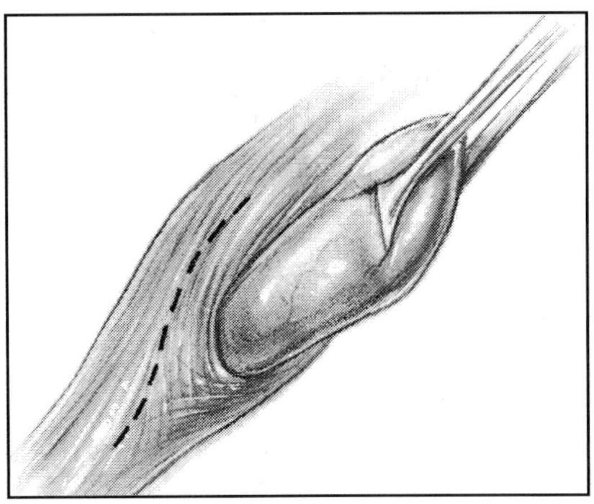

Fig. 11-7

POSTOPERATIVE CARE

Remove the drain by postoperative day 4. Initiate a liquid diet on the first postoperative day and progress to a full diet over the next 2–3 days. Continue perioperative antibiotics for a second dose.

COMPLICATIONS

Esophageal fistula. When the fistula is small and drains primarily saliva, it generally closes after a week of intravenous feeding if the patient's operative site has been drained as described above.

Recurrent laryngeal nerve palsy. It is generally temporary, secondary to excessive traction on the thyroid cartilage or to direct trauma to the nerve

Persistent dysphagia. This is due to inadequate myotomy.

REFERENCES

Belsey R. Functional disease of the esophagus. J Thorac Cardiovasc Surg 1966;52:164.

Bremner CG. Zenker diverticulum. Arch Surg 1988; 133:1131.

Crescenzo DG, Trastek VF, Allen MS, Deschamps C, Pairolero PC. Zenker's diverticulum in the elderly: is operation justified? Ann Thorac Surg 1998;66:347.

Ellis FH Jr, Crozier RE. Cervical esophageal dysphagia; indications for and results of cricopharyngeal myotomy. Ann Surg 1981;194:279.

Henderson RD, Hanna WM, Henderson RF, Maryatt G. Myotomy for reflux-induced cricopharyngeal dysphagia. J Thorac Cardiovasc Surg 1989;98:428.

Huang B, Payne WS, Cameron AJ. Surgical management for recurrent pharyngoesophageal (Zenker's) diverticulum. Ann Thorac Surg 1984;37:189.

Rocco G, Deschamps C, Martel E, et al. Results of reoperation on the upper esophageal sphincter. J Thorac Cardiovasc Surg 1999;117:28.

Worman LW. Pharyngoesophageal diverticulum excision or incision? Surgery 1980;87:236.

12 Esophagomyotomy for Achalasia and Diffuse Esophageal Spasm

INDICATIONS

Achalasia

Extended myotomy sometimes performed for diffuse esophageal spasm

PREOPERATIVE PREPARATION

Obtain a barium swallow esophagram.

Perform esophagoscopy with biopsy and brushings of the narrowed portion of distal esophagus if any mucosal abnormalities are noted.

Perform esophageal manometry.

For advanced cases, lavage the dilated esophagus with a Levine tube and warm saline for 1–2 days prior to operation to evacuate retained food particles. Combine this with a liquid diet.

Pass a nasogastric tube into the esophagus the morning of operation.

Administer perioperative antibiotics.

PITFALLS AND DANGER POINTS

Extending the myotomy too far on the stomach

Perforating the esophageal mucosa

Performing an inadequate circumferential liberation of the mucosa

Creating a hiatus hernia

OPERATIVE STRATEGY

Length of Myotomy for Achalasia

Ellis et al. (1980) attributed their low incidence of postoperative gastroesophageal regurgitation (3% to the fact that the myotomy terminates only a few millimeters beyond the esophagogastric junction. At the esophagogastric junction, several veins run in a transverse direction just superficial to the esophageal mucosa. One does not encounter any other transverse vein of this size during myotomy of the more proximal esophagus. Once these veins are encountered, terminate the myotomy. In no case should more than 1 cm of gastric musculature be divided. Continue the myotomy in a cephalad direction for 1–2 cm beyond the point at which the esophagus begins to dilate. For early cases, where no significant esophageal dilatation is evident, the length of the myotomy should be 5–8 cm.

Choice of Operative Approach

Laparoscopic myotomy is an excellent alternative for patients with achalasia in whom the narrow segment is limited to the distal esophagus (see Chapter 13). Open esophagomyotomy may be performed through a thoracotomy incision (as shown here) or transabdominally. The thoracic approach allows excellent exposure without disrupting the phrenoesophageal ligaments, potentially contributing to postoperative gastroesophageal reflux. It facilitates a long myotomy in cases of diffuse esophageal spasm.

Mucosal Perforation

Mucosal perforation is easily repaired if recognized. It is advisable for the surgeon to test the integrity of the mucosal layer following myotomy by having the anesthesiologist insert 100–200 ml of a methylene blue solution through the nasogastric tube. When a mucosal perforation is identified during the operation, careful suturing of the mucosa generally avoids further difficulty. Some surgeons close the muscle over the perforation and then rotate the esophagus so the myotomy can be performed at a different point on the esophageal circumference. Closing the mediastinal pleura over the esophagus, as we do routinely, helps buttress a sutured perforation of the mucosa (see Figs. 14–1 to 14–3).

OPERATIVE TECHNIQUE

Incision and Exposure

Place the patient in the full left thoracotomy position. Make a skin incision along the course of the seventh intercostal space. Incise the serratus and latissimus muscles with electrocautery; then make an incision along the upper border of the eighth rib through the intercostal musculature (see Figs. 9-1 to 9-3). Open the pleura for the length of the eighth rib. Insert a Finochietto retractor and gradually increase the space between the seventh and eighth ribs. Divide the inferior pulmonary ligament and retract the left lung in a cephalad and anterior direction using large moist gauze pads and Harrington retractors. Make an incision in the mediastinal pleura overlying the distal esophagus **(Fig. 12–1)**. Then gently encircle the esophagus with the index finger, which is facilitated by the indwelling nasogastric tube. Encircle the esophagus with a latex drain. Be careful to identify and preserve the vagus nerves. Free the esophagus from surrounding structures to the level of the diaphragm but no lower **(Fig. 12–2)**.

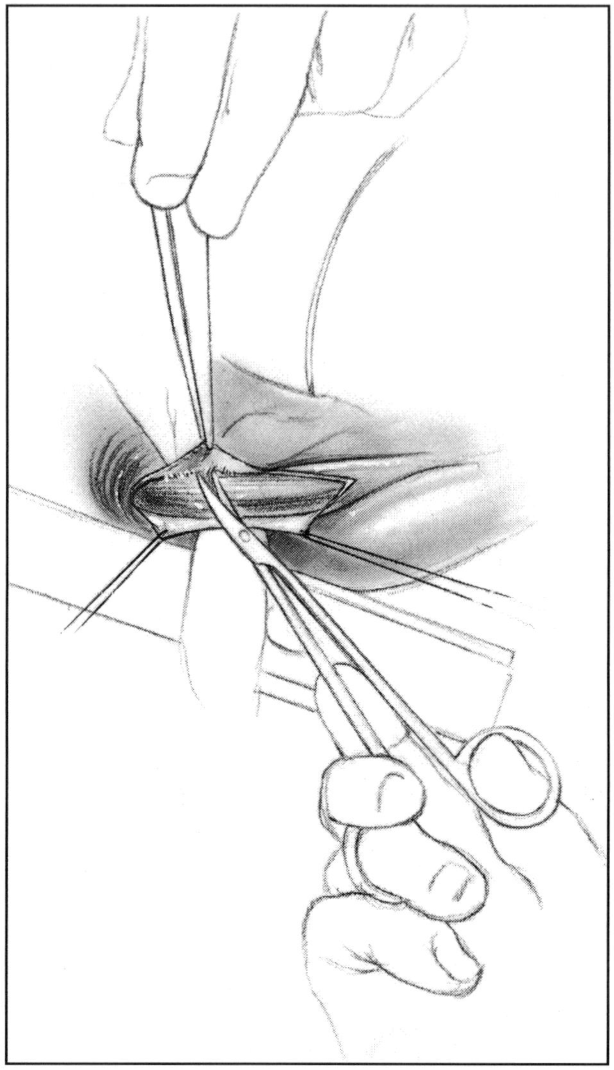

Fig. 12-1

Esophagomyotomy for Achalasia

Place the left index finger underneath the distal esophagus. Make a longitudinal incision through both the longitudinal and circular muscle layers of the esophagus until the muscosal surface is exposed **(Fig. 12–3)**. Continue this incision in a cephalad direction for a distance of about 2 cm above the point where the esophagus begins to dilate, or at least 5–7 cm.

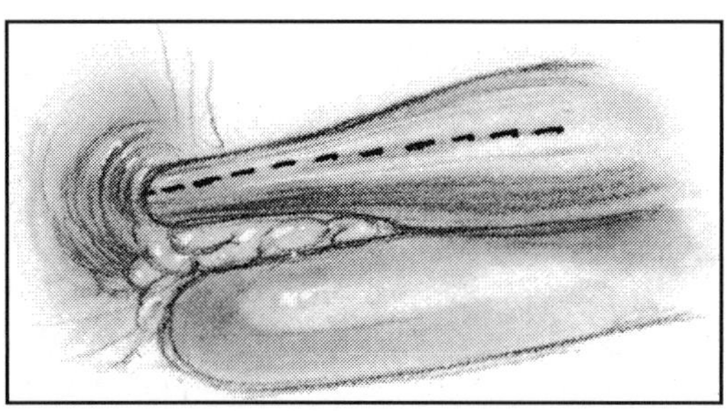

Fig. 12-2

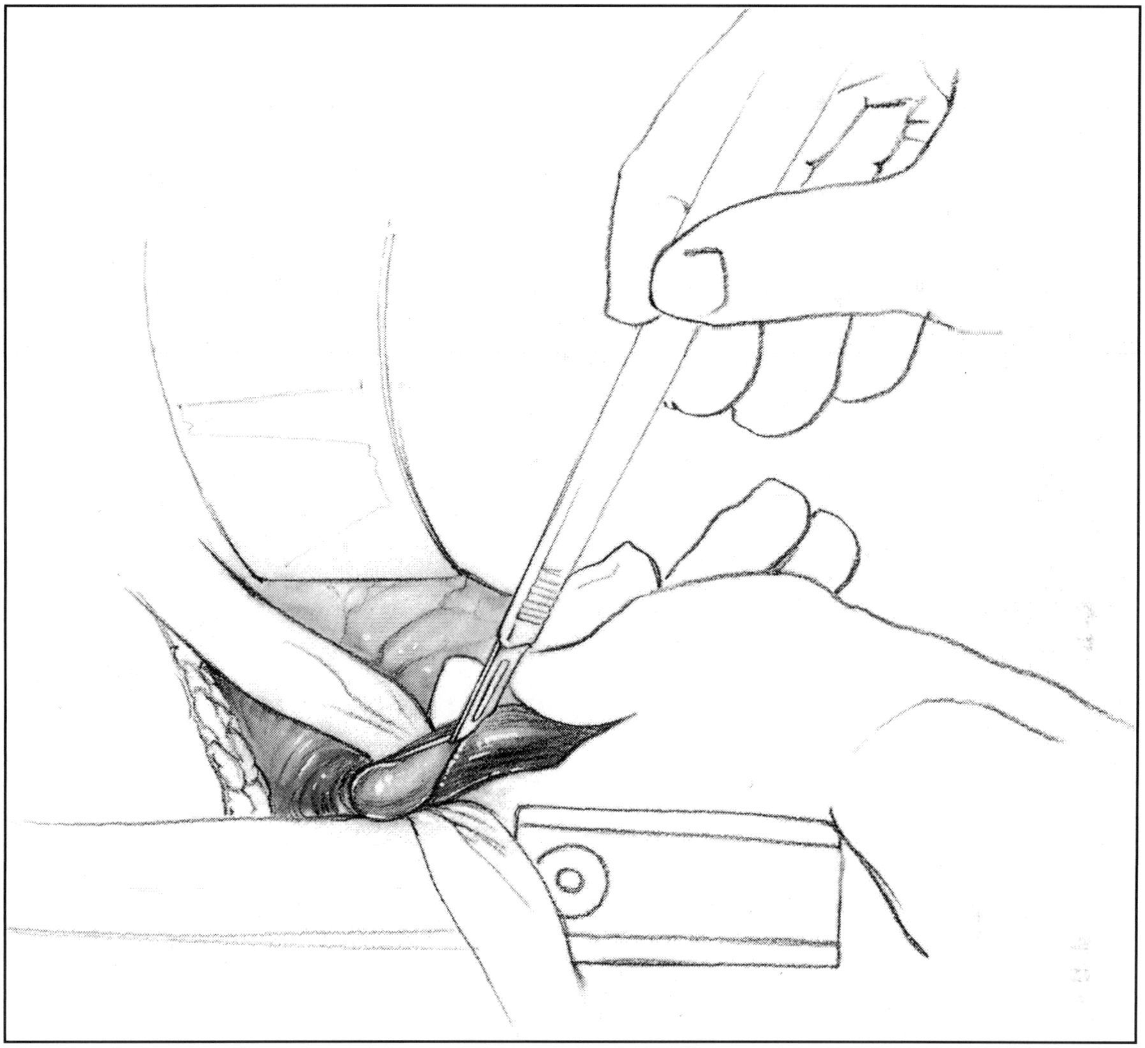

Fig. 12–3

Continue the myotomy in a caudal direction as far as the esophagogastric junction **(Fig. 12–4)**. This junction can be identified by noting one or two veins crossing transversely over the mucosa deep to the musculature. Do not continue the incision more than 1 cm into the gastric musculature. Another way to confirm the location of the esophagogastric junction is that the gastric musculature differs from that of the esophagus.

To prevent the muscle fibers from reuniting it is important to free at least 50% of the circumference of the mucosa from its muscular coat. This may be accomplished using Metzenbaum scissors to elevate the circular muscle from the underlying mucosa, proceeding medially and then laterally to the initial longitudinal myotomy until the mucosa bulges out, as seen in cross section in **Figure 12–5**. Achieve complete hemostasis by cautious electrocoagulation and fine suture-ligatures, especially in the incised esophageal muscle.

If the mucosa has been inadvertently incised, carefully repair the laceration with one or more 5-0 nonabsorbable sutures. At this point, ask the anesthesiologist to inject a solution of methylene blue into the esophagus to prove that there is no mucosal perforation.

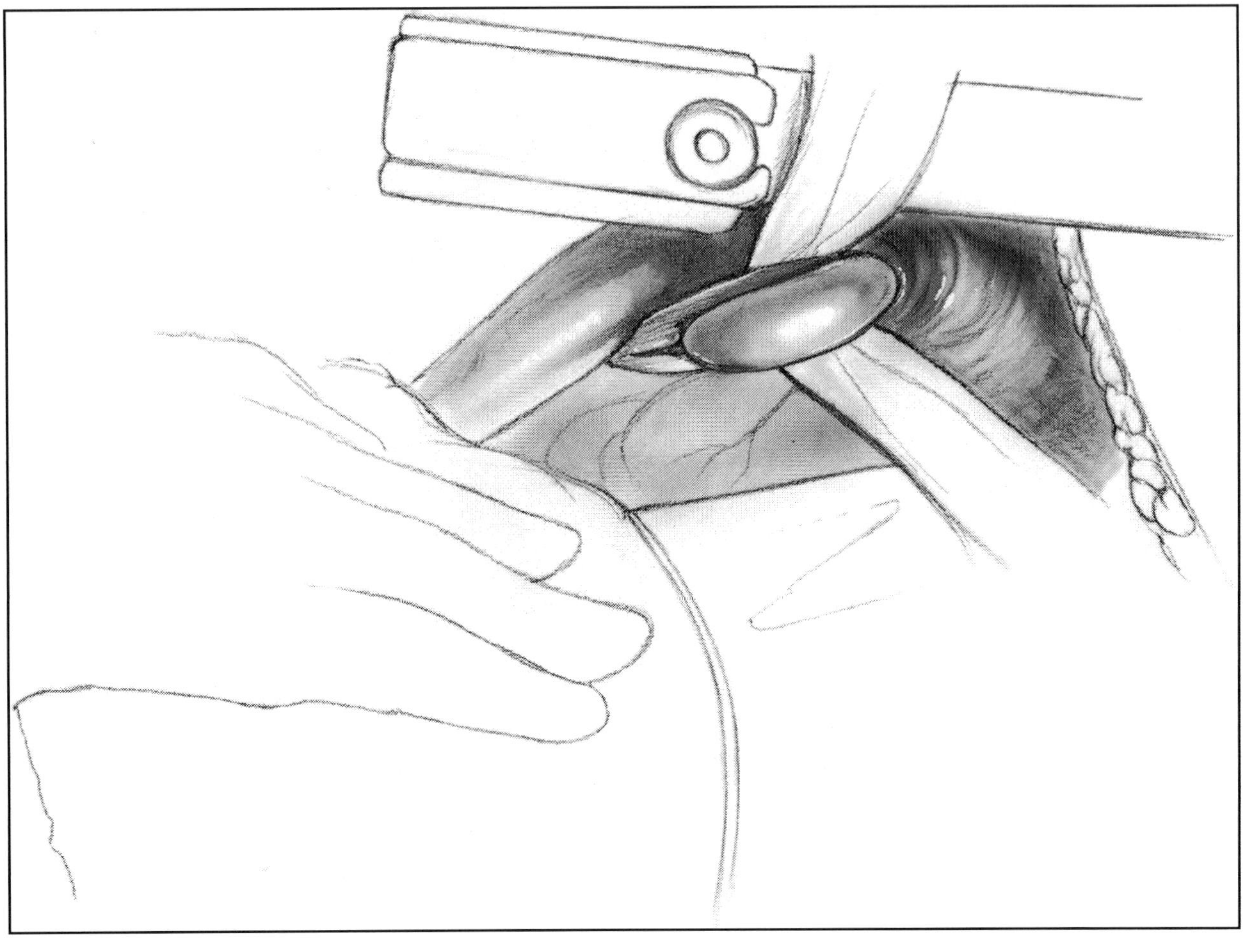

Fig. 12–4

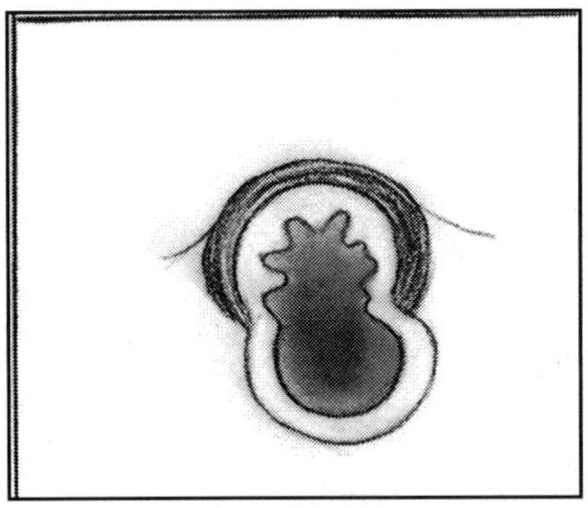

Fig. 12–5

Esophagomyotomy for Diffuse Esophageal Spasm

The technique for performing a myotomy to alleviate diffuse spasm differs from that described for achalasia only in the length of the myotomy. If the lower esophageal sphincter can relax normally when swallowing occurs, do not extend the myotomy to the terminal esophagus. The preoperative manometric assessment of the patient's esophageal contractions determines how far the esophagomyotomy should be extended.

Closure and Drainage

Bring a 30F chest tube out through a stab wound in the ninth intercostal space in the anterior axillary line. Approximate the ribs with two or three pericostal sutures of no. 2 PDS. Close the remainder of the wound in layers, as illustrated in Figures 3-42 to 3-44.

POSTOPERATIVE CARE

Remove the nasogastric tube the day following surgery.

Initiate oral intake of liquids on the first or second postoperative day, if tolerated.

Remove the chest tube as soon as the drainage becomes minimal, about the third or fourth postoperative day.

COMPLICATIONS

Persistent dysphagia. In some cases an inadequate myotomy for achalasia fails to relieve the patient's dysphagia. About 2 weeks following operation in such cases, esophageal dilatation with Maloney dilators may help. If reoperation is needed, consider laparoscopic myotomy, as the problem is generally at the distal end of the myotomy.

Recurrent dysphagia following initial relief of symptoms. It is possible that in these cases the muscular tissues have reunited. A trial of bougienage with Maloney bougies up to 50F may prove successful. Because esophageal carcinoma occasionally complicates long-standing achalasia, patients with recurrent dysphagia following a symptom-free interval after esophagomyotomy should have complete evaluation by radiography, esophagoscopy, and biopsy.

Reflux esophagitis. Although most patients with symptoms of reflux can be handled conservatively, an antireflux operation is required in severe cases.

Diaphragmatic hernia.

Empyema.

REFERENCES

Csendes A, Braghetto I, Mascaro J, Henriquez A. Late subjective and objective evaluation of the results of esophagomyotomy in 100 patients with achalasia of the esophagus. Surgery 1988;104:469.

Donohue PE, Schlesinger PK, Sluss KF, et al. Esophagocardiomyotomy~~flo~~ppy Nissen fundoplication effectively treats achalasia without causing esophageal obstruction. Surgery 1994;116:719.

Ellis FH. Esophagectomy for achalasia: who, when, and how much? Ann Thorac Surg 1989;47:334.

Ellis FH Jr. Oesophagomyotomy for achalasia: a 22 year experience. Br J Surg 1993;80:882.

Ellis FH Jr, Gibb SP, Crozier RE. Esophagomyotomy for achalasia of the esophagus. Ann Surg 1980;192:157.

Henderson RD, Ryder DE. Reflux control following myotomy in diffuse esophageal spasm. Ann Thorac Surg 1982;34:230.

Hunter JG, Richardson WS. Surgical management of achalasia. Surg Clin North Am 1997;77:993.

Murray GF, Battaglini JW, Keagy BA, et al. Selective application of fundoplication in achalasia. Ann Thorac Surg 1984;37:185.

Orringer MB, Stirling MC. Esophageal resection for achalasia: indications and results. Ann Thorac Surg 1989;47:340.

Pellegrini C, Wetter LA, Patti M, et al. Thoracoscopic esophagomyotomy: initial experience with a new approach for the treatment of achalasia. Ann Surg 1992;216:296.

Skinner DB. Myotomy and achalasia. Ann Thorac Surg 1984;37:183.

13 Laparoscopic Esophagomyotomy

INDICATIONS

Achalasia in which the high-pressure zone is localized to the distal esophagus

PREOPERATIVE PREPARATION

See Chapters 7 and 12.

PITFALLS AND DANGER POINTS

Inadequate myotomy. Careful review of preoperative studies (esophagoscopy, manometry, contrast esophagraphy) helps determine whether the high-pressure zone is limited to the distal esophagus and hence is accessible from the abdominal approach. Intraoperative endoscopy assists in ensuring that an adequate myotomy has been performed.

Esophageal perforation.

Creation of severe gastroesophageal reflux. Overzealous myotomy, extension of the myotomy too far down on the cardia, poor patient selection, and excessive mobilization of the esophagus contribute to postoperative reflux. Selective use of partial fundoplications (Dor and Toupet) is advocated by some surgeons. We believe this is not necessary routinely.

OPERATIVE STRATEGY

The first laparoscopic esophagomyotomies were done through the left chest using a thoracoscope in a manner analogous to the open Heller myotomy (see Chapter 12). As experience with laparoscopic Nissen fundoplication grew, it became obvious that access to the distal esophagus was better through the laparoscopic approach than through the thoracoscopic approach. For the typical patient with achalasia limited to the distal esophagus, laparoscopic approach is easiest. References at the end of the chapter describe the thoracoscopic approach, which is needed when a long myotomy is required for diffuse esophageal spasm. Most surgeons who perform this procedure are already facile in laparoscopic Nissen fundoplication (see Chapter 7).

Patient Position, Room Setup, Trocar Placement

Use the same patient position and room setup shown for the Nissen fundoplication (see Figs. 7–1, 7–2). Allow room at the head of the table for an esophagogastroduodenoscopy (EGD) scope, which is used at the end of the procedure to judge the adequacy of the myotomy. Typical trocar placement is shown in **Figure 13–1**. Generally five ports are required, and the general considerations discussed in Chapter 7 apply to trocar site placement for this procedure.

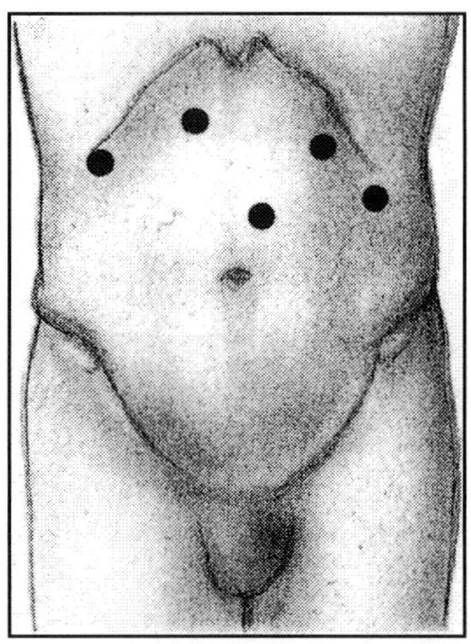

Fig. 13–1 Trocar placement. The supraumbilical trocar and the right subcostal trocar are placed 15 cm from the xiphoid, the left subcostal trocar about 10 cm from the xiphoid. The epigastric trocar is placed as high as the liver edge allows and as lateral as the falciform ligament allows. The left flank port is about 7 cm lateral to the left subcostal trocar.

Initial Exposure and Esophageal Mobilization

Place a liver retractor and obtain access to the hiatus in the usual fashion (see Figs. 7–3 through 7–5). Concentrate on the anterior dissection. It is not strictly necessary to mobilize the esophagus fully both anteriorly and posteriorly if the *narrowed segment and the dilated segment above it* are easily visualized once the hiatus has been cleared. Many surgeons believe that preserving the posterior attachments of the esophagus at the hiatus may decrease the incidence of postoperative reflux. Additional length may be gained, if necessary, by minimal additional dissection, sufficient to pass an articulating curved grasper behind the esophagus **(Fig. 13–2a)** and encircling the esophagus with a 6 inch segment of a 0.25-inch Penrose drain **(Fig. 13–2b)**. Grasp the drain and pull

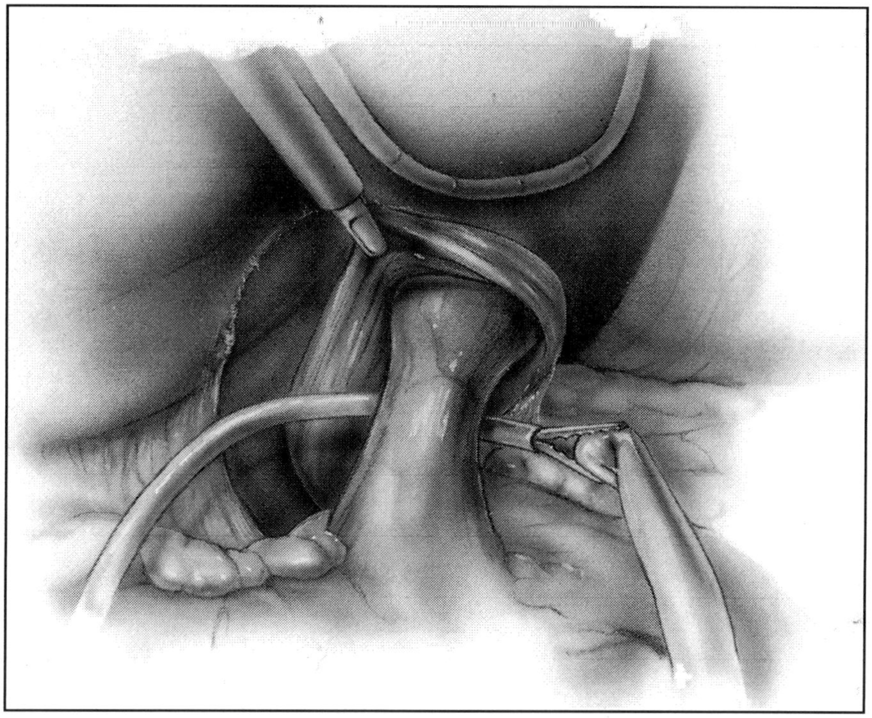

Fig. 13–2a

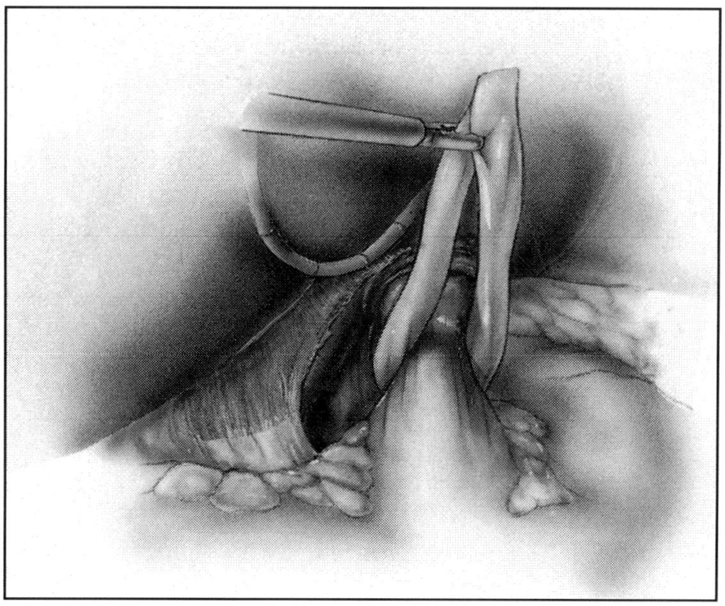

Fig. 13–2b

down toward the left lower quadrant to lengthen the segment of intraabdominal esophagus.

Myotomy

Begin the myotomy at a convenient location on the midportion of the thickened distal esophagus **(Fig. 13–3a)**. Curved scissors attached to electrocautery are useful for splitting, elevating, lightly cauterizing, and cutting parallel to the longitudinal muscle fibers.

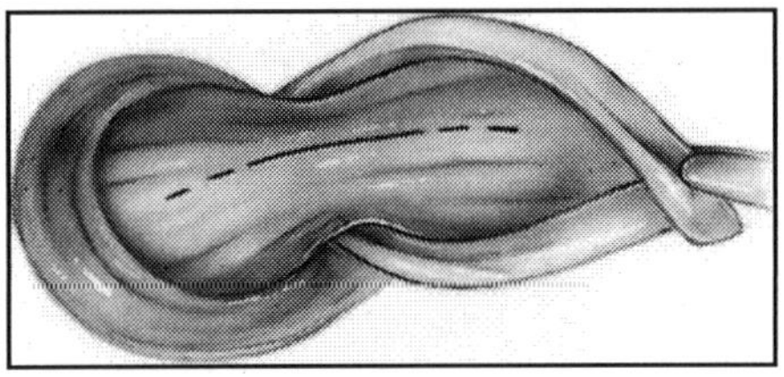

Fig. 13-3a

Use atraumatic graspers to elevate and pull down on the longitudinal muscle to improve exposure **(Fig. 13–3b)**. The underlying hypertrophied circular muscle fibers then come into view. Release the tension on the Penrose drain (if one was placed) to avoid pushing the walls of the esophagus together, which would increase the probability of injury to the epithelial tube.

Sequentially elevate the circular muscle fibers on the blade of the scissors, lightly cauterize, and cut. As the esophageal wall starts to open, place atraumatic graspers on the left and right cut edges of the muscular tube and pull gently apart and toward the patient's feet.

The epithelial tube is readily identified by its whitish color, smooth texture, and the small blood vessels that cross it. It may appear to balloon out into the field and is easily injured **(Fig. 13–4)**. Elevating the muscle edges helps minimize this tendency.

Extend the myotomy cephalad with the scissors until the circular muscle layer becomes thinner and the esophagus is dilated by sequentially lifting the

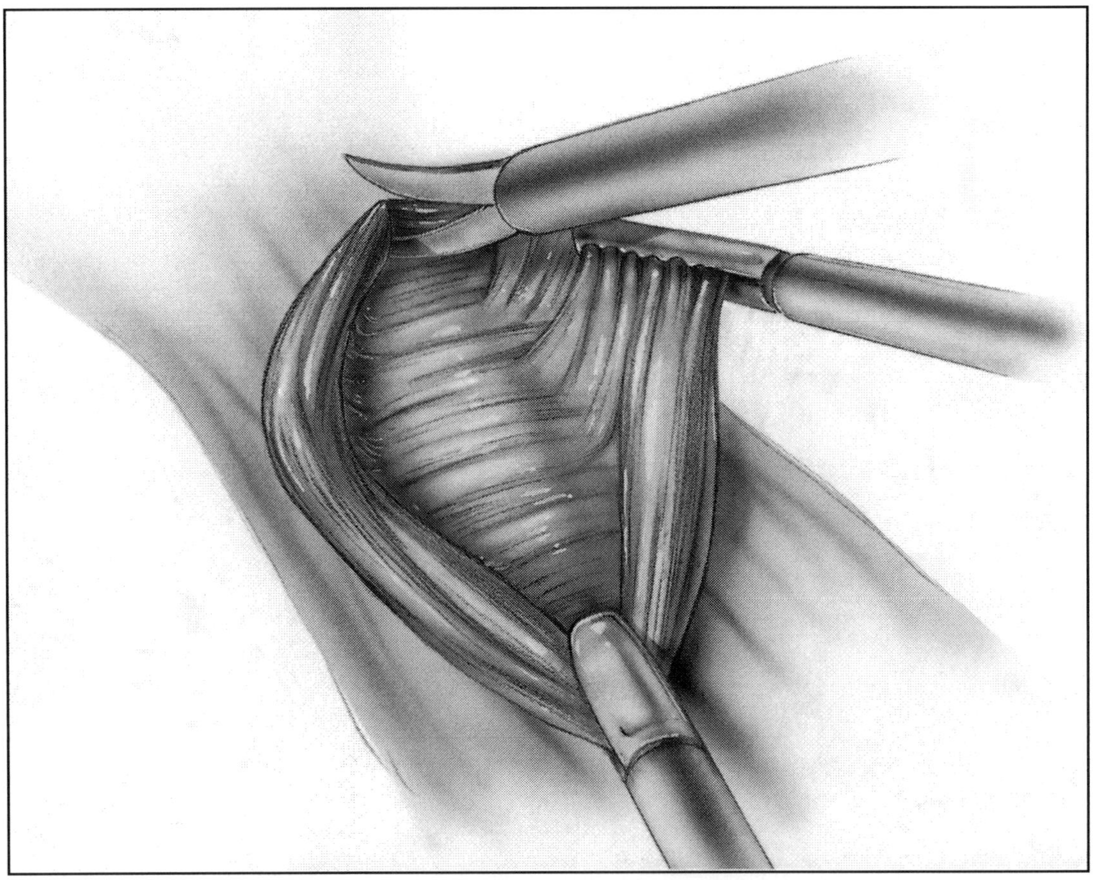

Fig. 13-3b

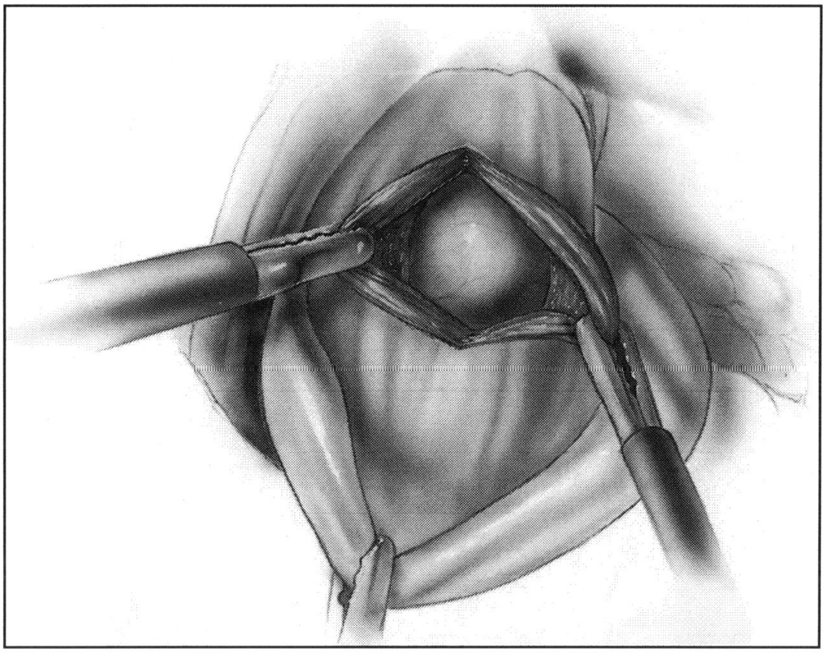

Fig. 13-4

circular muscle away from the epithelial tube with the blade of the scissors and cutting it **(Figs. 13–5a, 13–5b)**.

Complete the myotomy distally with hook cautery. Engage the hook under the circular muscle fibers; lift it up to avoid burning the underlying epithelial tube, and pull it down to cauterize and divide the muscle **(Fig. 13–6)**. Some surgeons pass a right-angle clamp under the circular muscle and use it to displace the epithelial tube deep, out of harm's way.

Generally, a complete myotomy must extend about 1 cm onto the stomach **(Fig. 13–7)**. Release all instruments from the esophagus. Pass an EGD scope into the distal esophagus and visualize the gastroesopha-

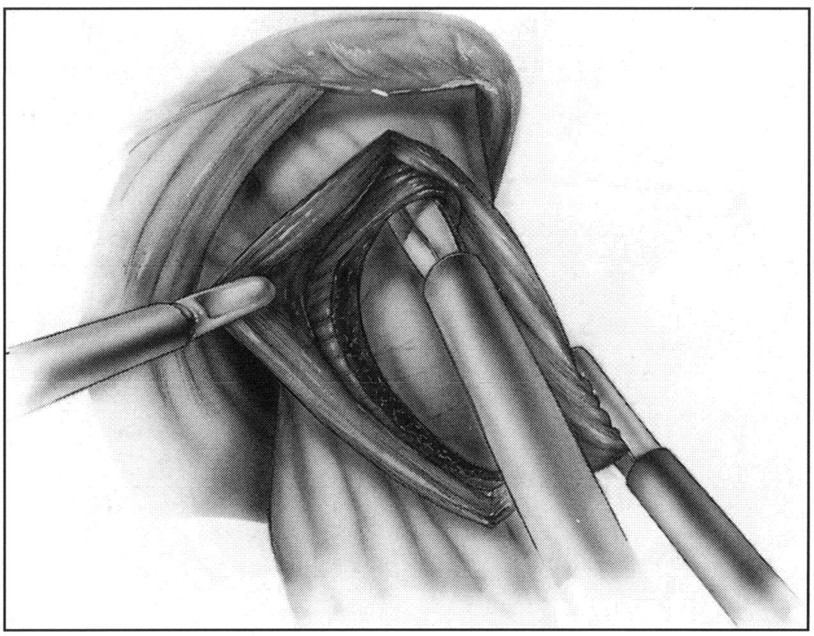

Fig. 13-5a

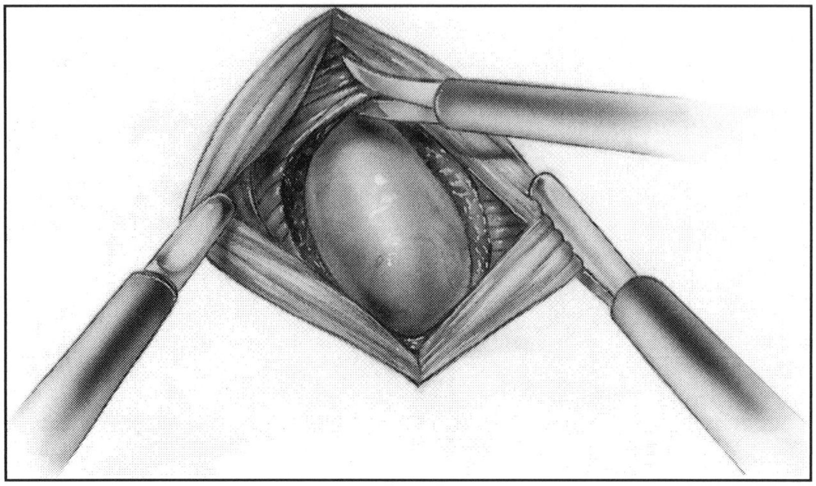

Fig. 13-5b

geal junction, identifiable by the Z-line where the color changes between whitish esophageal epithelium and pink gastric mucosa. The opening should be patulous if an adequate myotomy was performed.

Irrigate the abdomen with saline and fill the left upper quadrant. Insufflate with the EGD scope and watch for bubbles. The completed myotomy is shown in Figure 13-7.

Fundoplication

Some surgeons perform a partial fundoplication at the conclusion of the procedure. An anterior (Dor) fundoplication is a simple way to buttress a small (repaired) perforation. A posterior partial (Toupet) fundoplication is said to help keep their edges of the myotomy separate. We use a partial fundoplication selectively.

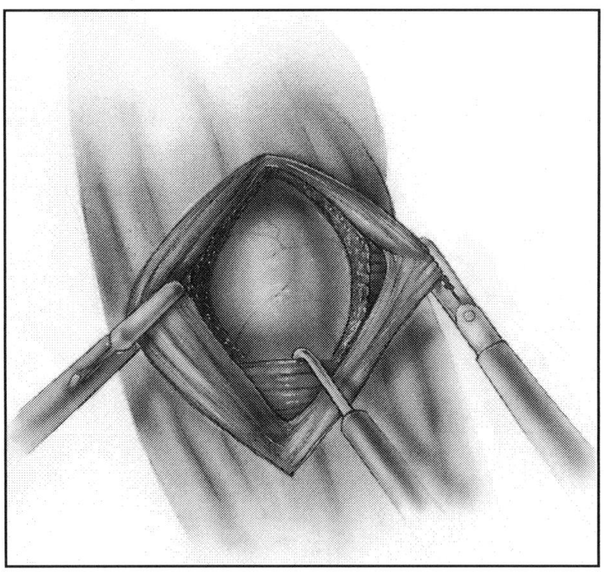

Fig. 13-6

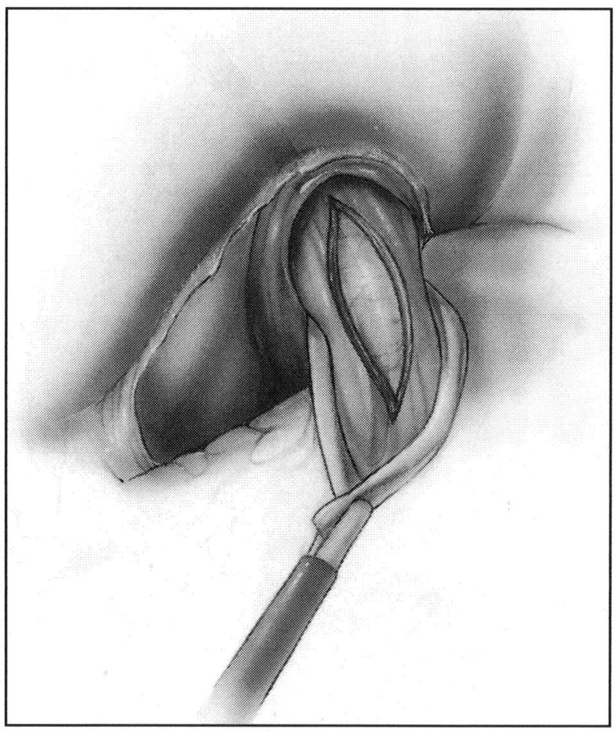

Fig. 13-7

COMPLICATIONS

Inadequate myotomy
Gastroesophageal reflux
Esophageal perforation

REFERENCES

Alves A, Perniceni T, Godeberge P, et al. Laparoscopic Heller's cardiomyotomy in achalasia: is intraoperative endoscopy useful and why? Surg Endosc 1999;13:600.

Dempsey DT, Kalan MM, Gerson RS, Parkman HP, Maier WP. Comparison of outcomes following open and laparoscopic esophagomyotomy for achalasia. Surg Endosc 1999;13:747.

Maher JW. Thoracoscopic esophagomyotomy for achalasia: maximum gain, minimal pain. Surgery 1997;122:836.

Oddsdottir M. Laparoscopic cardiomyotomy. In: Scott-Conner CEH (ed) The SAGES Manual: Fundamentals of Laparoscopy and GI Endoscopy. New York, Springer-Verlag, 1999, pp 213–220.

Patti MG, Pellegrini CA. Minimally invasive approaches to achalasia. Semin Gastrointest Dis 1994;5:108.

Stewart KC, Finley RJ, Clifton JC, et al. Thoracoscopic versus laparoscopic modified Heller myotomy for achalasia: efficacy and safety in 87 patients. J Am Coll Surg 1999;189:169.

14 Operations for Esophageal Perforation and Anastomotic Leaks

INDICATIONS

Instrumental or emetogenic esophageal perforation
Postoperative leak

PREOPERATIVE PREPARATION

Confirm perforation with diagnostic studies such as chest radiography; for suspected cervical perforations, lateral neck films in hyperextension; computed tomography (CT) scan or esophageal contrast radiographs.

Administer nasoesophageal suction proximal to perforation of the thoracic esophagus.

Insert a thoracostomy tube for pneumothorax.

Maintain fluid resuscitation.

Administer appropriate systemic antibiotics.

Insert appropriate central venous or pulmonary artery pressure monitors.

Control the airway with endotracheal intubation.

PITFALLS AND DANGER POINTS

Delayed diagnosis of the perforation

Inadequate attention to pulmonary function

Inadequate surgery to control continuing contamination

Inadequate drainage

Depending on sutured closure of inflamed esophagus

Suturing a perforated esophagus proximal to an obstruction

Inadequate pleural toilet and lung decortication

OPERATIVE STRATEGY

Visualize and thoroughly explore the region of the perforation. What appears to be a 1 cm perforation may prove to be three to four times that length after it is mobilized from the mediastinal pleura. Débride necrotic material around the perforation if suturing is anticipated. When the defect appears too large or the tissues too inflamed for suturing, it may be possible to apply a roof patch consisting of a flap of muscle pedicle, pleura, or pericardium that is sutured over the perforation. Otherwise, a diversion-exclusion operation or thoracic esophagectomy is necessary.

OPERATIVE TECHNIQUE

Pleural Flap Repair of Thoracic Esophageal Perforation

Incision

Make an incision in the left or right thoracic cavity depending on which side the perforation appears to present on the contrast esophageal radiograph. Generally, the lower half of the esophagus is approached through a left sixth or seventh intercostal space thoracotomy. The uncommon perforations of the upper esophagus are better approached through the right chest.

Exposure; Locating the Perforation

Incise the mediastinal pleura above and below the area of suspected perforation. Free to the mediastinal pleura from the esophagus so the esophagus can be elevated from its bed for thorough exploration. Sometimes the perforation is obscured by a layer of necrotic tissue. If the perforation is not immediately apparent, ask the anesthesiologist to instill air or a solution of methylene blue into the nasoesophageal tube and look for bubbling or the area of blue staining on the esophageal wall. Most patients have a pleural and a significant mediastinal infection with necrosis. Complete débridement of the mediastinum and decortication of the lung with removal of both parietal and visceral peels are used to control infection and ensure maximal lung function. Complete expansion of the lung is the best secondary defense against breakdown of an esophageal repair and helps control any fistula that develops.

Repair

When operation is performed soon (8 hours) after perforation, it may be possible to débride the tissues around the esophagus if marked edema and inflammation have not yet occurred; a viable tissue buttress should always be added to the repair. For suture closure, close the mucosal layer with interrupted sutures of 4-0 or 5-0 nonabsorbable synthetic suture and approximate the muscular layer with interrupted Lembert sutures of 4-0 silk or Prolene. In selected cases, a stapled closure may work. There must be sufficient good tissue to achieve an everted stapled closure without narrowing the lumen. Mobilize the edges of the effect and use Allis clamps to bring the full thickness of the esophageal wall within the jaws of a linear thick tissue stapler. Cover the suture line with a pleural flap. If the perforation is located in the lateral aspect of the esophagus, a simple rectangular flap of pleura is elevated and brought over the suture line. Use many interrupted 4-0 nonabsorbable sutures to fix the pleural flap around the sutured perforation.

When the perforation is not suitable for a sutured closure due to marked edema and inflammation, employ a pleural flap, an intercostal muscle flap, or some other viable buttress as a roof patch over the open defect in the esophagus. First débride the obvious necrotic tissue around the perforation. When the esophagus is too inflamed to hold sutures, it is advisable to exclude the upper esophagus from the gastrointestinal tract by one of the methods described below to supplement the pleural roof patch. With an extensive defect in the esophagus or one located on the posterior surface, outline a large rectangular flap of pleura as illustrated in **Figure 14–1**. In the presence of mediastinitis, the pleura is thickened and easy to mobilize from the posterior thoracic wall. Leave the base of the pedicle attached to the adjacent aorta. Slide the pedicle flap underneath the esophagus **(Fig. 14–2)** so it surrounds the entire organ. Insert multiple 4-0 interrupted nonabsorbable sutures deep enough to catch the submucosa of the esophagus around the entire circumference of the perforation as well as the entire circumference of the esophagus above and below the perforation, as illustrated in **Figure 14–3**.

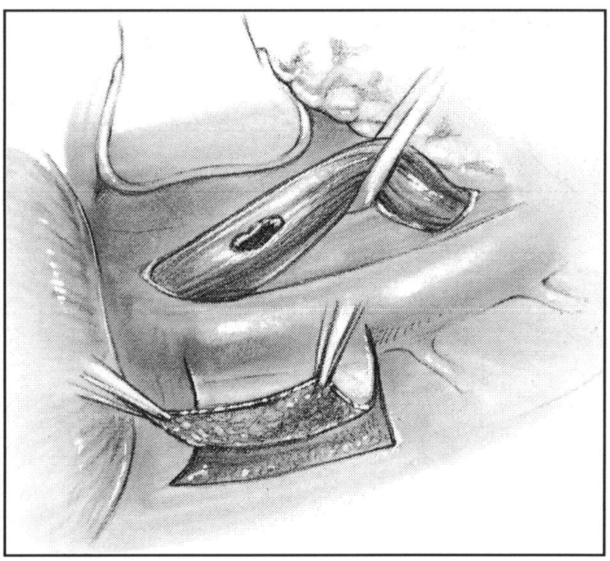

Fig. 14-1

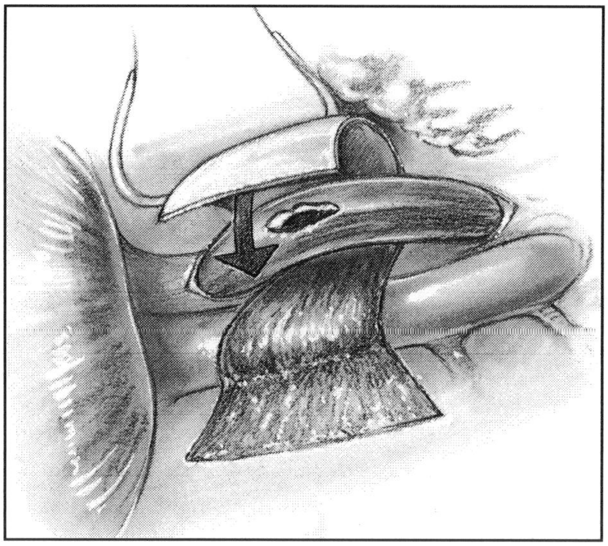

Fig. 14-2

Drainage

Place the tip of a 36F chest tube near the site of the esophageal perforation. Suture it to the mediastinal tissues with a catgut stitch. Bring this tube out through a small incision through the ninth or tenth interspace in the anterior axillary line. Place a smaller chest tube in the posterior portion of the apex of the chest and bring it out through a second stab wound. Attach both to underwater suction drainage.

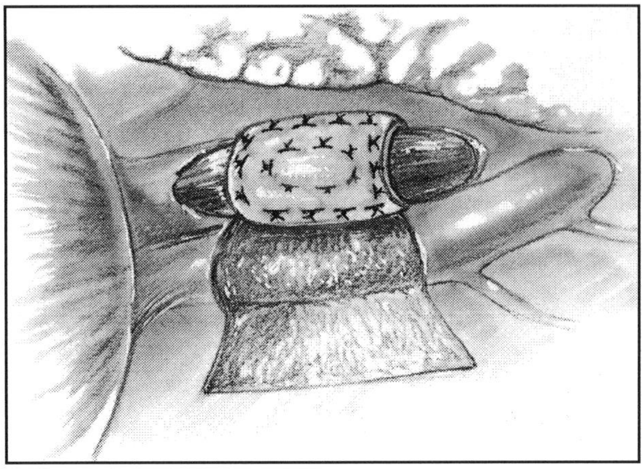

Fig. 14-3

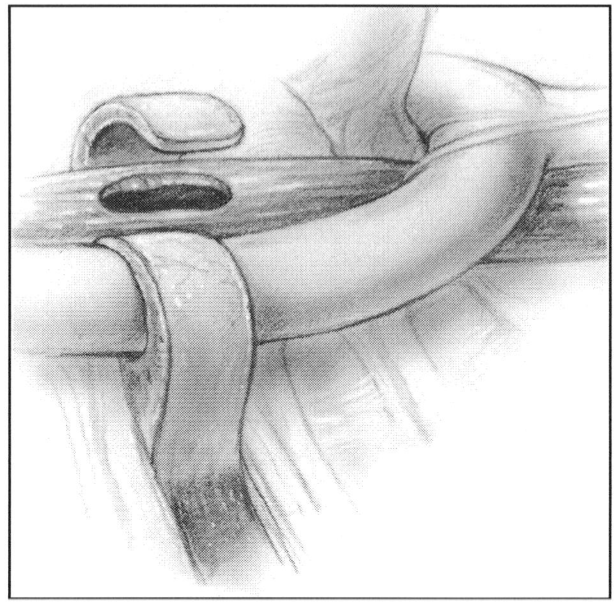

Fig. 14-5

Intercostal Muscle Flap Repair of Esophageal Perforation

Another method for bringing viable tissue to the site of an esophageal perforation is to create a vascularized flap of the appropriate intercostal muscle with which to wrap the perforation of the esophagus. If the patient undergoes surgery within the first 8 hours after a perforation, minor débridement and primary suturing generally remedy the situation. However, for perforations that have been leaking for a longer interval before surgery is undertaken, débridement of necrotic tissue and primary suturing may not be adequate; in these situations wrapping with a viable muscle flap may help achieve primary healing. In cases where the perforation is too large for suture closure, a roof patch consisting of viable intercostal muscle sutured to the intact esophagus around the perforation may be effective. Richardson et al. have reported remarkable success with this technique for esophageal defects due to penetrating trauma.

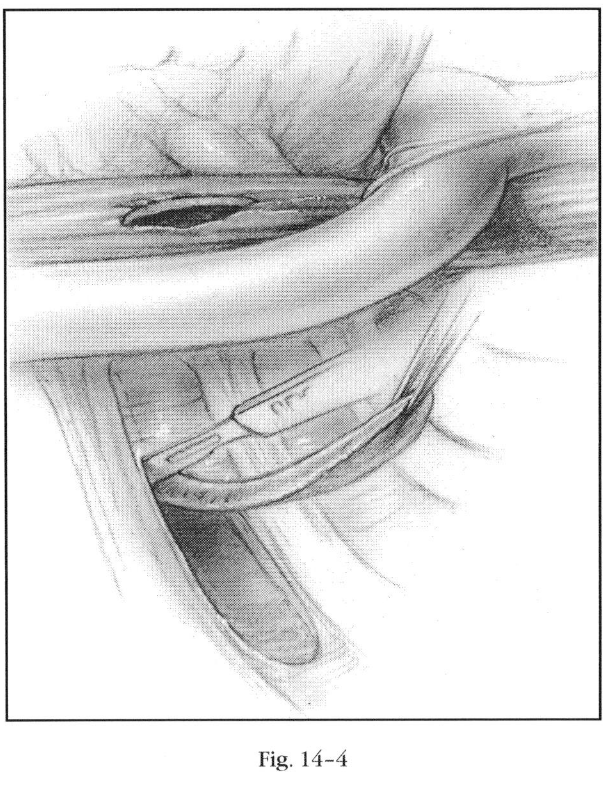

Fig. 14-4

To achieve a viable muscle flap, care must be taken to preserve the intercostal vessels. These vessels must be left attached to the muscle as it is being dissected away from the upper and lower rib borders. **Figure 14–4** illustrates dissection of the full thickness of the intercostal muscle from its attachments to the adjacent ribs. **Figures 14–5**, **14–6**, and **14–7** illustrate application of the intercostal muscle flap as a roof patch over a perforation that was not suitable for sutured closure. Large perforations (longer than the width of the muscle flap) may be difficult to repair by this technique. Drain the mediastinum and chest as described above. If the repair proves to be of poor quality, do not hesitate to resect the esophagus or to apply a temporary occlusion technique to the esophagus, as described below.

Esophageal Occlusion Methods Without Cervical Esophagostomy

When cervical esophagostomy is used for diversion in the neck, it is sometimes difficult to reconstruct the esophagus after the perforation heals. An alternative but less secure method is staple occlusion of the proximal esophagus. Avoid capturing the vagus nerves when stapling the lower esophagus. It is possible to occlude the esophagus above a thoracic perforation through the exploratory chest incision if the thoracic esophagus above the perforation is healthy. A sump-type nasoesophageal suction catheter is placed above the staple line.

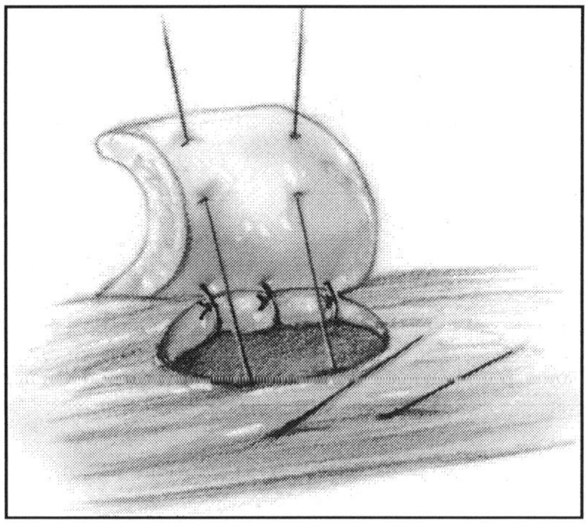

Fig. 14-7

Esophageal Diversion by Cervical Esophagostomy

Incision and Exposure

With the patient's head turned toward the right, make an incision along the anterior border of the sternomastoid muscle beginning 2–3 cm below the level of the mandibular angle and continuing down to the clavicle (see Fig. 2-27). Liberate the anterior border of the sternomastoid muscle. Divide the omohyoid muscle if it crosses the operative field. Retract the sternomastoid muscle and carotid sheath laterally and retract the prethyroid muscles medially, exposing the thyroid gland (see Fig. 2-29). Carefully divide the areolar tissue between the thyroid gland and the carotid sheath to expose the inferior thyroid artery and the recurrent laryngeal nerve. In some cases it is necessary to divide the inferior thyroid artery. Preserve the recurrent nerve. Identify the tracheoesophageal groove. Begin the dissection on the prevertebral fascia and free the esophagus posteriorly. Then encircle the esophagus with the index finger or a right angle clamp, but keep the plane of dissection close to the esophagus; otherwise, it is possible to traumatize the *opposite* recurrent laryngeal nerve or injure the membranous posterior wall of the trachea. After the esophagus has been encircled, pass a latex drain around the esophagus for purposes of traction. Mobilize the esophagus from the level of the hypopharynx down to the upper mediastinum.

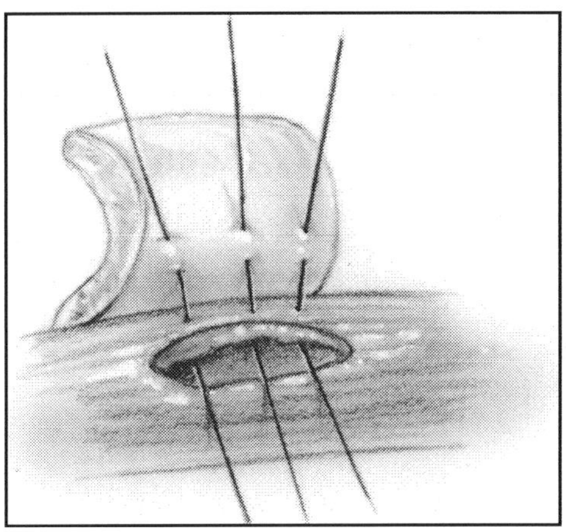

Fig. 14-6

Suturing the Esophagostomy

After mobilization is satisfactory, suture the sternomastoid muscle back in place by means of several interrupted 4-0 synthetic absorbable stitches. Close the platysma muscle with interrupted sutures of the same material, leaving sufficient space to suture the esophagostomy to the skin. Then insert interrupted 4-0 PG subcuticular sutures to close the skin, leaving a 3- to 4-cm gap in the closure for the esophagostomy.

Now make a transverse incision across the anterior half of the circumference of the esophagus. Suture the full thickness of the esophagus to the subcuticular layer of skin with interrupted 4-0 absorbable synthetic sutures **(Fig. 14–8)**.

In one case we found that, despite thorough mobilization of the esophagus, the incised esophagus could not be sutured to the skin without tension. A subtotal thyroid lobectomy was carried out. The incised esophagus was then sutured to the platysma muscle with interrupted sutures, leaving the skin in this area open. These steps produced a satisfactory result. As an alternative, mobilize the proximal thoracic esophagus and staple it closed with the

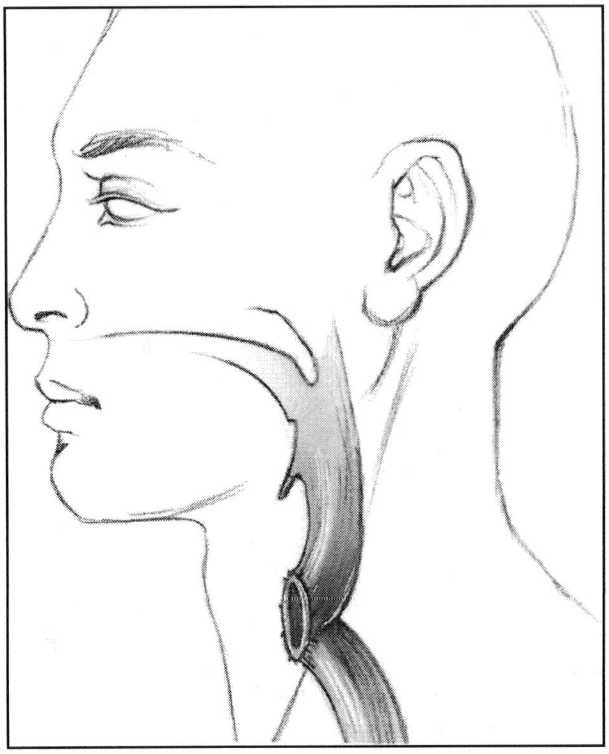

Fig. 14-8

linear stapler. Then either return it to its bed and decompress the closed esophageal remnant with a nasoesophageal tube or a lateral pharyngostomy tube or explant it to a subcutaneous position and create a stoma as described below.

Anterior Thoracic Esophagostomy

When a thoracic esophagectomy (Orringer and Stirling 1990) is carried out in these patients, an incision is made in the neck along the anterior border of the sternomastoid muscle. After the esophagus has been delivered through this incision, excise the segment that is nonviable and preserve all the viable esophagus. Make a subcutaneous tunnel from the incision in the neck over the anterior thorax. This tunnel should equal the length of the preserved esophagus. Make the esophagostomy on the anterior wall of the chest by making an incision in the skin and suturing the full thickness of the esophagus to the subcuticular layer of skin with interrupted 5-0 Vicryl sutures. It is much easier to apply stoma collection bags to the anterior chest than to a cervical esophageal stoma.

Excluding the Esophagus from the Gastrointestinal Tract

Perform a thoracotomy as described for the pleural flap operation. Incise the mediastinal pleura and liberate the esophagus from its bed **(Fig. 14–9)**. The perforation may be sutured or covered with a pleural flap (Fig. 14-3).

Then free the esophagus around its entire circumference distal to the perforation. Urschel et al. occluded the esophagus by surrounding it with a strip of Teflon that was sutured to itself to form a circumferential constricting band. Do not make this band so tight it strangulates the tissue. An umbilical tape may be passed around the Teflon band and tied to ensure the proper degree of constriction. Try to avoid including the vagus nerves in the constricting band. An alternative method of occluding the lower esophagus is to ligate it with a Silastic tube, such as the Jackson-Pratt catheter **(Figs. 14–10, 14–11)**. This material appears to be less irritating to the tissues than Teflon or umbilical tape. Another alternative is to use the TA-55 stapling device *with 4.8mm staples* to occlude the esophagus. When applying the staples, separate the vagus nerves from the esophagus so they are not trapped in the staple line. Use staples only if the esophagus is not markedly thickened or inflamed. Otherwise, the thickened tissues may be strangulated by the staples. After a period of 3–4 weeks a gap often appears in this staple line. This gap can usually be dilated by gentle passage of Maloney dilators. If the gap is small, the interventional radiologist can pass a guidewire over which dilating devices may be passed.

Another reported method for occluding the esophagus is passage of no. 2 chromic catgut or PG twice around the esophagus, which is then tied in a snug but not strangulating knot. The esophagus should respond easily to dilatation by the end of 2–4 weeks. It has been reported that even with delayed operations in patients who suffer large lacerations of the thoracic esophagus spontaneous healing occasionally occurs over a period of weeks, so esophageal replacement with either colon or stomach is not necessary.

This technique should be used if the patient has significant reflux. In other circumstances, we eliminate this step altogether because it is a distal obstruction and can prevent healing of a fistula.

To decompress the stomach and prevent pressure against the esophageal closure, a Stamm gastrostomy should be performed. In contrast to the usual location shown in Figure 14-11, it is wise to place this gastrostomy near the lesser curvature of the stomach if possible. In this way, if a gastric pull-up operation

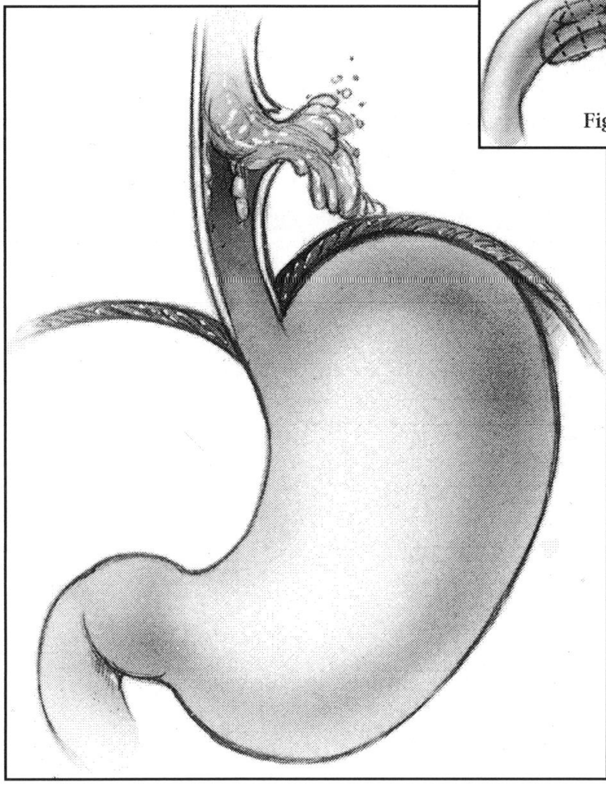

Fig. 14-9

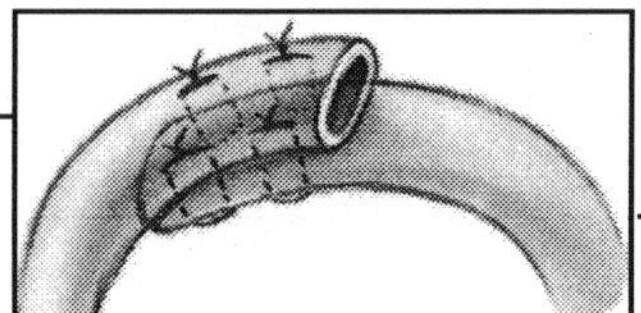

Fig. 14-10

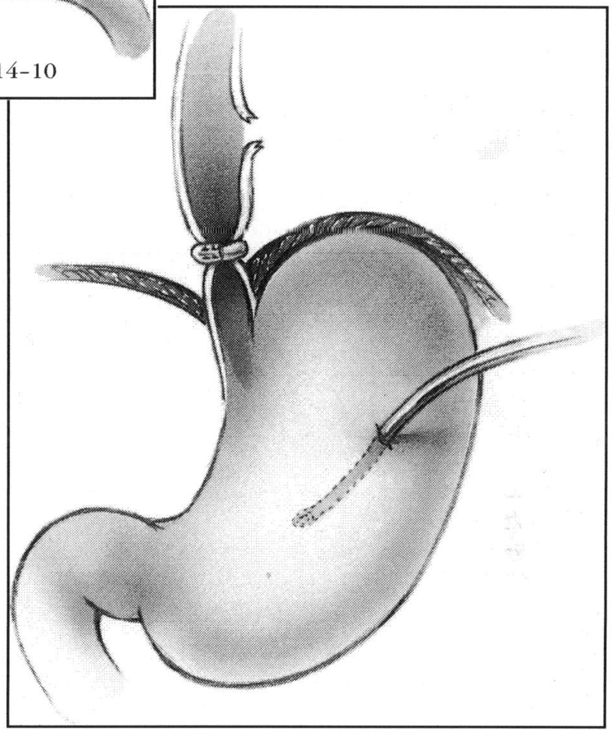

Fig. 14-11

is to be performed to replace the esophagus, the gastrostomy defect can be included in the segment of the lesser curvature that is customarily excised when preparing the stomach for advancement into the neck. It does not interfere with the blood supply to the greater curvature.

Finally, place proper drainage tubes to the area of perforation and close the thoracic incision. All of these patients require a tube gastrostomy to decompress the stomach; after the esophageal perforation has healed, the gastrostomy tube is used for purposes of feeding.

POSTOPERATIVE CARE

Most of these patients require *ventilatory support* for several days. Careful *cardiopulmonary monitoring* is a necessity.

Paste a small *drainage* bag or ileostomy bag over the esophagostomy to collect saliva. In patients without an esophagostomy, maintain nasoesophageal sump suction postoperatively.

These patients require intensive *antibiotic* treatment, depending on bacterial cultures of the mediastinum.

Do not remove the thoracotomy drainage tubes until drainage has ceased.

Total parenteral nutrition is necessary until the gastrostomy tube can be used for feeding.

Obtain frequent *chest radiographs* or *CT scans* in a search for loculated collections of pus.

COMPLICATIONS

Esophagocutaneous fistula

Uncontrolled sepsis including empyema or mediastinal abscess

Subphrenic abscess

Limited expansion of lung, requiring surgical decortication after active infection has subsided

REFERENCES

Alexander PV, Hollands M, O'Roaurke IC, Tait N. Intercostal pedicle flap for thoracic esophageal perforations. Aust NZ J Surg 1997;67:133.

Altorjay A, Kiss J, Voros A, Sziranyi E. The role of esophagectomy in the management of esophageal perforations. Ann Thorac Surg 1998;65:1433.

Bardini R, Bonavina L, Pavanello M. Temporary double exclusion of the perforated esophagus using absorbable staples. Ann Thorac Surg 1992;54:1165.

Goldstein LA, Thompson WR. Esophageal perforations: a 15 year experience. Am J Surg 1983;143:495.

Gouge TH, Depan HJ, Spencer F. Experience with the Grillo pleural wrap procedure in 18 patients with perforation of the thoracic esophagus. Ann Surg 1989;209:612.

Iannettoni MD, Vlessis AA, Whyte RI, Orringer MB. Functional outcome after surgical treatment of esophageal perforation. Ann Thorac Surg 1997;64:1609.

Mansour KA, Wenger RK. T-Tube management of late esophageal perforations. Surg Gynecol Obstet 1992;175:571.

Maroney TP, Ring EJ, Gordon RL, et al. Role of interventional radiology in the management of major esophageal leaks. Radiology 1989;170:1055.

Michel L, Grillo HC, Malt RA. Operative and nonoperative management of esophageal perforations. Ann Surg 1981; 194:57.

Orringer MB, Stirling MC. Esophagectomy for esophageal disruption. Ann Thorac Surg 1990;49:35.

Paramesh V, Rumisek JD, Chang FC. Spontaneous recanalization of the esophagus after exclusion using nonabsorbable staples. Ann Thorac Surg 1995;59:1214.

Pate JW, Walker WA, Cole FH Jr, et al. Spontaneous rupture of the esophagus: a 30-year experience. Ann Thorac Surg 1989;47:689.

Richardson JD, Tobin GR. Closure of esophageal defects with muscle flaps. Arch Surg 1994;129:541.

Richardson JD, Martin LF, Borzotta AP, Polk HC Jr. Unifying concepts in treatment of esophageal leaks. Am J Surg 1985;149:157.

Sarr MG, Pemberton JH, Payne WS. Management of instrumental perforations of the esophagus. J Thorac Cardiovasc Surg 1982;84:211.

Skinner DB, Little AG, DeMeester TR. Management of esophageal perforation. Am J Surg 1980;139:760.

Thai AP, Hatafuku T. Improved operation for esophageal rupture. JAMA 1964;188:826.

Triggiani E, Belsey R. Oesophageal trauma: incidence, diagnosis, and management. Thorax 1977;32:241.

Urbani M, Mathisen DJ. Repair of esophageal perforation after treatment for achalasia. Ann Thorac Surg 2000;69: 1609.

Urschel HC Jr, Razzuk MA, Wood RE, et al. Improved management of esophageal perforation: exclusion and diversion in continuity. Ann Surg 1974;179:587.

Whyte RI, Iannettoni MD, Orringer MB. Intrathoracic esophageal perforation: the merit of primary repair. J Thorac Cardiovasc Surg 1995;109:140.

Wilson SE, Stone R, Scully M, et al. Modern management of anastomotic leak after esophagogastrectomy. Am J Surg 1982;144:94.

Wright CD, Mathisen DJ, Wain JC, et al. Reinforced primary repair of thoracic esophageal perforation. Ann Thorac Surg 1995;60:245.

Index

FSC
www.fsc.org
MIX
Papier | Fördert gute Waldnutzung
FSC® C083411

Kolibri 360 GmbH
Ferdinand-Jühlke-Straße 7
99095 Erfurt, Deutschland
produktsicherheit@kolibri360.de